The Emerging Role of Advanced Technologies in Neurological Diseases

Adnène Arbi
National Institute of Applied Sciences and Technology, University of Carthage, Tunisia & Laboratory of Mathematical Engineering, Tunisia Polytechnic School, University of Carthage, Tunisia

Walid Ben Ameur
https://orcid.org/0009-0000-5046-7408
Faculty of Sciences of Gabes, Tunisia

IGI Global
Scientific Publishing
Publishing Tomorrow's Research Today

Vice President of Editorial	Melissa Wagner
Director of Acquisitions	Mikaela Felty
Director of Book Development	Jocelynn Hessler
Production Manager	Mike Brehm
Cover Design	Jose Rosado

Published in the United States of America by
IGI Global Scientific Publishing
701 East Chocolate Avenue
Hershey, PA, 17033, USA
Tel: 717-533-8845 | Fax: 717-533-7115
Website: https://www.igi-global.com E-mail: cust@igi-global.com

Library of Congress Cataloging-in-Publication Data

LCCN: 2025014131 (CIP Data Pending)
ISBN13: 9798337327068
Isbn13Softcover: 9798337327075
EISBN13: 9798337327082
British Cataloguing in Publication Data
A Cataloguing in Publication record for this book is available from the British Library.

Table of Contents

Detailed Table of Contents

Over the past decade, AI has transformed multiple sclerosis (MS) research and care, enhancing diagnosis, prognosis, and disease monitoring. From 2015 to 2025, AI evolved from basic image classification to advanced multi-modal models predicting disease progression and treatment response. Deep learning improved lesion detection and brain atrophy assessment via MRI, while machine learning enabled MS subtype identification and prognostic modeling. Researchers leveraged diverse datasets—MRI repositories, clinical trials, and EHRs—to train CNNs, RNNs, ensembles, and transformers. These advances improved diagnostic precision and supported disease trajectory prediction. AI tools now aid radiologists in tailoring treatments, though challenges like model generalizability, data harmonization, and regulatory approval persist. The future lies in federated learning, explainable AI, and real-time decision support to realize precision medicine in MS care.

This chapter investigates the recent advances in Convolutional Neural Networks for breast cancer detection in mammography. The survey reviews how emerging progress in CNN architectures are reshaping mammography interpretation and diagnostics. State-of-the-art and evaluation of optimization techniques are provided. A dedicated use case is analyzes and recommendations for model training optimization are revealed. The study is conducted on the Mammogram Mastery dataset which comprises 745 original images and 9,685 augmented images. Furthermore, the chapter addresses deep learning's potential to enhance mammographic assessment by improving diagnostic accuracy and reducing false errors. The insights presented aim to guide researchers and practitioners towards developing robust, reliable, and clinically impactful AI for breast cancer detection, highlighting key requirements for achieving advanced trustworthy and equitable outcomes.

Akash Saxena, Compucom Institute of Technology and Management, Jaipur, India
Satish Kumar Alaria, Government of Rajasthan, India
Ashish Raj, Poornima University, India
Apoorva Sharma, Poornima University, India
Arpita Sharma, Swami Keshvanand Institute of Technology, Management, and Gramothan, Jaipur, India

This study explores various machine learning and deep learning approaches to classify normal and arrhythmic heartbeats using the MIT-BIH Arrhythmia dataset. Feature extraction techniques, including Discrete Fourier Transform, Discrete Wavelet Transform, and Continuous Wavelet Transform, were employed to enhance signal representation. Machine learning classifiers were tested, along with deep learning-based models and a custom Convolutional Neural Network (CNN) trained on CWT-generated scalograms. The results indicate that deep learning models significantly outperform traditional machine learning classifiers, with the custom CNN achieving the highest accuracy of 82.76% when trained on augmented CWT scalogram images. While KNN (97.76%) and SVM (98%) performed well, their dependency on feature engineering and computational limitations restricted their scalability. This study underscores the potential of AI-driven ECG classification to revolutionize automated arrhythmia detection, enabling real-time monitoring and early intervention in clinical settings.

Affaan Shaikh, Neuratia Labs, UAE
Ravi Teja Kothuru, University of San Diego, USA
Khalid Shaikh, Prognica Labs, UAE

This chapter presents a theoretical overview of the integration of Electroencephalography (EEG) with smart devices, focusing on the technological developments, applications, and challenges in this rapidly evolving field. EEG, a non-invasive method of recording brain activity, has historically been limited to clinical and research environments. However, advancements in wearable technology, wireless communication, and signal processing have paved the way for EEG to be utilized in consumer-grade smart devices such as smartphones, smartwatches, and other IoT-connected systems. This chapter explores the theoretical underpinnings of EEG technology and how recent innovations have facilitated its incorporation into portable and wearable devices. Key applications discussed include mental health monitoring, cognitive state tracking, neurofeedback, and enhanced human-computer interactions. Additionally, the chapter addresses the technical, ethical, and privacy challenges associated with EEG-smart device integration, particularly concerning data accuracy, user comfort, and data security.

The accelerating global prevalence of neurological diseases such as Alzheimer's, Parkinson's, epilepsy, stroke, and multiple sclerosis has created an urgent demand for advanced technologies that can improve diagnostic precision, treatment personalization, and long-term patient outcomes. This chapter explores the transformative role of neural networks—computational systems inspired by the structure and function of the human brain—in revolutionizing the diagnosis, treatment, and management of neurological disorders. Beginning with foundational principles in deep learning, including key architectures like convolutional neural networks, recurrent neural networks, and long short-term memory networks, the chapter outlines how these models process complex, high-dimensional neurological data. Practical applications are examined across neuroimaging analysis, signal interpretation, and brain-computer interface systems, showcasing their ability to detect early disease markers, predict therapeutic responses, and support neurorehabilitation.

This monograph explores the intersection of robotics and neuroscience in the field of motor neurorehabilitation, focusing on the development and application of brain-computer interface (BCI) systems. Emphasizing principles of neuroplasticity, it examines how technologies such as EEG-based BCI, functional electrical stimulation (FES), virtual reality (VR), and robotic exoskeletons can be integrated into closed-loop, feedback-rich rehabilitation platforms. Special attention is given to hybrid systems combining multiple sensory modalities to enhance user engagement and therapeutic outcomes. The monograph also discusses current challenges in clinical translation, including signal variability, training demands, and hardware limitations, while highlighting promising advances in AI-driven algorithms, wearable EEG solutions, and co-adaptive control strategies. Overall, it argues for a shift toward personalized, home-based rehabilitation technologies that empower patients with motor impairments to achieve greater autonomy and functional recovery.

Interpreting human emotional states is crucial for advanced AI in human-computer interaction. Addressing this need, we propose a comprehensive methodology centered on facial Electromyography (fEMG) signals. fEMG offers a direct, objective measure of muscle activation for genuine emotional responses. We detail a complete pipeline: from fEMG acquisition to advanced time-frequency analysis using Continuous Wavelet Transform (CWT). This robust feature extraction integrates with machine learning models for emotion classification and prediction. Leveraging fEMG's temporal dynamics, we aim to enhance emotion recognition system accuracy and real-time capability. This chapter addresses the methodology and demonstrates its effectiveness through the rigorous validation of its evaluation framework, rigorously validated, demonstrating exceptionally consistent performance in both continuous regression and discrete classification tasks with simulated data. This strong alignment between predicted and ground truth confirms the reliability and correctness of the pipeline depoloyed.

Neurological conditions include traumatic brain injury, Parkinson's disease, stroke, multiple sclerosis and spinal cord injuries frequently cause cognitive and movement impairments. Traditional rehabilitation methods can result in patient disengagement, limited accessibility, and inadequate functional recovery. Virtual reality has become a powerful instrument in neurorehabilitation due to its interactive, immersive, and flexible therapeutic environment for cognitive and motor recovery.Virtual reality-based exergames optimize functional recovery and improve motor development by fusing mental difficulties with physical exercise.

Preface

Neurological disorders represent one of the most complex and burdensome challenges for global healthcare systems. They affect millions of people worldwide, impacting cognition, mobility, emotional well-being, and overall quality of life. Over the past decade, rapid advancements in artificial intelligence (AI), machine learning (ML), neuroimaging, robotics, wearable systems, and immersive technologies have reshaped how clinicians, researchers, and engineers understand and address these conditions. What was once the domain of speculative innovation is now moving firmly into clinical translation, transforming diagnosis, prognosis, treatment personalization, and long-term rehabilitation.

This edited volume brings together diverse perspectives from international scholars and practitioners working at the intersection of technology and neuroscience. Each chapter offers an in-depth exploration of how advanced computational and engineering tools are redefining neurological healthcare, ranging from AI-driven diagnostics to neuroprosthetic rehabilitation, EEG-enabled smart devices, VR-based recovery platforms, and emerging sensing modalities such as facial electromyography.

The collection reflects three core ambitions:

1. To document the scientific and technological progress of the past decade, highlighting breakthroughs in AI architectures, signal processing, human–computer interaction, and robotics.
2. To integrate multidisciplinary insights from computer science, biomedical engineering, neuroscience, and clinical practice.
3. To identify future pathways for clinically meaningful, ethically responsible innovation, especially as these technologies become more ubiquitous and embedded in everyday life.

Together, the chapters illustrate not only how far the field has come but also how much untapped potential remains. As the neurological disease burden rises globally, the integration of advanced technologies will play an increasingly central role in enabling earlier diagnosis, personalized care, continuous monitoring, and accessible rehabilitation.

This volume is intended for researchers, clinicians, graduate students, and innovators seeking a comprehensive overview of emerging computational and engineering solutions shaping the future of neurological health. We hope that the work presented here stimulates deeper interdisciplinary collaboration and accelerates the translation of technological progress into tangible patient benefit.

CHAPTER OVERVIEW

Chapter 1: A Decade of Progress — Artificial Intelligence in Multiple Sclerosis (2015–2025)

Jyoti Kumari, Santi Behera, and Prabira Kumar Sethy chart the remarkable transformation of AI applications in Multiple Sclerosis (MS) research over the past ten years. By tracing developments from early image-based classifiers to modern multimodal transformer and deep learning systems, this chapter demonstrates how AI enhances lesion detection, subtype classification, and prognostic modeling. It reviews the diverse datasets fueling these advancements, including MRI repositories and EHRs, and highlights both clinical benefits and remaining challenges such as data harmonization and regulatory readiness. The chapter concludes by outlining future directions in explainable AI, federated learning, and real-time clinical decision support.

Chapter 2: Advances in CNN-Based Breast Cancer Detection

Sana Salhi, Nour Fakhfakh, and Malak Sayeb present an in-depth survey of recent breakthroughs in convolutional neural networks for mammographic breast cancer detection. Drawing on experiments using the Mammogram Mastery dataset, the authors analyze how evolving CNN architectures, optimization techniques, and data-augmentation strategies improve diagnostic accuracy and reduce false detections. The chapter offers a dedicated use case illustrating practical training considerations and concludes with recommendations for building equitable and trustworthy AI systems capable of supporting real-world clinical workflows.

Chapter 3: Automated Detection of Cardiovascular Arrhythmias Using ML and DL on ECG Signals

In this chapter, Akash Saxena, Satish Alaria, Ashish Raj, Apoorva Sharma, and Arpita Sharma examine machine learning and deep learning approaches to arrhythmia detection using the MIT-BIH dataset. The authors provide a rich comparison of feature extraction techniques—including DFT, DWT, and CWT—and evaluate both classical ML classifiers and deep CNN architectures. Their custom CWT-based CNN achieves significant performance improvements, underscoring the power of deep learning for real-time ECG monitoring. The findings highlight the potential for scalable, automated arrhythmia detection to support early intervention in clinical and telemedicine settings.

Chapter 4: Integrating EEG with Smart Devices — A Theoretical Overview

Affaan Shaikh, Ravi Teja Kothuru, and Khalid Shaikh explore how recent progress in wearable sensors, wireless communication, and signal processing has enabled EEG to move beyond traditional laboratory environments and into smart consumer devices. This chapter explains the theoretical foundations of EEG acquisition and processing, and discusses emerging applications such as mental health tracking, neurofeedback, cognitive state monitoring, and enhanced human-computer interaction. It also offers an important discussion of ethical and privacy challenges, including data security and accuracy, associated with integrating sensitive neurophysiological data into everyday technologies.

Chapter 5: Neural Networks Transforming the Diagnosis and Treatment of Neurological Diseases

S. Ida Evangeline offers a comprehensive overview of how neural network architectures, ranging from CNNs and RNNs to LSTMs, are being deployed across neuroimaging analysis, electrophysiological interpretation, and brain-computer interfaces. By detailing applications in conditions such as Alzheimer's, Parkinson's disease, epilepsy, stroke, and MS, the chapter illuminates how neural networks enable early detection, therapeutic response prediction, and personalized treatment pathways. It emphasizes the growing role of deep learning in improving diagnostic precision and supporting neurorehabilitation strategies.

Chapter 6: Robotics and Neuroscience in Rehabilitation — Modern Approaches to Motor Disorders

Alexander Zakharov and colleagues present a monograph-style examination of robotic and neurotechnological innovations in motor rehabilitation. Emphasizing neuroplasticity and closed-loop design, the chapter explores EEG-based BCIs, functional electrical stimulation, VR environments, and robotic exoskeletons as synergistic tools for motor recovery. The authors discuss hybrid systems combining multimodal sensory input, and address barriers to clinical translation, such as signal variability and hardware limitations. The chapter advocates for personalized, home-based rehabilitation ecosystems supported by wearable EEG and AI-powered adaptive control.

Chapter 7: Leveraging Facial Electromyography for Enhanced Emotion Recognition in AI Systems

Khaoula Ben Ali and Adnène Arbi introduce a comprehensive methodology for using facial electromyography (fEMG) to improve emotion recognition in artificial intelligence systems. The chapter details a complete pipeline from acquisition to CWT-based feature extraction and machine-learning-driven classification and highlights fEMG's ability to capture genuine muscle-based emotional responses. Rigorous validation demonstrates high consistency between predicted and real emotional states, illustrating the promise of fEMG for next-generation affective computing, human-robot interaction, and adaptive user interfaces.

Chapter 8: VR in Rehabilitation — A New Frontier for Cognitive and Motor Recovery

Kirthika Ramesh, Rajalaxmi V., Veenakirthika S., and Mohan Kumar G. conclude the volume by examining how virtual reality (VR) is transforming rehabilitation for patients with neurological disorders such as stroke, TBI, MS, Parkinson's disease, and spinal cord injuries. The chapter explains how immersive VR environments and exergames enhance motivation, accessibility, and functional recovery by blending cognitive engagement with physical activity. It underscores VR's potential to overcome limitations of traditional rehabilitation and promote more adaptive, personalized therapeutic strategies.

Collectively, the contributions in this book highlight a future in which neurological healthcare becomes increasingly preventive, personalized, and participatory. Advanced technologies will not replace clinicians; instead, they will augment expertise, expand diagnostic capabilities, and empower patients with tools that offer unprecedented insight into their neurological well-being. As research continues and interdisciplinary collaboration deepens, the boundary between engineering and medicine will further dissolve, giving rise to a new era of intelligent neurology marked by greater precision, accessibility, and humanity.

This volume serves as both a snapshot of current progress and a roadmap for what lies ahead. We hope it inspires further inquiry, collaboration, and innovation at the intersection of technology and brain health, and strengthens the global effort to improve outcomes for individuals living with neurological diseases.

Chapter 1
A Decade of Progress: Artificial Intelligence in Multiple Sclerosis (2015–2025) – Diagnostic Innovations, Prognostic Modeling, and Future Pathways

Jyoti Kumari
https://orcid.org/0009-0005-4853-8963
Veer Surendra Sai University of Technology, India

Santi Kumari Behera
https://orcid.org/0000-0003-4857-7821
Veer Surendra Sai University of Technology, India

Prabira Kumar Sethy
https://orcid.org/0000-0003-3477-6715
Sambalpur University, India

ABSTRACT

Over the past decade, AI has transformed multiple sclerosis (MS) research and care, enhancing diagnosis, prognosis, and disease monitoring. From 2015 to 2025, AI evolved from basic image classification to advanced multi-modal models predicting disease progression and treatment response. Deep learning improved lesion detection and brain atrophy assessment via MRI, while machine learning enabled MS subtype identification and prognostic modeling. Researchers leveraged diverse datasets—MRI repositories, clinical trials, and EHRs—to train CNNs, RNNs, ensembles, and transformers. These advances improved diagnostic precision and supported disease trajectory prediction. AI tools now aid radiologists in tailoring

DOI: 10.4018/979-8-3373-2706-8.ch001

treatments, though challenges like model generalizability, data harmonization, and regulatory approval persist. The future lies in federated learning, explainable AI, and real-time decision support to realize precision medicine in MS care.

1. INTRODUCTION

Multiple Sclerosis (MS) is an immune-mediated, chronic neurodegenerative condition of the central nervous system (CNS) that strikes millions of people across the globe. MS is marked by inflammation, demyelination, and neurodegeneration, resulting in numerous physical and cognitive disabilities (Ramaglia et al., 2021). Primary progressive MS (PPMS), secondary progressive MS (SPMS), and relapsing remitting MS (RRMS) are some of the other forms of MS, which have their own respective clinical issues and disease courses. Treatment at an early stage for the delay of the course of the disease is dependent on early and proper diagnosis, but MS remains difficult to diagnose because of its heterogeneity, symptom variability, and requirement for proper integration of clinical, radiological, and laboratory evaluations (Ghasemi et al., 2016). Challenges in discrimination between multiple sclerosis and other neuroinflammatory diseases, discrimination of disease subtypes, prediction of long-term outcomes, and assessment of response to therapy remain undeterred notwithstanding advances in clinical and radiological assessment, including magnetic resonance imaging (MRI) (Rose et al., 2021). Because of their deep dependence on experienced doctors, classical diagnostic and prognosis methods impose subjectivity, inter-observer variability, and time lag in decision-making. Exploration into advanced technology, particularly artificial intelligence (AI), has been motivated by the growing complexity in MS diagnosis and treatment. AI has the potential to tackle grand challenges in MS clinical practice by enhancing disease stratification, enhancing diagnostic precision, and providing predictive value (Nabizadeh et al., 2022). AI has the ability to assist doctors in identifying patterns that may be difficult for human vision to detect using vast amounts of clinical and imaging information. This can assist in the detection of early MS, accurate subtype classification, and prediction of disease progression. This decade review strives to present the key advances in AI applications in MS research during the period 2015-2025. Besides predicting the future direction and emerging trends, this research tries to evaluate the impact of these advances in MS diagnostics, prognostics, and clinical management. This review is targeted at presenting a systematic understanding of the progress in application of AI in MS by integrating the current status of integration of AI in MS and indicating any loopholes and areas where research can be extended. An extensive literature search was conducted to identify relevant studies that were published between 2015 and 2025. A PRISMA-type architecture guided the search, ensuring complete inclusion criteria for conference proceedings, peer-reviewed journals, and clinical trials. The search terms were "Multiple Sclerosis," "Artificial Intelligence," "Machine Learning," "MRI," "Diagnosis," "Prognosis," and also "Subtypes." All major databases such as PubMed, IEEE Xplore, Scopus, and Google Scholar were searched. Studies that provided valuable information on the evolving role of AI in MS research and clinical practice were selected following eligible studies were screened for quality, relevance, and utility to AI in MS.

2. FOUNDATIONS: AI TECHNIQUES AND CLINICAL NEEDS IN MS

Machine Learning (ML): A subfield of artificial intelligence that enables computers to predict or decide without explicit programming by extracting patterns from data. Used to identify patterns, categorize, and forecast data from imaging and clinical formats.
Deep Learning (DL): A technical branch of ML employing multi-layer neural networks to represent advanced patterns in big data. Particularly useful in image analysis (e.g., lesion detection, segmentation) through Convolutional Neural Networks (CNNs).
Radiomics: A method that pulls a high volume of quantitative features from medical images to detect patterns not perceptible to the naked eye. Helpful in determining disease progression and treatment response prediction.
Natural Language Processing (NLP): An AI technique dedicated to processing and interpreting human language in text format. Utilized to pull useful information from clinical notes, radiology reports, and electronic health records.

Mapping Clinical Needs of MS to AI Applications

Imaging Segmentation: Deep Learning (e.g., CNNs) of AI performs the segmentation of spinal cord and brain lesions in MRI scans automatically. This enhances consistency, minimizes manual labor, and increases detection of disease activity.
Progression Prediction: Machine Learning models process longitudinal clinical and imaging data to predict disease progression. These predictions enable clinicians to track worsening disability and plan interventions on time.
Cognitive Impairment Modeling: AI integrates imaging biomarkers, neuropsychological evaluation, and clinical information to predict and model cognitive decline. It facilitates early identification and cognitive rehabilitation planning.

DMT Response Prediction: AI algorithms evaluate patient-specific variables (e.g., imaging, genomics, treatment) to predict disease-modifying therapy response. This allows for improved personalized and efficient treatment planning.

3. CHRONOLOGICAL MILESTONES (2015–2025)

3.1 Early Phase (2015–2018): Foundation and Exploration

Automated Lesion Detection: CNNs have been extensively applied to detect and localize white matter lesions from MS patients' MRI scans, minimizing the requirement for radiologists' manual annotations.
Lesion Volume Estimation: CNN-based models precisely estimate lesion volumes over time, essential for tracking disease progression and treatment efficacy.
Multi-Modal MRI Integration: CNNs seamlessly integrate various MRI sequences (e.g., T1-w, T2-w, FLAIR) to improve lesion contrast and segmentation accuracy.
Cascaded and Ensemble Models: Sophisticated architectures such as cascaded CNNs and ensemble networks enhance accuracy by removing false positives and sharpening lesion edges.
Transfer Learning and Few-Shot Learning: Large amounts of training data can be used to train CNNs, which can then be transferred to new datasets with very few labeled examples, overcoming the problem of data scarcity in MS imaging.
Clinical Decision Support: CNN predictions are increasingly being incorporated into clinical workflows to aid neurologists in diagnosis, disease monitoring, and treatment planning.

Here are several recent research papers (2015–2018) that align with the themes of clinical integration and innovation in multiple sclerosis (MS) research, focusing on transformer-based models, AI integration with genomics and wearable sensor data, early clinical deployment tools, and federated learning for privacy-preserving research:

Zaltzhendler et al. (2015) presents a solidly structured and extensive study of the application of convolutional neural networks (CNNs) to detect and segment Multiple Sclerosis (MS) lesions from brain MRIs. The multi-scale CNN solution successfully combines local and contextual features of the image with good generalization over diverse clinical conditions. The research is based on robust experimental validation on two large-scale clinical trials with encouraging sensitivity and Dice values, especially for large lesions. In summary, the research shows a remarkable advancement in automated pathology segmentation with possible extension to other 3D medical image tasks. Valverde et al. (2017) presents a new automated technique for white matter lesion segmentation in Multiple Sclerosis employing a cascaded 3D patch-wise CNN architecture. The two-stage network improves the sensitivity of detecting lesion candidates followed by refining the outputs to limit false positives. Its strength lies in its ability to work with few labeled samples a typical difficulty with medical images. The approach showcases best-in-class performance on the public MICCAI2008 data, beating all MRI inputs with a ranking of first and third with fewer inputs. The approach also illustrates good generalizability on private clinical datasets with high correlation ($r \geq 0.97$) with ground truth lesion volumes, highlighting its strength and utility in clinical practice. Inglese et al. (2018), this paper introduce well captures the increasing significance of 7 Tesla (7T) MRI in the diagnosis and research of Multiple Sclerosis (MS). It summarizes the benefits of 7T MRI as enhanced detection of lesions, increased spatial resolution, and enhanced diagnostic specificity. The article also underscores its wider implications for neuroimaging and recent approval in the clinic, further cementing its capability to improve MS diagnosis, monitoring, and treatment planning. Eshaghi et al. (2018), this work presents a comprehensive longitudinal examination of grey matter atrophy development in multiple sclerosis (MS), based on a large, multi-center database and a data-driven event-based model. It discloses a uniform pattern of atrophy in MS phenotypes and demonstrates significant correlations between disease duration, disability accumulation, and atrophy progression—particularly in relapsing-remitting MS. The results provide useful information on MS pathophysiology and identify possible markers for monitoring disease, although the absence of observed treatment effects provokes further research. Yoo et al. (2018), this study provides an exhaustive set of deep learning methods for multimodal neuroimaging analysis in Multiple Sclerosis (MS). Overcoming issues with minor annotations and high data dimensionality, the research presents new unsupervised and supervised strategies for lesion segmentation, early pathology detection, conversion prediction, and differential diagnosis. A key feature is the application of unlabeled data and hierarchical multimodal fusion, which are valuable contributions. The models present a major improvement in the automated analysis of neuroimaging for multiple sclerosis and demonstrate strong performance, indicating high clinical utility even with minor datasets. Pawlitzki et al. (2017) suggested it gives strong evidence that even without white matter lesions or brain atrophy, the integrity of the corticospinal tract (CST) is disrupted in early multiple sclerosis (MS).With the use of diffusion tensor imaging (DTI), the authors prove that, compared to normal controls, patients with relapsing-remitting multiple sclerosis (RRMS) and clinically isolated syndrome (CIS) have prominent microstructural anomalies. These results prove the sensitivity of DTI in detecting early neurodegenerative changes and highlight the utility of DTI as a diagnostic tool for early identification of MS. Zhang et al. (2018), employing a new convolutional neural network (CNN) structure, this paper reports a paradigm-shifting deep learning method for the MS brain slice classification. The proposed model is shown to exhibit outstanding performance with 98.22% sensitivity, 98.24% specificity, and 98.23% accuracy through parametric rectified linear unit (PReLU) and dropout. The outcome reveals that, compared to conventional methods, both PReLU and dropout significantly enhance model accuracy. The model's superiority compared to current methods indicates that it has excellent potential for clinical use in MS diagnosis. Manogaran et al. (2016), in evaluating axonal and neuronal loss in Multiple Sclerosis (MS) and Neuromyelitis Optica Spectrum Disorder (NMOSD), the utility of structural magnetic resonance imaging (MRI) and optical coherence tomography (OCT) is emphasized by this review. Given specific attention to the visual pathway, providing a singular method for CNS damage evaluation, the review highlights how the integration of OCT and MRI can elucidate important information regarding disease-specific injury, trans-synaptic degeneration, and the wider effects of MS and NMOSD on the central nervous system. There is considerable promise in distinguishing between these diseases and disentangling the course of neurodegeneration using this dual approach. Tsagkas et al. (2018), For relapse-onset multiple sclerosis (MS), this study offers informative long-term results on the amount of spinal cord (SCV) loss as a disease progression biomarker. Across 6 years, SCV loss emerged as a robust predictor of the course of disability, with secondary progressive multiple sclerosis (SPMS) being particularly well-predicted. In relapsing-remitting multiple sclerosis (RRMS), the findings show that SCV loss is associated with clinical relapses and is a better indicator of physical disability than other MRI measures such as total brain volume or T2 lesion volume. The findings highlight the utility of SCV loss as an important measure for assessing the severity and progression of MS. Birenbaum et al. (2017), This work proposes an independent, deep learning-based algorithm for MS lesion segmentation that overcomes the limitation posed by lesion heterogeneity in MR images. The algorithm utilizes priors and White Matter MR intensities to identify probable lesion voxels, which are subsequently segmented with Convolutional Neural Networks (CNN) once false positives are minimized. Employing longitudinal data to enhance segmentation accuracy is a new aspect. When evaluated on the 2015 Longitudinal MS Lesion Segmentation Challenge dataset, the approach achieves state-of-the-art performance comparable to that of experienced human raters. The proposed approach holds high promise in clinical diagnosis and follow-up of patients by reducing the need for lengthy manual segmentation.

3.2 Middle Phase (2019–2022): Model Sophistication and Dataset Growth

Here are several recent research papers (2019–2022) that align with the themes of clinical integration and innovation in multiple sclerosis (MS) research, focusing on transformer-based models, AI integration with genomics and wearable sensor data, early clinical deployment tools, and federated learning for privacy-preserving research:

Zhang et al. (2019), This work introduces RSANet, a novel deep network for automatically segmenting MS lesions from T2-weighted MRI. By considering 3D scans as sequential slice attention, RSANet employs recurrent attention mechanisms to learn more contextual information among slices. The approach outperforms existing state of the art on a 43-patient MS dataset, and its high potential use for more accurate and efficient lesion volume measurement in clinical work. . Hou et al. (2019), The novel deep architecture for MS lesion segmentation introduced in this paper, CA-DCN, incorporates an attentive cross-attention mechanism into traditional encoder-decoder networks. Spatial and channel attention are integrated into the model to enhance feature representation and reduce deep networks' interpretability issue. On the ISBI 2015 MS segmentation dataset, when evaluated, CA-DCN is one of the top-performing algorithms, not just proving to be clinically useful but also showing its efficacy. Vang et al. (2020), To improve performance for lesions of varying sizes, this paper presents Synergy-Net, a new MS lesion segmentation method that integrates global and local perspectives. The model successfully captures big as well as small lesions by merging U-Net for global segmentation with Mask R-CNN for local segmentation. When these methods are integrated into one framework, segmentation accuracy is greatly enhanced, as evidenced by higher Dice scores, decreased true positive rates, and fewer false positives on two datasets. The results showcase how the combination of stronger lesion segmentation can be obtained through the integration of local and global contextual information. Chen et al (2021), To overcome the challenges of distributed lesions and non spherical lesion shapes, this paper proposes DAG-Net, a new MS lesion segmentation method that works synergistically by fusing attention mechanisms and graph-based learning. To efficiently discriminate lesions in various locations and induce global contour definition, DAG-Net combines spatial correlations and global context into one framework. Dynamic graphs allow the model to be explained, and that provides confidence to the segmentation outcome. Experiment results on the ISBI2015 and an in-house dataset indicate that DAG-Net is superior to current methods and proves its ability to segment fragmented and heterogeneous MS lesions. Zhang et al. (2021), This work proposes DAG-Net, a new method of MS lesion segmentation to solve issues of disparate lesion morphologies and spread-out lesions. DAG-Net represents geospatial relationships and strikes a balance between global outline definition through graph-guided networks and attention mechanisms. The model's dynamic graphs and spatial-channel attention module facilitate better feature aggregation and offer explainable learning. DAG-Net surpasses current state-of-the-art methods both in geometrical and in clinical measures with regards to segmenting lesions of various sites, as shown by measurements on the ISBI 2015 dataset and an internal dataset. Sadeghibakhi et al. (2022), This research provides a faster alternative to multimodal methods through the description of a new MS lesion segmentation technique based solely on FLAIR MRI scans. Inspired by spatial-channel attention mechanisms and 3D-ResNet, the researchers propose a patch-based Convolutional Neural Network (CNN). The proposed technique involves preprocessing steps in the form of edge detection and CLAHE, patch selection, and attention-based segmentation. The efficacy of one-modality lesion segmentation is evidenced in our approach, which, when compartmentalized on the ISBI challenge database, provides better dice similarity and absolute volume difference than currently offered by those methods. Essa et al. (2020), This work proposes a patch-wise 3D R-CNN-based method for unsupervised MS lesion segmentation from FLAIR and T2-weighted MRI scans. The first step of the two-phase framework construction is lesion segmentation employing R-CNN. The results of both modalities are subsequently fused using fusion via an adaptive neuro-fuzzy inference system (ANFIS).The technique competes favorably with an average total score of 83.25 and a sensitivity of 61.8% when evaluated on the MICCAI 2008 MS challenge dataset. For enhanced MS lesion segmentation, the outcomes demonstrate the capability to merge deep learning with neuro-fuzzy systems. Krishnamoorthy et al. (2022), This paper presents a CNN-based approach for MS lesion segmentation with a pretrained VGG19 encoder and a VGG-UNet model. The proposed approach performs significantly better on axial, coronal, and sagittal 2D slices of the FLAIR modality when validated on 30 patient images. The accuracy (>98%), dice (>92%), and jaccard (>85%) values of the new strategy highlight its better performance compared to conventional methods like UNet, SegNet, and other VGG versions. These encouraging findings emphasize just how well the VGG-UNet model performs in identifying MS lesions in brain MRI with precision. Zeng et al. (2020), this paper provides a systematic review of automatic MS lesion segmentation using deep learning-based methods, bridging the gap in previous research that had not comprehensively explored CNN-based methods. The authors classify the reviewed algorithms into two categories based on CNN type and their strengths and limitations. Quantitative comparison between methods is performed with metrics such as Dice Similarity Coefficient (DSC) and Positive Predictive Value (PPV). The paper concludes with the mention of future possibilities regarding the use of deep learning for MS lesion segmentation, offering valuable suggestions to researchers. Sarica et al. (2022), the present work introduces a deep neural network pipeline involving U-Net, attention gates, and residual learning for better segmentation of new MS lesions using baseline and follow-up 3D FLAIR MRI scans. The architecture uses residual units for better training and performance with fewer parameters, and attention gates focus on salient lesion features. Evaluated on the MSSEG-2 challenge dataset, the approach described herein achieved similar lesion-wise F1 and Dice scores and ranked 8th in a competition, beating 22 other methods. The results obtained demonstrate the effectiveness of the approach described herein for longitudinal MS lesion tracking.

3.3 Recent Phase (2023–2025): Clinical Integration and Innovation

Here are several recent research papers (2023–2025) that align with the themes of clinical integration and innovation in multiple sclerosis (MS) research, focusing on transformer-based models, AI integration with genomics and wearable sensor data, early clinical deployment tools, and federated learning for privacy-preserving research:

Bučková et al. (2023), this research employs statistical and machine learning methods to model multimodal neuroimaging data to classify multiple sclerosis (MS) patients and healthy controls, and to predict motor disability in MS patients. The methods used include fractional anisotropy, grey matter volumes, and functional connectivity and had high classification accuracy (96.1%) with support vector machines. The low-dimensional logistic regression model yielded more consistent results in predicting motor impairment. The research points out the association between white and grey matter alterations and motor disability, and shows the promise of quantitative MRI metrics for precise classification and understandable machine learning models in MS research. Andorra et al. (2024), this research investigates the application of machine learning models to forecast disease activity and disability development in patients with multiple sclerosis (MS) by combining clinical, imaging, and omics information. Examined on a multi-centric cohort of 322 patients with MS and 98 controls, the research suggests predictors of disability accumulation, disease activity, and treatment intensification with intermediate to high accuracy. Combination of clinical and imaging information produced robust results, and inclusion of omics information marginally increased performance. The method was applied to an independent cohort and shown to have utility in identifying patients with MS who are at risk of worsening disability. Noteboom et al. (2024), this research examines the application of machine learning (ML) models for the classification of clinical impairment and prediction of worsening in individuals with multiple sclerosis (pwMS) based on clinical and MRI information from two MS cohorts. It was discovered that ML models classified clinical impairment at baseline accurately, especially for cognitive impairment and high disability, and support vector machines (SVM) performed the best. However, long-term clinical deterioration prediction at 2- and 5-year follow-ups was still an unsolved challenge. The findings indicate that although ML can contribute to pwMS classification and the identification of appropriate biomarkers, more effort should be made to advance predictions of disease progression. Bai et al. (2024), this paper tackles a key challenge in automatic segmentation of Multiple Sclerosis (MS) lesions based on deep learning models, i.e., the lack of well-annotated data. The authors design a federated learning framework that facilitates collaboration among several clinical sites without compromising data privacy, an essential aspect in medical studies. They introduce two new approaches: the Decoupled Hard Label Correction (DHLC) and Centrally Enhanced Label Correction (CELC). These methods efficiently resolve label noise and imbalanced distributions by enhancing the quality of annotations via prediction confidence and central model direction. The experiments, conducted with large-scale multi-site datasets, show the efficacy and resilience of these techniques for training deep learning models. The suggested framework not only enhances model performance but also decreases the cost and complexity of data annotation and collection, which makes it extremely applicable for clinical use. De Rosa et al. (2024), this work presents a consensus strategy for enhancing MS lesion segmentation in brain MRI imaging, a vital diagnostic and follow-up task which has long been labor-intensive. Through the combining of the predictions of several contemporary state-of-the-art deep-learning algorithms without having to retrain them, the approach takes the best from all algorithms. Used on both public and private data, the method demonstrated evident gains in segmentation accuracy—4–8% improvement in Dice scores and 3–4% in precision. The strong correlation with true lesion volume and number validates its reliability. This ensemble-type framework works well to improve performance and consistency, providing a feasible and scalable solution for clinical application. Zhang et al. (2024), this work addresses the problem of domain generalization in deep learning-based MS lesion segmentation of MR images. Acknowledging the shortcoming of one-shot domain adaptation in the face of limited labeled data, the authors present a new approach that combines one-shot adaptation examples with *contrast-harmonized* training examples to more closely resemble the target domain. Their approach greatly enhances segmentation accuracy, illustrating that harmonized data alone can at times outperform standard one-shot methods. Notably, the adaptation procedure is effective, and only minimal fine-tuning is needed. The method presents a useful and efficient solution for model generalization improvement across varied clinical environments. Chaves et al. (2024), the present research introduces an exhaustive analysis of a DL model for MS lesion segmentation with the comparison of its performance with both DL and non-DL competitors. Cross-tested on a wide variety of Latin American and European datasets, the model beat all others with regard to Dice coefficient and reliability. The model proved to be robust and generalizable and stable on rescanned patients. Most importantly, it surpassed inter-human annotator agreement and reached high consistency across scans. The findings underscore the model's clinical promise for precise, cost-effective, and generalizable MS lesion segmentation in diverse real-world scenarios. Tahghighi et al. (2024), this work presents a new self-supervised pre-training method augmented with synthetic lesion data to enhance novel MS lesion segmentation. Based on the MSSEG-2 challenge dataset, the model achieved a Dice score of 56.15 ± 7.06% and an F1 score of 56.69 ± 9.12%, a 2.06% and 3.3% improvement over existing methods respectively. The approach successfully combines real and synthetic data to enhance model generalizability and robustness against limitations of limited annotated data and inter-expert variations in lesion tracking. Wiltgen et al. (2024), LST-AI is an AI-powered, open-source successor of the classical LST white matter lesion segmentation tool in Multiple Sclerosis (MS). It ensembles three trained 3D U-Nets on 491 expert-annotated in-house T1-weighted and FLAIR MRI scans. With 0.65 Dice and 0.63 F1 on MSSEG-1 challenge data set, LST-AI achieves higher results compared to proven software like nnUNet, SAMSEG, and LST (< 0.56 all of them). It also encompasses lesion-type annotation according to McDonald criteria. LST-AI provides better performance, high rates of lesion detection (>75% for lesions of 10–100 mm^3), and adjustable deployment through Python, Docker, or CLI, which makes it a good candidate for clinical and research applications. Madduri et al. (2024), this paper introduces a visionary solution toward achieving a Learning Healthcare System (LHS) through the incorporation of Privacy-Preserving Federated Learning (PPFL). PPFL allows for collaborative, decentralized multimodal patient data analysis with strict privacy, overcoming key obstacles in sharing data. The introduced framework aligns with the Institute of Medicine's vision and provides a scalable and secure road toward ongoing healthcare improvement through self-learning systems.

4. DOMAIN-WISE REVIEW OF AI IN MS

4.1 AI in MRI Lesion Segmentation and Quantification

The application of AI for MRI lesion segmentation has come a long way. Initial approaches used patch-based Convolutional Neural Networks (CNNs), which analyzed small image patches separately. As time passed, more advanced architectures such as U-Net3D that can capture the entire volumetric context appeared. This was further optimized by nnU-Net, a self adjusting framework that adjusts to new data sets, and by Transformer-based hybrids, which integrate global attention mechanisms to improve feature learning. Comparative analyses on public benchmarks like BRATS, ISLES, and MSSEG have revealed that nnU-Net tends to establish state-of-the-art performance, although Transformer models are now catching up, particularly in intricate lesion tasks. Moreover, AI methods now automatically perform brain atrophy measurement, essential for conditions like multiple sclerosis and Alzheimer's. Such approaches offer reliable, reproducible volumetric measurements, enhancing clinical decision making..

4.2 MS Subtype Classification and Disease Course Prediction

AI techniques for multiple sclerosis (MS) are aimed at subclassifying types such as Relapsing-Remitting MS (RRMS), Secondary Progressive MS (SPMS), and Primary Progressive MS (PPMS). Conventional classifiers such as random forests and SVMs have been employed using clinical, imaging, and biomarker information. Time-series models such as RNNs and LSTMs have recently emerged for identifying patterns of disease progression over time. One of the key research objectives is forecasting the shift from RRMS to SPMS, in order to intervene earlier and provide tailored therapy.

Here's a simple and clean comparison table:

Table 1.

Subtype	Imaging Features	Clinical Features	Demographic Features
RRMS (Relapsing-Remitting MS)	New/enlarging lesions during relapses	Relapses with partial or full recovery	Onset: 20–40 years; more common in women
SPMS (Secondary Progressive MS)	Progressive brain atrophy; fewer new lesions	Gradual worsening after initial RRMS phase	Develops after 10–20 years of RRMS
PPMS (Primary Progressive MS)	Diffuse spinal cord damage; brain atrophy; fewer lesions	Steady decline from onset, without clear relapses	Onset: around 40 years; affects men and women equally

4.3 Prognostic Modeling and Relapse Prediction

Machine learning (ML) models are commonly employed to predict relapse counts and future burden of lesions among MS patients. The models analyze trends in prior MRI scans, clinical visits, and treatment courses. Prognostic models are usually blended with EDSS (Expanded Disability Status Scale) progression curves that monitor worsening of disability over a period of time to enhance the prediction of long-term outcomes. One of the most important breakthroughs is data fusion, in which heterogeneous sources such as MRI imaging, clinical history, and cognitive test scores are integrated to create more precise, individualized models for relapse risk and disease progression.

4.4 AI for Therapeutic Response Prediction

Artificial Intelligence (AI) models are trained to forecast individual MS patients' response to disease-modifying treatments (DMTs). Some of the algorithms employed to model DMT success from patient information (MRI, clinical presentation, demographics) include XGBoost, Support Vector Machines (SVM), and deep neural networks. These models enable personalized treatment protocols, choosing the therapy with the greatest likelihood of succeeding for every patient. Further, AI can undertake longitudinal outcome prediction, forecasting the trajectory of disability and lesion burden with different treatments, optimising long-term management.

4.5 Multimodal and Multitask Learning in MS

MS multimodal learning constructs better and more detailed models by taking advantage of diverse forms of data. This involves consolidating cerebrospinal fluid (CSF) biomarkers, electronic health records (EHR), and neuroimaging data (e.g., MRI). The diversity of the data provides a wider perspective of the status of the patient as well as improving understanding of the disease course. Multimodal models, in contrast to single-modality models, can predict cognitive decline, lesion burden, and relapse risk more reliably through integrating structural and functional imaging and clinical and biochemical information. Alternatively, training models that can perform a few related tasks simultaneously is referred to as multitask learning. Such tasks in MS typically involve prognosis (estimating disease progression, relapse frequency, and functional impairment) as well as diagnosis (identifying the MS subtype, e.g., RRMS, SPMS, or PPMS). Because they provide knowledge exchange across activities, multitask models are particularly advantageous as they improve the model's performance across all tasks. For example, predicting neuroimaging features and assessing cognitive outcomes or functional test performance (e.g., hand function or mobility) gives clinicians a more complete picture of the condition and helps them make better treatment decisions. These techniques can also be used with longitudinal data, which allows models to forecast future illness progression in addition to the current state, improving patient monitoring and care over time.

5. KEY DATASETS AND BENCHMARKS IN THE DECADE

Over the last ten years, a number of important datasets and benchmarks have helped AI applications for multiple sclerosis (MS) get better. The MSSEG challenges in 2016 and 2021 were important because they gave researchers standardised datasets to use to test how well lesion segmentation works. The ISBI Longitudinal MS Lesion Challenge gave researchers a way to look at how lesions change over time, which helped them create models that predict the future. MICCAI datasets have been very helpful for comparing algorithms and analysing multi-modal MRI data. Also, many important studies have used in-house information from clinical centres, which has made it possible to create models that are specific to each study. Even with these resources, there are still problems with data diversity, built-in biases, and the lack of standardised imaging methods. These problems make it hard to compare and generalise models across investigations. For wider use in clinical settings, it is important to fix these problems through harmonisation and federated learning.

6. EXPLAINABILITY, VALIDATION, AND CLINICAL TRANSLATION

Explainability, validation, and clinical translation are essential components for the integration of AI into multiple sclerosis (MS) care. Explainable AI (XAI) tools, including SHAP, Grad-CAM, and LIME, are utilised to interpret model decisions, allowing clinicians to comprehend feature significance and visualise lesion-based predictions in MRI scans. Validation frameworks that evaluate performance across different centres and scanners are essential for ensuring model robustness and generalisability in various clinical environments. Initial pilot trials and clinical acceptance studies indicate a positive integration of AI tools within diagnostic workflows, facilitating personalised treatment planning. Regulatory compliance presents a significant challenge, as agencies such as the FDA prioritise safety and efficacy, while GDPR and HIPAA establish frameworks for data privacy and ethical utilisation. Understanding these frameworks is crucial for integrating AI developments into standard clinical practice.

7. CHALLENGES OVER THE DECADE

Although the past decade has witnessed unprecedented advances in the use of AI for managing multiple sclerosis (MS), various obstacles persist and must be overcome for the ongoing success and expansion of AI technologies in this context.

- Dataset Constraints (Size, Annotating Cost, Heterogeneity):

A key problem with AI research in MS is the small dataset size. Medical datasets, especially those of neuroimaging data, are usually small because collecting data from many patients is challenging. Also, annotating medical images and clinical data is costly and time-consuming, involving expert clinicians and radiologists. MS heterogeneity, with different subtypes, disease stages, and responses to treatment, makes dataset construction more complicated. These aspects may restrict the diversity and representativeness of training data for AI models, hence their performance across various patient groups and clinical settings.

- Generalizability and Model Robustness:

AI models tend to suffer from issues regarding generalizability the capacity to perform optimally on data that were not part of the training group. A model that has been trained on data from one institution can have difficulty functioning when used with data from another institution because of differences in imaging protocol, patient populations, or practice patterns. Robustness to a variety of patient populations, imaging modalities, and healthcare systems is a major challenge. Models need to be trained and tested on large sets of datasets so that they can be assured to work in real-world, clinical settings.

- Interpretability vs. Complexity Trade-Off:

As AI models, particularly deep learning methods, increase in complexity, they tend to become "black-box" systems that are hard to interpret. Though such models may offer high performance, their un-transparency becomes a significant limitation in clinical settings, where knowing the reasoning behind a decision is imperative. The interpretability complexity trade-off is a basic problem—simple models are more interpretable but might not capture the full predictive capability of complex models. Balancing good predictions and comprehensible decision-making is vital when integrating AI into clinical practice, where there must be trust and belief in the model's outputs.

- Challenges with Reproducibility and Benchmarking:

Repeatability of results is another important issue in the MS field that relies on AI. Most research fails to replicate results on other datasets or with different software tools because there is either a lack of standardized protocols or transparent methods. In addition, benchmarking of AI models on consistent large datasets is problematic because publicly available datasets tend to be small, incomplete, or without adequate clinical annotations.

This model can result in a lack of ability to accurately capture the performance of a model and its comparison with current methods. Setting standardized datasets and methods for benchmarking would be a key step towards solving these issues of reproducibility. Each one of these is an area of continued research and cooperation needed in order to increase the performance and clinical utility of AI models applied to MS. To overcome all of these is the key to achieving the greatest potential of the use of AI in the care and treatment of MS.

8. FUTURE OUTLOOK (2025–2030)

The decade to come for AI in MS research and clinical practice is extremely promising, with numerous major advancements in the making to redefine precision neurology and live MS tracking.

- Large Multimodal Models (e.g., Med-PaLM, BioGPT, MONAI):

Big multimodal models, such as Med-PaLM, BioGPT, and MONAI, are likely to transform MS research and care. These models combine different types of data—clinical, imaging, genetic, and even electronic health records—enabling a more thorough understanding of MS. Through the strength of newer deep learning, these models not only will increase diagnostic accuracy but also provide predictive information on disease progression and response to treatment. With the development of these models, they will be instrumental in personalized treatment plans, providing individualized interventions based on individual patient profiles.

- Combining Patient-Reported Outcomes and Wearable Data:

In the future, the combination of patient-reported outcomes (PROs) and wearable data will become extremely important in MS management. Wearable devices monitoring actual physiological metrics (e.g., activity, heart rate, or sleep) will offer real-time feedback on the patient's status. Combined with PROs, which provide subjective measures of symptoms and quality of life, these streams of data will enable more accurate, dynamic monitoring of the disease. This change will permit clinicians to make more informed decisions in near real-time, modifying treatment protocols and interventions as a result.

- Rise of Federated Learning in Neuroimaging:

Federated learning, a method in which models are trained on decentralized datasets without exchanging sensitive patient information, is making waves in neuroimaging and MS research. This method will allow collaboration among medical institutions globally without patient privacy breaches, resulting in more powerful and diverse AI models. By aggregating information from different sources, federated learning will enable cross-institutional studies that increase the generalizability of AI algorithms, making them more accurate and useful for a global MS population.

- Vision for AI in Precision Neurology and Real-Time MS Monitoring:

The future of AI in MS will be closely interlinked with precision neurology, where AI-based tools monitor and analyze patient information in real time. By 2030, artificial intelligence-driven systems will most likely be a part of tailored treatment plans, adjusting drug options and dosing on the basis of continuous surveillance. This future is imagined as one of easy coordination among imaging, genetic information, wearable technology, and patient feedback, so clinicians can monitor disease activity, forecast relapses, and evaluate treatment response in real time. These developments will result in a move towards preventive care, as AI picks up early indicators of disease progression much earlier than clinical symptoms are apparent.

In short, from massive multimodal AI models to live MS monitoring, the future for MS research and treatment is bright. By joining innovative technologies with patient-orientation, the coming decade will witness AI revolutionizing not just the way we comprehend MS but also the way we treat and manage it, opening the door to a future of more accurate, tailored, and efficient care.

9. CONCLUSION

AI in MS has witnessed a revolution in the last decade with strong advancements in personalized medical methods, early detection, and prognosis of disease progression. Techniques based on AI, particularly machine learning-based algorithms that are complex, have enhanced the precision and speed of lesion segmentation, facilitated the prediction of relapse, and allowed multimodal data integration. These advances have enhanced our understanding of multiple sclerosis and how to treat MS, leading to precision medicine in the clinic. Yet, only through collaboration among doctors, AI scientists, and policymakers will the full promise of AI in MS research and treatment be fulfilled. Physicians bring essential medical expertise, and AI scientists create the tools and algorithms to analyze complex information. It is essential for policymakers to ensure legal frameworks that facilitate the ethical and pervasive use of AI technology in health. Standardized AI pipelines for MS research and clinical practice are urgently required to drive this field forward. By guaranteeing that AI models are tested, reproducible, and portable across institutions, standardization would facilitate collaboration and allow more pervasive, standardized clinical use. AI can revolutionize MS care and better the lives of patients with these collaborative efforts.

REFERENCES

Andorra, M., Freire, A., Zubizarreta, I., de Rosbo, N. K., Bos, S. D., Rinas, M., Høgestøl, E. A., de Rodez Benavent, S. A., Berge, T., Brune-Ingebretse, S., Ivaldi, F., Cellerino, M., Pardini, M., Vila, G., Pulido-Valdeolivas, I., Martinez-Lapiscina, E. H., Llufriu, S., Saiz, A., Blanco, Y., & Villoslada, P. (2024). Predicting disease severity in multiple sclerosis using multimodal data and machine learning. *Journal of Neurology, 271*(3), 1133–1149. DOI: 10.1007/s00415-023-12132-z

Bai, L., Wang, D., Wang, H., Barnett, M., Cabezas, M., Cai, W., Calamante, F., Kyle, K., Liu, D., Ly, L., Nguyen, A., Shieh, C.-C., Sullivan, R., Zhan, G., Ouyang, W., & Wang, C. (2024). Improving multiple sclerosis lesion segmentation across clinical sites: A federated learning approach with noise-resilient training. *Artificial Intelligence in Medicine, 152*, 102872. DOI: 10.1016/j.artmed.2024.102872

Birenbaum, A., & Greenspan, H. (2017). Multi-view longitudinal CNN for multiple sclerosis lesion segmentation. *Engineering Applications of Artificial Intelligence, 65*, 111–118. DOI: 10.1016/j.engappai.2017.06.006

Chaves, H., Serra, M. M., Shalom, D. E., Ananía, P., Rueda, F., Osa Sanz, E., Stefanoff, N. I., Rodríguez Murúa, S., Costa, M. E., Kitamura, F. C., Yañez, P., Cejas, C., Correale, J., Ferrante, E., Fernández Slezak, D., & Farez, M. F. (2024). Assessing robustness and generalization of a deep neural network for brain MS lesion segmentation on real-world data. *European Radiology, 34*(3), 2024–2035. DOI: 10.1007/s00330-023-10093-5

Chen, Z., Wang, X., Huang, J., Lu, J., & Zheng, J. (2021). Deep attention and graphical neural network for multiple sclerosis lesion segmentation from MR imaging sequences. *IEEE Journal of Biomedical and Health Informatics, 26*(3), 1196–1207. DOI: 10.1109/JBHI.2021.3109119

De Rosa, A. P., Benedetto, M., Tagliaferri, S., Bardozzo, F., D'Ambrosio, A., Bisecco, A., Gallo, A., Cirillo, M., Tagliaferri, R., & Esposito, F. (2024). Consensus of algorithms for lesion segmentation in brain MRI studies of multiple sclerosis. *Scientific Reports, 14*(1), 21348. DOI: 10.1038/s41598-024-72649-9

Eshaghi, A., Marinescu, R. V., Young, A. L., Firth, N. C., Prados, F., Jorge Cardoso, M., Tur, C., De Angelis, F., Cawley, N., Brownlee, W. J., De Stefano, N., Laura Stromillo, M., Battaglini, M., Ruggieri, S., Gasperini, C., Filippi, M., Rocca, M. A., Rovira, A., Sastre-Garriga, J., & Ciccarelli, O. (2018). Progression of regional grey matter atrophy in multiple sclerosis. *Brain, 141*(6), 1665–1677. DOI: 10.1093/brain/awy088

Essa, E., Aldesouky, D., Hussein, S. E., & Rashad, M. Z. (2020). Neuro-fuzzy patch-wise R-CNN for multiple sclerosis segmentation. *Medical & Biological Engineering & Computing*, *58*(9), 2161–2175. DOI: 10.1007/s11517-020-02225-6

Ghasemi, N., Razavi, S., & Nikzad, E. (2016). Multiple sclerosis: Pathogenesis, symptoms, diagnoses and cell-based therapy. *Cell Journal (Yakhteh)*, *19*(1), 1.

Hou, B., Kang, G., Xu, X., & Hu, C. (2019, November). Cross attention densely connected networks for multiple sclerosis lesion segmentation. In *2019 IEEE International Conference on Bioinformatics and Biomedicine (BIBM)* (pp. 2356-2361). IEEE. DOI: 10.1109/BIBM47256.2019.8983149

Inglese, M., Fleysher, L., Oesingmann, N., & Petracca, M. (2018). Clinical applications of ultra-high field magnetic resonance imaging in multiple sclerosis. *Expert Review of Neurotherapeutics*, *18*(3), 221–230. DOI: 10.1080/14737175.2018.1433033

Krishnamoorthy, S., Zhang, Y., Kadry, S., & Yu, W. (2022). Framework to segment and evaluate multiple sclerosis lesion in MRI slices using VGG-UNet. *Computational Intelligence and Neuroscience*, *2022*(1), 4928096. DOI: 10.1155/2022/4928096

Madduri, R., Li, Z., Nandi, T., Kim, K., Ryu, M., & Rodriguez, A. (2024, October). Advances in Privacy Preserving Federated Learning to Realize a Truly Learning Healthcare System. In *2024 IEEE 6th International Conference on Trust, Privacy and Security in Intelligent Systems, and Applications (TPS-ISA)* (pp. 273-279). IEEE. DOI: 10.1109/TPS-ISA62245.2024.00039

Manogaran, P., Hanson, J. V., Olbert, E. D., Egger, C., Wicki, C., Gerth-Kahlert, C., Landau, K., & Schippling, S. (2016). Optical coherence tomography and magnetic resonance imaging in multiple sclerosis and neuromyelitis optica spectrum disorder. *International Journal of Molecular Sciences*, *17*(11), 1894. DOI: 10.3390/ijms17111894

Nabizadeh, F., Masrouri, S., Ramezannezhad, E., Ghaderi, A., Sharafi, A. M., Soraneh, S., & Moghadasi, A. N. (2022). Artificial intelligence in the diagnosis of multiple sclerosis: A systematic review. *Multiple Sclerosis and Related Disorders*, *59*, 103673. DOI: 10.1016/j.msard.2022.103673

Noteboom, S., Seiler, M., Chien, C., Rane, R. P., Barkhof, F., Strijbis, E. M., Paul, F., Schoonheim, M. M., & Ritter, K. (2024). Evaluation of machine learning-based classification of clinical impairment and prediction of clinical worsening in multiple sclerosis. *Journal of Neurology*, *271*(8), 5577–5589. DOI: 10.1007/s00415-024-12507-w

Pawlitzki, M., Neumann, J., Kaufmann, J., Heidel, J., Stadler, E., Sweeney-Reed, C., Sailer, M., & Schreiber, S. (2017). Loss of corticospinal tract integrity in early MS disease stages. *Neurology Neuroimmunology & Neuroinflammation*, *4*(6), e399. DOI: 10.1212/NXI.0000000000000399

Ramaglia, V., Rojas, O., Naouar, I., & Gommerman, J. L. (2021). The ins and outs of central nervous system inflammation—Lessons learned from multiple sclerosis. *Annual Review of Immunology*, *39*(1), 199–226. DOI: 10.1146/annurev-immunol-093019-124155

Rehák Bučková, B., Mareš, J., Škoch, A., Kopal, J., Tintěra, J., Dineen, R., Řasová, K., & Hlinka, J. (2023). Multimodal-neuroimaging machine-learning analysis of motor disability in multiple sclerosis. *Brain Imaging and Behavior*, *17*(1), 18–34. DOI: 10.1007/s11682-022-00737-3

Rose, D. R., Amin, M., & Ontaneda, D. (2021). Prediction in treatment outcomes in multiple sclerosis: Challenges and recent advances. *Expert Review of Clinical Immunology*, *17*(11), 1187–1198. DOI: 10.1080/1744666X.2021.1986005

Sadeghibakhi, M., Pourreza, H., & Mahyar, H. (2022). Multiple sclerosis lesions segmentation using attention-based CNNs in FLAIR images. *IEEE Journal of Translational Engineering in Health and Medicine*, *10*, 1–11. DOI: 10.1109/JTEHM.2022.3172025

Sarica, B., & Seker, D. Z. (2022). New MS lesion segmentation with deep residual attention gate U-Net utilizing 2D slices of 3D MR images. *Frontiers in Neuroscience*, *16*, 912000. DOI: 10.3389/fnins.2022.912000

Tahghighi, P., Zhang, Y., Souza, R., & Komeili, A. (2024, October). Enhancing New Multiple Sclerosis Lesion Segmentation via Self-supervised Pre-training and Synthetic Lesion Integration. In *International Conference on Medical Image Computing and Computer-Assisted Intervention* (pp. 263-272). Cham: Springer Nature Switzerland. DOI: 10.1007/978-3-031-72111-3_25

Tsagkas, C., Magon, S., Gaetano, L., Pezold, S., Naegelin, Y., Amann, M., Stippich, C., Cattin, P., Wuerfel, J., Bieri, O., Sprenger, T., Kappos, L., & Parmar, K. (2018). Spinal cord volume loss: A marker of disease progression in multiple sclerosis. *Neurology*, *91*(4), e349–e358. DOI: 10.1212/WNL.0000000000005853

Valverde, S., Cabezas, M., Roura, E., González-Villà, S., Pareto, D., Vilanova, J. C., Ramió-Torrentà, L., Rovira, À., Oliver, A., & Lladó, X. (2017). Improving automated multiple sclerosis lesion segmentation with a cascaded 3D convolutional neural network approach. *NeuroImage*, *155*, 159–168. DOI: 10.1016/j.neuroimage.2017.04.034

Vang, Y. S., Cao, Y., Chang, P. D., Chow, D. S., Brandt, A. U., Paul, F., . . . Xie, X. (2020, April). SynergyNet: a fusion framework for multiple sclerosis brain MRI segmentation with local refinement. In *2020 IEEE 17th international symposium on biomedical imaging (ISBI)* (pp. 131-135). IEEE. DOI: 10.1109/ISBI45749.2020.9098610

Wiltgen, T., McGinnis, J., Schlaeger, S., Kofler, F., Voon, C., Berthele, A., Bischl, D., Grundl, L., Will, N., Metz, M., Schinz, D., Sepp, D., Prucker, P., Schmitz-Koep, B., Zimmer, C., Menze, B., Rueckert, D., Hemmer, B., Kirschke, J., & Wiestler, B. (2024). LST-AI: A deep learning ensemble for accurate MS lesion segmentation. *NeuroImage. Clinical*, *42*, 103611. DOI: 10.1016/j.nicl.2024.103611

Yoo, Y. (2018). *Deep learning for feature discovery in brain MRIs for patient-level classification with applications to multiple sclerosis* (Doctoral dissertation, University of British Columbia).

Zaltzhendler, M. (2015). *A deep-learning convolutional neural network framework for mulitple sclerosis lesion detection and segmentation in patient brain images.* McGill University.

Zeng, C., Gu, L., Liu, Z., & Zhao, S. (2020). Review of deep learning approaches for the segmentation of multiple sclerosis lesions on brain MRI. *Frontiers in Neuroinformatics*, *14*, 610967. DOI: 10.3389/fninf.2020.610967

Zhang, H., Zhang, J., Li, C., Sweeney, E. M., Spincemaille, P., Nguyen, T. D., Gauthier, S. A., Wang, Y., & Marcille, M. (2021). ALL-Net: Anatomical information lesion-wise loss function integrated into neural network for multiple sclerosis lesion segmentation. *NeuroImage. Clinical*, *32*, 102854. DOI: 10.1016/j.nicl.2021.102854

Zhang, H., Zhang, J., Zhang, Q., Kim, J., Zhang, S., Gauthier, S. A., & Wang, Y. (2019). RSANet: recurrent slice-wise attention network for multiple sclerosis lesion segmentation. In *Medical Image Computing and Computer Assisted Intervention–MICCAI 2019: 22nd International Conference, Shenzhen, China, October 13–17, 2019* [Springer International Publishing.]. *Proceedings*, *22*(Part III), 411–419.

Zhang, J., Zuo, L., Dewey, B. E., Remedios, S. W., Hays, S. P., Pham, D. L., . . . Carass, A. (2024, April). Harmonization-enriched domain adaptation with light fine-tuning for multiple sclerosis lesion segmentation. In *Medical Imaging 2024: Clinical and Biomedical Imaging* (Vol. 12930, pp. 635-641). SPIE. DOI: 10.1117/12.3011291

Zhang, Y. D., Pan, C., Sun, J., & Tang, C. (2018). Multiple sclerosis identification by convolutional neural network with dropout and parametric ReLU. *Journal of Computational Science*, *28*, 1–10. DOI: 10.1016/j.jocs.2018.07.003

Chapter 2
Advances in CNN-Based Breast Cancer Detection

Sana Salhi
https://orcid.org/0000-0001-6569-0952
Tunis El Manar University, Tunisia

Nour Fakhfakh
National School of Advanced Science and Technologies in Borj Cedria, Tunisia

Malak Sayeb
National School of Advanced Science and Technologies in Borj Cedria, Tunisia

ABSTRACT

This chapter investigates the recent advances in Convolutional Neural Networks for breast cancer detection in mammography. The survey reviews how emerging progress in CNN architectures are reshaping mammography interpretation and diagnostics. State-of-the-art and evaluation of optimization techniques are provided. A dedicated use case is analyzes and recommendations for model training optimization are revealed. The study is conducted on the Mammogram Mastery dataset which comprises 745 original images and 9,685 augmented images. Furthermore, the chapter addresses deep learning's potential to enhance mammographic assessment by improving diagnostic accuracy and reducing false errors. The insights presented aim to guide researchers and practitioners towards developing robust, reliable, and clinically impactful AI for breast cancer detection, highlighting key requirements for achieving advanced trustworthy and equitable outcomes.

DOI: 10.4018/979-8-3373-2706-8.ch002

1. INTRODUCTION

Breast cancer (BC) is the most prevalent cancer affecting women and has cancer-related mortality in women worldwide (Freddie, et al., 2024). Effective BC treatment poses a significant public health challenge. Early and accurate detection plays a crucial role in improving survival rates and treatment outcomes (Xiong, et al., 2025). Expert interpretation remains an essential step in current diagnostic methods such as mammography and biopsy. However, due to its perceptual nature, this process can be subject to variability besides being time-consuming. Cutting-edge progress in deep learning, notably Convolutional Neural Networks (CNNs) have offered a promising solution for automated and precise breast cancer classification and demonstrated tremendous success in medical image analysis.

This chapter presents an overview of the recent related works and highlights the existing deep learning approaches for breast cancer classification, with a special focus on CNNs. The study reports on the common methodologies and experimental outcomes, assessing each approach's efficacy and limits in accurately distinguishing benign from malignant breast tumors. The survey concludes by investigating the critical role of balanced datasets in the performance development of Convolutional Neural Networks (CNNs) for breast cancer detection in mammography. The review provides a case study that emphasizes the implications of training CNN models without applying data balancing techniques. Furthermore, this chapter reviews a bunch of deep learning techniques for breast cancer detection, emphasizing recent advances in hybrid architectures and sequence-based models. The implementation results of a case study using a CNN on the Mastery Mammogram dataset are also presented to evaluate practical performance and suggest areas for further optimization.

The organization of the rest of the chapter is as follows. The first section is dedicated to a general description of CNNs architecture and operating metrics. The second section gives an insight into current techniques for Breast Cancer (BC) detection. The Third section reviews and analyzes the recent CNNs based BC diagnosis approaches. The fourth section benchmarks recent optimization advances in CNNs and their impact on BC detection. The last section showcases a Case Study about pretrained CNN model Using the Mammogram Mastery Dataset. Results and possible optimization perspectives are given at the end of the chapter.

2. CONVOLUTIONAL NEURAL NETWORKS AND LEARNING

Tailored for image data analysis, Convolutional Neural Networks (CNNs) represent a class of deep learning models inspired by the visual cortex of the human brain. Their design incorporates concepts like local receptive fields and weight sharing to allow effective learning and extraction of image features. CNNs remarkable performance was demonstrated in a variety of computer vision challenges, mainly in image recognition and object detection and segmentation (Gao, et al., 2018), (Balasubramaniam, Velmurugan, Jaganathan, & Dhanasekaran, 2023) (Balasubramaniam, Velmurugan, Jaganathan, & Dhanasekaran, 2023).

2.1 Structure of CNNs for Image Recognition

The structure of a CNN comprises convolutional layers, pooling layers, and fully connected layers. These elements establish hierarchical representations for image classification. Convolutional layers extract features through using a set of adjustable filters applied to the input image. Identification of each pattern or characteristic within the image is performed by a specific filter. Feature maps are generated through convolutional operations by translating filters across the image, carrying out element-by-element products and summations. Then, integrating pooling layers into CNNs reduces computational complexity and enhances dominant features retaining. For instance, Max pooling layers extract the maximum value from a specific image area allowing decrease in the spatial dimensions of feature maps while conserving relevant information. Final classification decision is performed by fully connected layers. Features extracted through the convolutional and pooling layers are received then mapped to the specified classes number. Common activation functions like ReLU or sigmoid are then employed to allow the model to recognize non-linear patterns (Meha & Manan, 2021), (Abunasser, Al-Hiealy, Zaqout, Abu-Naser, & S. S, 2023).

2.1.1 Building Blocks of CNN

As previously mentioned, CNN consists of three essential layers. The convolution Layer is the most important layer in CNN. It is always the first layer of the network. The convolution layers are made up of filters. These filters are arrays of values called feature maps. Each convolution layer considers an image as input and produces a feature map. Each feature map is obtained by filter application to the image. For example, if the image is 5x5 and the filter is 3x3, the feature map will be 3x3. The convolution layer thus gets diverse images as input and computes the convolution of each with each filter. The filters are designed to extract the specific features that the user wants to detect.

The activation function is a technique to solve a major problem related to the backpropagation process in the neural network. Indeed, the CNN learns by forward propagation (learning from input to output layer) and backward propagation (backpropagation of the error from the output layer to the input layer). During these passes, the connection weights are updated to correctly learn the label of an image. However, two major problems may occur during backpropagation errors:

- Gradient vanishing: gradients become very small, making weight updates ineffective.
- Gradient explosion: gradients may instead grow excessively, causing model instability.

The Pooling Layer is generally placed between two convolution layers: it has several feature maps as input and employs the pooling operation to each. A pooling layer acts as a reduction layer. It divides the image into blocks and keeps only the maximum of each block. This reduces the image dimension while preserving the most important features. The output has the same number of feature maps as the input, but they are much smaller. In practice, there are two common pooling methods:

- Max Pooling: calculates the maximum value for each window of the feature map, i.e., keeps the maximum pixel value in that region.
- Average Pooling: determines the average of the values in each region, providing a smoother representation of the image.

Usually, the last layer of each CNN architecture (used for classification) is made up of Fully Connected layers. The input to the fully connected layer corresponds to the last pooling layer. As the name suggests, this layer is fully connected, meaning all neurons are connected to each other, allowing the learning of non-linear combinations between the feature maps of the last layer of the neural network. As with convolution layers, fully connected layers are generally associated with an activation function. The common uses in this context are of the softmax and sigmoid functions. Their role is to assign to each output a score that is then converted into a probability of belonging to a given image class.

After exploring the individual functions of various neural network layers, this paragraph moves to the interpretation of their ultimate outputs. Activation functions serve as mathematical operators that introduce controlled nonlinear transformations between neural network layers, enabling hierarchical feature abstraction (Goyal, et al., 2020). The role of activation functions in deep learning models is fundamental, serving as the crucial link between inputs and outputs across various layers. As data propagates through the network, from initial input layers to hidden processing layers, activation functions introduce non-linearity, enabling the model to learn complex patterns and relationships within the data. That is to say that these functions are essential to map the affine combination of inputs and weights at each neuron into a bounded or regularized output, which becomes the input signal for subsequent layers.

2.1.2 Softmax: Activating Probabilities in Multi-Class Layers

The softmax function converts an array of K values (z) into a vector of probabilities, where the probabilities of each value are proportional to the relative scale of each value in the vector according to its mathematical expression in (5) (Minghong, et al., 2023). This subsection examines the Softmax function, a crucial component typically integrated into the final layer, responsible for transforming raw numerical outputs called logits, into a probability distribution. In simpler terms, it takes a set of numbers and converts them into probabilities that sum to 1.

In the context of neural networks, softmax is generally applied to the last layer of a network designed for multi-class classification. When there are several possible categories and the model must indicate the probability of each, the softmax activation function is the standard choice. However, it performs poorly as the input size grows as its ability to maintain sharpness decreases dramatically.

$$\sigma\left(z\right) = \frac{e^{z_k}}{\sum_{k=1}^{K} e^{z_k}} \tag{5}$$

This transformation is critical because simple linear compositions of layers collapse into a single linear transformation, fundamentally limiting representational capacity. This intricate processing allows deep learning models to excel in diverse applications, including the analysis of large datasets with numerous parameters, accurate forecasting, and specialized tasks such as image processing, natural language processing, object recognition, and financial prediction. Furthermore, the development of activation functions has been driven by the need to optimize the learning process, ensuring its stability, preventing overfitting, enhancing predictive accuracy, and simultaneously minimizing computational demands (Kiliçarslan, Adem, & Celik, 2021). Thus, the inputs of a network are processed using activation functions to generate the output corresponding to these inputs.

2.1.3 Sigmoid: Activating Probability Functions in Multi-Class Layers

Sigmoid functions are mathematical equations that squash all values of x to an output ranging between 0 and 1 thus creating an S-shaped graph. Sigmoid is a non-linear activation function. Although it was assessed as a great step in neural networks since it improved aligning the outputs of these functions with standard probability situations, it is constrained to its diminishing gradient in the deep layers based on a chain rule. The gradient of sigmoid values based on a chain rule vanishes during backpropagation as the gradients are repeatedly multiplied, ultimately diminishing in deep networks. The most common form of sigmoid functions that is typically found in artificial neural networks is (Anirban Dutta, Rohan, Sanjay, & Arpan, 2022):

$$\sigma\left(X\right) = \frac{1}{1 + e^{-X}} \tag{6}$$

All these steps allow the CNN to progressively understand the content of a medical image, such as a mammogram, first identifying simple shapes (edges, textures), then combining these elements to recognize more complex structures.

Therefore, thanks to this information hierarchy, the network can distinguish normal areas from potentially pathological regions. When trained on a large number of annotated images, i.e., with precise indications of the presence and location of anomalies, the model learns to recognize the characteristic visual signatures of certain pathologies, such as masses or microcalcifications associated with breast cancer. Thus, deep learning is not limited to indicating whether an image is normal or suspicious, but can also precisely locate the affected region, highlighting the area of interest on the mammogram. This detection and automatic localization capability is a valuable aid for radiologists, especially in early screening, where speed and reliability of diagnosis are essential. That is why using a comprehensive and well-annotated database is very important. Mammogram Mystery stands out in this regard for its image quality, annotation precision, and clinical relevance, making it particularly suitable for training and evaluating breast cancer detection models.

2.2 The Role of Pre-Trained Models in Transfer Learning

Transfer learning is a deep learning technique based on applying knowledge obtained from one model to another. Which means using already trained models on large-scale datasets, like those for ImageNet classification, on a different related problem. Transfer learning concept aims at improving computation time and generalization results based on the valuable learned representations offered by pre-trained models as baseline for novel tasks. This method offers considerable advantages, for small target datasets, as it prevents overfitting and raises the model's generalization ability. To adapt to the higher-level features, the pre-trained models can be fine-tuned on the target dataset mainly for breast cancer images classification task (Ziyang, Yong, Shih-Chi, & Junghua, 2025).

2.3 Training Strategy and Hyperparameter Optimization

Training encompasses inputting training data and continually tuning the model's weights to lower the defined loss function. Effective adjustment of model's parameters is performed through optimization algorithms like Stochastic Gradient Descent

(SGD) or Adam. This process is heavily influenced by hyperparameter tuning, which is critical for optimizing the model's overall outcomes. Number of epochs, learning rate, regularization parameters, number of epochs, and batch size are among the key hyperparameters that need careful adjustment. Different combinations are explored using random search techniques or grid search to define the optimal configuration (Marouene, Malek, Mokhles, & Mouadh, 2025). Model performance is tracked during the training progress through metrics such as accuracy, loss, precision, recall, and F1-score, which are crucial for understanding its recognition capacity. Model checkpoints may be retained to record progress. The best-performing model selection is then established based on validation metrics.

2.4 Metrics of Evaluation and Validation

As mentioned before, the trained model performance evaluation is assessed using various metrics. Equations of commonly considered quantifiers are outlined in this section (Musthafa, 2024).

- **Accuracy** is a direct measure of classification correctness of the model. It is represented by the ratio of how many samples the model performed right classification versus the total number of classified samples.

$$Accuracy = \frac{TP + TN}{TP + FP + TN + FN} \quad (1)$$

- **Precision** is a metric that quantifies the capacity of a classifier to identify all positive instances from the hole number of positive instances. It is the ratio of true positives to the sum of true positives and false positives.

$$Precision = \frac{TP}{TP + FP} \quad (2)$$

- **Sensitivity** (also called Recall), it evaluates a model's ability to identify negative cases through measuring the proportion of true negatives that are correctly identified.

$$Sensitivity = Recall = \frac{TP}{TP + FN} \quad (3)$$

- **F1-score** is the harmonic mean of precision and recall. It combines both of them into a single metric.

$$F1\ score = 2 . \frac{Recall. Precision}{Precision + Recall} \quad (4)$$

- **AUC** or the **Area Under the Receiver Operating Characteristic** (ROC) Curve, is derived from the area beneath a curve plotted considering the False Positive Rate on the X-axis and the True Positive Rate on the Y-axis. It quantifies a model's overall performance over all classification cut-off points. A perfect classifier has the closest AUC to 1.

3. BREAST CANCER DIAGNOSIS TECHNIQUES

Breast cancer diagnosis entails abnormal cells or tumors identification and classification. Clinically, a range of techniques are employed, including mammography, ultrasound, biopsy and magnetic resonance imaging (MRI). Mammography is recognized as the most prevalent breast cancer screening method. However, its effectiveness is still limited to the presence of false-positive and false-negative outcomes. MRI and ultrasound offer complimentary information, enabling the detection of tumors missed by mammography. While biopsy represents the definitive diagnostic standard involving removing tissue for analysis, its interpretation relies highly on the subjective expertise of radiologists and pathologists. This reliance underscores a growing need for accurate, automated approaches to breast cancer diagnosis.

3.1 Medical Image Analysis Based on Deep Learning

Convolutional Neural Networks (CNNs) have advanced medical image analysis through providing tools for automated feature classification. They demonstrated strong ability in acquiring hierarchical representations directly from images and deriving pertinent features to enable precise classification. In Breast Cancer detection context, Deep Learning can enhance earlier detection and better patient outcomes as it significantly improves diagnosis accuracy and efficiency. Thus, medical images like histopathological images and mammograms are analyzed to classify tumors as benign or malignant (Darshini, 2023). ResNet, Inception and VGG16 are three deep learning models for breast cancer detection highlighted in the latter reference. The study offers a benchmarking insight into the different architectures; however, no interpretability techniques were addressed. These techniques include tools like attention mechanisms, visualizations, and saliency maps (Yongshu, et al., 2023), allowing understanding how AI models make decisions. They unveil specific features and areas of interest that influence a model's predictions, enabling clinicians to validate predictions and ensure trustworthy diagnostics (Ibomoiye et al., 2024).

3.2 Main Challenges in Deep Learning-Based BC Diagnosis

Despite the advantages of using Deep Learning for BC detection, several challenges still need to be addressed. Firstly, the limited availability of diverse and well-annotated datasets restricts the process for training accurate models. Robust model establishment requires large and well-labeled data. A second essential factor is the interpretability of these models, which is crucial for their endorsement in medical context. Finally, explicit decision-makings based on proven robustness and reliability on varied datasets, raise faith among clinicians and generalize practical applications considering population-specific disease characteristics (K, et al., 2025). Mapping these research gaps guides future efforts to refine breast cancer models, ensuring a coherency between the dual demands of algorithmic performance and clinical adoption (Aqdar, et al., 2024).

Nevertheless, a fundamental challenge within this axis stems from imbalanced datasets. Based on the predominance of benign presentations, malignant cases are observed as a distinct minority. This severe imbalance biases detection models, make them tend to non-cancerous results, which reduces their capacity to identify true cancer instances. Addressing this limitation needs complex training methodologies, such as synthetic data generation, data augmentation, or cost-sensitive learning, to yield improved results (K, et al., 2025), (Alderman, et al., 2025), (Laws, et al., 2025).

Accordingly, the interpretability of model decisions retains its critical importance in the realm of medical diagnostics. Healthcare practitioners often display a significant reluctance to adopt machine learning systems that operate as opaque processes. The integration of AI-based diagnoses into clinical practice remains difficult, primarily because doctors require clear expositions of how algorithms arrive at their conclusions. When the operational mechanisms of AI systems remain opaque, their trustworthiness suffers, impeding their widespread adoption despite promising accuracy metrics

The challenges posed by data heterogeneity, class imbalance, and the limited sensitivity of traditional CNNs in detecting nuanced malignant features raise the necessity of systematically assessing existing recent methodological approaches. The aim is to establish a foundation for advancing the field, the following section critically examines contemporary methodologies in breast cancer classification. A comprehensive review of recent advancements in CNN-based breast cancer detection is presented, evaluating deep learning structures, feature extraction techniques, and optimization strategies. A comparative analysis of different CNNs based approaches highlights their strengths, limitations, and applicability in medical image classification.

By analyzing architectural innovations and algorithmic refinements proposed in recent literature, this review identifies key strategies to address the mentioned technical challenges while mapping the evolution of deep learning applications in the BC domain.

4. RELATED WORKS

This section is dedicated to comparative analysis based on a review and evaluation of prevalent breast cancer classification approaches. This section highlights the distinct advantages and drawbacks of each method, Giving guidance on their most effective application scenarios. An insight into the research landscape of the application of CNNs in relation to existing literature is fostered by this section.

4.1 Object Detection Models for Mammogram Recognition

The main challenge for current CNNs' detection methods of breast cancer is the lack of training data sets that represent different types of breast cancer manifestations specific to each population characteristics. Improving models to allow boosting diagnosis accuracy and tackling error rates would lead to earlier breast cancer detection resulting in improved patient survival and reduced diagnosis expenses. Reference (K, et al., 2025) illustrates optimized robust algorithms developed for specific breast cancer features. These algorithms integrate multiple models, encompassing factors such as medical history age, breast density and age to enhance diagnosis performance and improve interpretability. Integrating four models allows achieving a drastic improvement in diagnosis performance, leading to an AUC of 0.98. Simulation results give a sensitivity value of 86.7% and a specificity of 96.1%. These findings underscore the potential of advanced deep learning techniques to boost diagnostic accuracy and reduce false errors.

4.1.1 Detection and Classification

Mammogram image processing is held through an end-to-end machine assisted detection system based on YOLO V3 which identifies abnormal regions and delivers simultaneously both bounding boxes and class labels. YOLO V3 allows simultaneous detection of suspicious regions (such as masses and microcalcifications) in full-field digital mammograms and pathology classification as benign or malignant. YOLOv3 uses three detection scales (13×13, 26×26, 52×52) to capture objects of varying sizes, addressing the limitation of YOLOv2's single-scale detection. This is critical for detecting masses in mammograms, which vary in size and appearance (Aly, Mareley, El-Sayed, & Tolba, 2021). Small lesion detection posed significant challenges for YOLOv1 and v2 architectures, since their fundamental grid structures limited resolution required for precise localization.

4.1.2 Anchors and Data Augmentation

The model uses anchor boxes generated via k-means clustering tailored to the specific dataset, improving detection accuracy, especially for challenging cases. Data augmentation methods are also applied to improve model robustness (C, et al., 2023). Performance: The system demonstrates high accuracy in both detection and classification tasks, achieving detection rates above 89% and classification precision rates above 84% on benchmark datasets such as INbreast and CBIS-DDSM.

4.1.3 Dataset Preprocessing

A merged dataset of AIIMS and DDSM comprising 2700 mammograms is used for model training. The impact of extensive data augmentation techniques such as angle rotation, saturation variation, exposure adjustment, horizontal and vertical flipping and random cropping is proven through the drastic enhancement of model robustness. Hue augmentation was excluded given the grayscale nature of mammograms. The input images were sized at 416 x 416 pixels.

4.1.4 Main Results

The proposed framework demonstrates robust generalization in breast cancer detection across heterogeneous datasets (AIIMS, INbreast) and external validation cohorts. Comparative analysis reveals YOLOv3 and RetinaNet outperform conventional architectures (AlexNet, CNN, BCDNet) across key metrics:

- YOLOv3 achieves 98.8% accuracy, 98.5% sensitivity, and AUC greater than 0.96 through optimized anchor box scaling and Darknet-53 backbone.
- RetinaNet synergizes Feature Pyramid Networks (FPN) for multi-scale tumor detection with Focal Loss to address class imbalance, improving small-lesion sensitivity by 12% over Faster R-CNN.

Moreover, the study introduces Perturbation Analysis as an interpretable AI tool to substitute CAM/Grad-CAM. The contribution clearer and more explainable features for extended instances.

4.2 CNN-LSTM Hybrid Models

Recently, the accuracy of BC detection has greatly increased thanks to Deep Learning and powerful artificial intelligence. The main objective of using deep neural networks, mainly CNNs in medical image context, is to raise their ability to recognize and extract characteristics without needing human implication (Geert, et al., 2017).

4.2.1 CNNs Key Features

The study addressed CNNs trained on video data. Standardized scan planes in mid-pregnancy fetal ultrasound were then determined. CNNs models have demonstrated significant precision outcomes in problems related to images classifications like for BC detection. Their great performances have been validated at spatial feature extraction on identifying local and global patterns in breast cancer images. However, despite their effectiveness in reducing dimensionality through maintaining critical features via convolutional and pooling layers, these models have restricted capacity to simulate sequential data which are essential in medical context. A saliency map was derived from input features after a specific plane's presence was detected. The analysis of this XAI tool in CNNs revealed its limitation to providing only rough localization rather than detailed segmentation.

4.2.2 LSTMs Key Features

LSTMs (Long Short-Term Memory networks), stand for a sort of Recurrent Neural Network that are specifically promising for sequence prediction and time-series analysis based on their strength in capturing temporal dynamics and acquiring long-term dependencies within data. This hybrid process tackles the limitations of using separately CNNs or LSTMs. The memory units of LSTM maintain the critical features by preventing problems like vanishing gradients.

4.2.3 DL Model Hybridization Approach

(Kaddes, Ayid, Elshewey, & et al, 2025) provides an approach to mitigate the gaps of short generalization over diverse datasets and limited consideration of spatial and temporal features for medical image recognition through developing a hybrid DL Long Short-Term Memory network model (CNN-LSTM) that concentrates on breast cancer classification. The approach employs the advantages of both LSTMs and CNNs to enhance classification capacity. Simulation was performed on two Datasets obtained from Kaggle repository. Also, the model integrated tailored preprocessing techniques, performed advanced hyperparameter adjustment through grid search, and assessed computational efficiency, which highlights its applicability in practical clinical context.

4.3.3 Main Results

The proposed model emphasizes an optimized combination of CNN and LSTM layers for improved feature extraction and increased sequential analysis. Validation on different datasets (IDC and BreaKHis) confirm robustness, and optimized performance with accuracies of 99.17% and 99.90%, advancing existing models. However, more computational resources are needed due to sequential dependencies. The use of saliency maps or other XAI techniques with LSTM based models was not specified in this reference.

4.3 Hybrid bi-LSTM and EfficientNet-B0 Model

The research study in (Lilhore, Sharma, Shukla, & et al, 2025) suggests an advanced Adam optimized hybrid CNN-LSTM model integrating both spatial and temporal features to enhance breast cancer image prediction. The investigation aims to improve computational efficiency and interpretability.

Key contributions include:

- Improved CNN structure: extra convolutional layers and advanced pattern extraction are used to better retain intricate spatial features in breast cancer mammograms, leading to more precise feature representation and overall better model performance.
- Improved Bi-LSTM combined Transfer Learning: Long Short-Term Memory (Bi-LSTM) has an improved bidirectional structure that allows better representation of sequential data relationships, optimizing the consideration of temporal aspects for higher recognition accuracy and model stability. Additionally, transfer learning is applied using the pre-trained EfficientNet-B0 CNN, which was trained on ImageNet.
- Optimized hyperparameter adjustment: Adam optimization is employed for hyperparameter tuning to mitigate overfitting and underfitting problems, leading to more reliable and faster predictions and enhanced model efficiency.
- Superior prediction accuracy: The proposed model demonstrates higher accuracy compared to existing models like VGG-16, VGG-19, ResNet-50, DenseNet169 and DenseNet201) on prevalent breast cancer datasets like MIAS and CBIS-DDSM.

The proposed hybrid model revealed a sensitivity of 95.00% and an astounding accuracy of 99.00%. Model sensitivity and specificity were then improved by data pre-processing. Thus, the hybrid model attained a remarkable accuracy of 99.40% for benign, 98.50% for malignant, and 97.80% for normal cases.

Still, the deployed AI models offered enhanced feature visualization interpretability. However, the study explicitly recommends further methodological advancements in order to improve the explainability of AI-driven decisions to medical practitioners through boosting future explanatory algorithms.

4.4 CNN-MLPs model

CNN-MLP models leveraged hierarchical feature extraction with deep, fully connected layers to refine classification accuracy, Optimized MLP (Multi-Layer Perceptron) models using Adam and Stochastic Gradient Descent (SGD) optimizers, achieve an accuracy of around 89%. (Nasir, Rahman, & Nasir, 2025) highlights the further enhanced performances of Hybrid models combining CNNs with MLP classifiers yielding an accuracy of up to 98%. The same reference stipulates that federated learning approaches are estimated to achieve accuracy improvements of up to 2% while preserving data privacy, making them a high-potential technique for future AI-driven medical imaging solutions. **XAI techniques** like Grad-CAM and SHAP **are recommended at the end of the study** to enhance model interpretability.

4.5 HybMNet: Fusion of Swin Transformer and CNN

Deploying AI for breast cancer diagnosis is constrained to the lack of labeled and high-quality medical training data. Developing deep learning models for analyzing mammograms and recognizing abnormalities like masses or micro-calcifications demands extensive collections of labeled mammograms which is costly and time-consuming. To overcome this limitation, (Chen & Martel, 2025) developed a new method. The approach utilizes self-supervised learning (SSL) in conjunction with a hybrid deep model named HybMNet. This approach integrates local self-attention to fine-grained pattern captions to improve the accuracy of breast cancer recognition in screening mammograms. The method's efficacy in BC detection was assessed through its capacity to distinguish benign from malignant mammograms. By combining pretrained SSL to the HybMNet network. The resulting model has an area under the ROC curve (AUC) value of 0.864 on the Chinese Mammogram Database (CMMD) and 0.889 on the INbreast dataset, demonstrating stronger performances that Swin-T, CNN, and fusion prediction modules. The saliency maps in highlights the model ability to localize critical regions using only image-level labels without pixel level supervision.

This section presented a comprehensive review of deep learning trends for breast cancer diagnosis, analyzing strengths and limitations of existing CNNs and hybridized models in medical image prediction. The review demonstrated that hybrid CNN-based architectures achieve superior predictive accuracy by effectively capturing both spatial and sequential dependencies in tumor features, supporting their potential for clinical adoption. However, challenges such as high-dimensional data, class imbalance, and model interpretability remain critical barriers. By integrating temporal and spatial analysis while tackling dataset limitations, AI-driven diagnostic tools can significantly reduce errors and enhance early detection rates. Moving forward, interdisciplinary collaboration will be essential to refine these models, ensuring robustness, scalability, and real-world applicability against breast cancer. Table 1 summarizes the main findings of the above-mentioned studies.

Table 1. Main Reviewed Studies

Reference	Authors	Year of Publication	Main results
(K, et al., 2025)	K. Puttegowda et Al.	2025	YOLOv3 achieves high accuracy (98.8%) and AUC (>0.96) with optimized anchors and Darknet-53, while RetinaNet boosts small-lesion sensitivity by 12% using FPN and Focal Loss.
(Lilhore, Sharma, Shukla, & et al, 2025)	Lilhore, et al.	2025	The proposed hybrid Bi-LSTM with EfficientNet-B0 achieved outstanding performance, reaching 99.40% accuracy for non-cancer, 98.50% for cancer and 97.80% for normal cases, with a sensitivity of 95.00%
(Nasir, Rahman, & Nasir, 2025)	Nasir F, Rahman S and Nasir N	2025	Hybrid models combining CNNs with MLP classifiers achieved up to 98% accuracy, while federated learning approaches offer an additional ~2% improvement and ensure data privacy.
(Chen & Martel, 2025)	Chen, H., & Martel, A. L.	2025	The HybMNet model, enhanced with self-supervised learning, combines local self-attention and fine-grained pattern extraction, achieving strong breast cancer detection performance with AUCs of 0.864 (CMMD) and 0.889 (INbreast)

Table 2 recapitulates key performance metrics of the previous studies. Comparative summary between key approaches can then be derived. This comparison enables an overview of the different approaches investigated in terms of model architecture, accuracy, sensitivity, along with further relevant evaluation criteria.

Table 2. Benchmark of performance metrics

Method	Accuracy	Sensitivity	AUC	Small lesion sensitivity	Datasets
YOLOv3, RretinaNet	98.8%	98.5%	0.99	+12% (for RetinaNet)	AIIMS, INbreast datasets
Bi-LSTM + EfficientNet-B0	99.08%	96.05	0.98	--	CBIS-DDSM
CNN + MLP, Federated Learning	96.4%	97.5%	0.98	--	Kaggle (569 instances 33
HybMNet (Swin Transformer + CNN)	83%	--	0.889	--	INbreast test set

4.6 Challenges and Limitations

Despite high overall accuracy achieved by these different models, several limitations persist. For instance, elusive breast cancer histology such as Invasive Lobular Carcinoma (ILC) and Invasive Ductal Carcinoma (IDC) stands for a crucial challenge hindering subtype-specific detection. In this context, an AI-based computer-aided detection technique is developed by (Chang, et al., 2025) and aiming at screening mammograms in a real-world showed promising values of cancer detection rates (CDRs) and recall rates (RRs) of radiologists. Furthermore (Romania, et al., 2025) underscores how variable breast density obstructs mammography sensitivity challenging AI models leading to higher false-positive rates. The study addresses the need for AI tools to adapt to image artifacts for more clinical reliability. Moreover, the limited availability of large, balanced and diverse datasets that represent real-world heterogeneity remains a key limitation in Breast Cancer AI based approaches. However, harmonizing and standardizing multiple cohorts stands for a key progress in tackling this gap. Still, bringing together various datasets and ensuring effective generalization of models for diverse populations raises new challenges as mentioned in (Yizhou, Xiaoliang, Kuangyu, Axel, & Federico, 2025)

Still, to ensure ethical and equitable consideration of diverse populations, according to the WHO's 2025 AI ethics guidelines (TEAM, 2025) crucial challenges like algorithmic bias should be mitigated. For instance, Artificial Intelligence/Machine Learning (AI/ML)-Based Software as a Medical Device (SaMD) Action Plan (Health, 2021) is supporting regulatory framework for robust validation across heterogenous datasets.

In a related context, a scoping review implemented by (Masooma, Andre, & Elizabeth, 2024) emphasizes overcoming inherent infrastructure challenges and their related expenses. The study incorporates both sociotechnical and technical considerations influencing workflow transition from algorithmic research to routine clinical practice.

The following section explores use case performance and reliability analysis. This case study sets the stage for future enhancements aiming at improving diagnostic accuracy.

5. CNN TRAINING: A CASE STUDY USING THE MAMMOGRAM MASTERY DATASET

Deep learning shows great promise in mammographic image analysis, aiming to provide more accurate and automated diagnoses. This chapter evaluates the performance of a CNN model trained on the Mammogram Mastery dataset (745 original + 9,685 augmented images). Training results are analyzed through accuracy and loss metrics across epochs. The objective is to assess the model's learning behavior and generalization ability. Special focus is given to hyperparameter tuning and validation methods. These elements are crucial for ensuring training stability and minimizing overfitting. Results demonstrate that optimized configuration would improve model reliability. The study highlights the value of systematic performance evaluation. It also encourages further refinement for clinical applicability. Future work will explore more advanced tuning and validation strategies.

5.1 Description and Justification of Dataset Choice

The choice of dataset played a central role in the model's performance. In this case study, the Mini-MIAS dataset was first tested, which contains a very limited number of images. This lack of data prevented effective model training, making the results barely usable. Then the investigation moved to the CBIS-DDSM dataset, which is richer in images and well annotated. However, despite several attempts, performances remained low, with a maximum accuracy of 0.7, which is insufficient in the medical context. For these reasons, the Mammogram Mystery dataset was adopted. This one stands out for the quality of its images, the richness of its annotations, and a sufficient volume for deep learning. Trained with this database, the model achieved an accuracy exceeding 0.9, with a very low loss value, confirming the relevance of this choice for precise and reliable breast cancer detection. Hower some limitations are revealed based on classification results.

5.2 Working Environment

For the development and training of our model, a work environment suitable for deep learning should be set up, based mainly on the Python language. The implementation is performed on Google Colab, which is programmed with Python.

This coding language is mainly adopted for machine and deep learning for its ease of use and the libraries that come pre-installed.

The libraries relevant to current case study are:

- TensorFlow: Created by the Google Brain team, TensorFlow is an open-source library for numerical computation, machine learning, and deep learning. The name comes from multidimensional arrays (tensors), which are regularly used in neural networks.
- Keras.layers and Keras.models: Keras is a deep learning API written in Python, considered an open-source library, using TensorFlow. It allows the construction of neural networks simply and intuitively. These modules define the CNN model architecture, including convolution, pooling, flattening, and fully connected layers.
- ImageDataGenerator (tensorflow.keras.preprocessing.image): This class generates real-time batches of images with data augmentation. It is used to load images from folders, apply transformations (augmentation, resizing, etc.), and automatically generate batches for training and validation.
- matplotlib.pyplot: A set of command-style functions to visualize learning curves (accuracy/loss) and medical images, and to generate graphics for performance analysis.
- OS: Standard Python library for interacting with the file system. It allows manipulation of folder paths containing images and checking for the presence of files needed for training.

5.3 Model Training and Evaluation

5.3.1 Step 1: Library Installation

TensorFlow is installed via pip install -q tensorflow, where -q reduces displayed messages. Figure 1 displays the considered scrip for libraries installation.

Figure 1. Libraries installation

```
!pip install -q tensorflow
import tensorflow as tf
from tensorflow.keras import layers, models
from tensorflow.keras.preprocessing.image import ImageDataGenerator
import matplotlib.pyplot as plt
import os
from google.colab import drive
import numpy as np
from sklearn.metrics import confusion_matrix, classification_report
import seaborn as sns
```

5.3.2 Step 2: Data Preparation

The dataset chosen for this study stands for a valuable resource for investigating breast cancer in the MENA region. Comprising 745 original and 9,685 augmented breast cancer images, it provides a collection sourced from patients in Iraq. This dataset is meticulously curated by expert physicians, ensuring high quality and reliability through careful selection, verification, and categorization. Its distinct regional origin offers a fresh perspective on the prevalence and characteristics of breast cancer, making it an ideal choice for developing and rigorously testing deep learning algorithms for breast cancer detection and for various educational initiatives (Aqdar, et al., 2024). The organization of Mastery Mammogram is shown in figure 2.

Figure 2. Dataset organization (Aqdar et al., 2024)

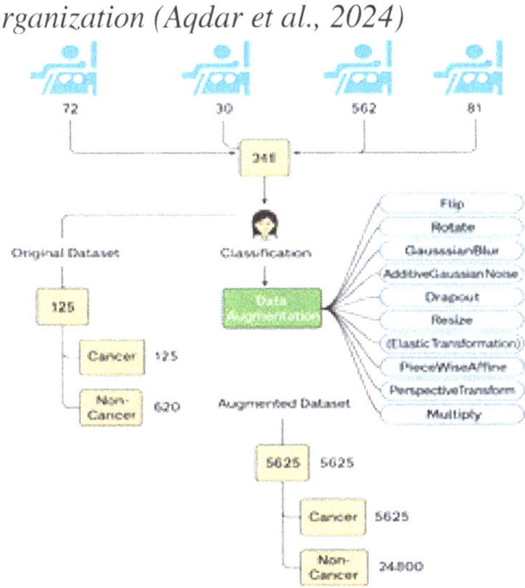

After accessing Google Drive, the local path to the folder containing the mammograms is defined for easy access from the execution environment. As figure 3 shows, images are then prepared using ImageDataGenerator, normalizing the pixels (dividing by 255) and applying various augmentation techniques such as rotation, zoom, horizontal and vertical shifts, and horizontal flipping. These transformations help make the model more robust to variations in real images. 20% of the data are set aside for validation.

Figure 3. Data preparation script

```
train_datagen = ImageDataGenerator(
    rescale=1./255,
    rotation_range=20,
    width_shift_range=0.2,
    height_shift_range=0.2,
    zoom_range=0.2,
    horizontal_flip=True,
    validation_split=0.2  # 20% pour la validation
)
```

5.3.3 Step 3: Data Generation

Two generators were created from the previously configured ImageDataGenerator object. First, train_generator mentioned in figure 4 provides training images shuffled randomly at each epoch, improving model learning. Secondly, val_generator mentioned in figure 5 is used for validation, where images are not shuffled to ensure consistent evaluation. Both generators automatically resize images to 224×224 pixels and organize them into batches, allowing more efficient model training.

Figure 4. Training data generation script

```
train_generator = train_datagen.flow_from_directory(
    os.path.join(data_dir, 'Original Dataset'), # Utilise seulement les originaux
    target_size=(224, 224),
    batch_size=32,
    class_mode='binary',
    color_mode='rgb',
    shuffle=True,
    subset='training'
)
```

Figure 5. Validation data generation script

```
val_generator = train_datagen.flow_from_directory(
    os.path.join(data_dir, 'Original Dataset'),
    target_size=(224, 224),
    batch_size=32,
    class_mode='binary',
    color_mode='rgb',
    shuffle=False,
    subset='validation'
)
```

5.3.4 Step 4: CNN Model Construction

This step refers to the design of a convolutional neural network (CNN) model suitable for binary classification of medical images (figure 6). The model consists of several Conv2D layers that automatically extract important visual features from mammograms. Then, a MaxPooling2D layer reduces image size and the number of parameters to learn. Once the features are extracted, they are flattened with the Flatten layer, then processed by Dense layers for the final prediction. The last layer uses sigmoid activation, for its efficiency in binary classification problems. Figure 6 gives a scope of how the model is compiled using the Adam optimizer. This optimizer is suitable for deep learning tasks thanks to its proven efficiency. The loss function used is binary cross entropy, ideal for binary classification. The metric tracked is accuracy, which measures the percentage of correct predictions during training and validation.

Figure 6. CNN Model Construction for Binary Classification

```
model = models.Sequential([
    layers.Conv2D(32, (3, 3), activation='relu', input_shape=(224, 224, 3)),
    layers.MaxPooling2D((2, 2)),
    layers.Conv2D(64, (3, 3), activation='relu'),
    layers.MaxPooling2D((2, 2)),
    layers.Conv2D(128, (3, 3), activation='relu'),
    layers.MaxPooling2D((2, 2)),
    layers.Flatten(),
    layers.Dense(128, activation='relu'),
    layers.Dense(1, activation='sigmoid')
])

model.compile(
    optimizer='adam',
    loss='binary_crossentropy',
    metrics=['accuracy']
)
```

5.3.5 Step 5: Model Training

The model is trained using the fit() method for 20 epochs and default settings was applied to the learning rate. During this phase, it learns to differentiate cancerous and non-cancerous images from the data generated by train_generator, while evaluating its performance on val_generator (figure 7).

Figure 7. CNN model training for 20 epochs

```
history = model.fit(
    train_generator,
    epochs=20,
    validation_data=val_generator
)
```

5.3.6 Step 6: Performance Visualization

The evolution curves of accuracy (figure 8) and loss (figure 9) are plotted for the training and validation phases. This allows tracking of:

- Learning progression and
- The detection of possible overfitting.

Figure 8. Accuracy progression

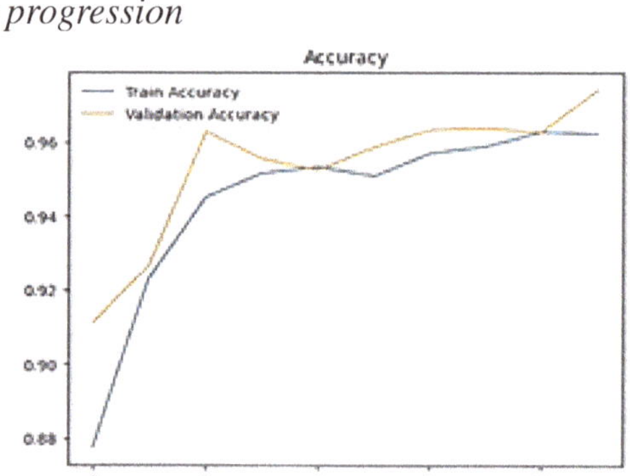

Figure 9. Loss progression

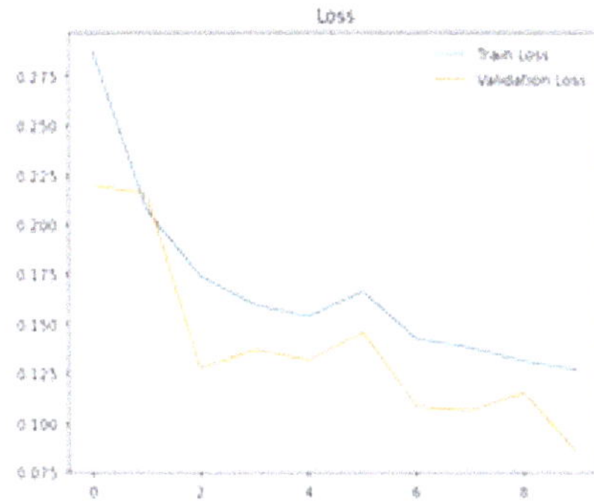

5.3.7 Step 7: Model Evaluation

The model evaluation is based on a confusion matrix and a classification report. These tools measure prediction quality (precision, recall, F1-score) and identify model errors on the validation data. The implementation of this step is shown in figure 10.

Figure 10. Model Evaluation Script

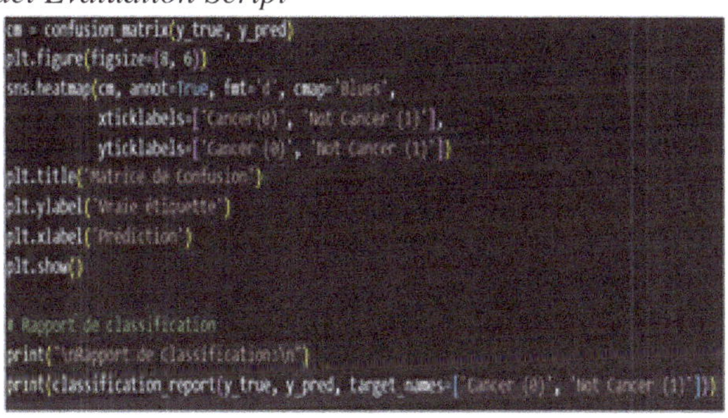

```
cm = confusion_matrix(y_true, y_pred)
plt.figure(figsize=(8, 6))
sns.heatmap(cm, annot=True, fmt='d', cmap='Blues',
            xticklabels=['Cancer(0)', 'Not Cancer (1)'],
            yticklabels=['Cancer (0)', 'Not Cancer (1)'])
plt.title('Matrice de Confusion')
plt.ylabel('Vraie étiquette')
plt.xlabel('Prédiction')
plt.show()

# Rapport de classification
print("\nRapport de Classification:\n")
print(classification_report(y_true, y_pred, target_names=['Cancer (0)', 'Not Cancer (1)']))
```

5.4 Results and Discussion

5.4.1 Training Results

The model was trained on preprocessed dataset. The learning curves illustrate the evolution of accuracy and loss over the training epochs for both the training and validation phases.

The learning curves (accuracy and loss), generated during training, provide insight into the model's behavior and performance. The accuracy curve increases steadily for both training and validation sets. The gap between training and validation accuracy remains small (less than 3%), indicating low variance and minimal overfitting. The loss curve decreases gradually, suggesting effective optimization without signs of stagnation or significant divergence. Overall, the plot results indicate a stable learning process and demonstrate the model's ability to generalize well with unseen data.

5.4.2 Performance Analysis

During the experimental phase, an initial evaluation was conducted using a pre-trained EfficientNetB0 model. Despite its known robustness across diverse datasets, its performance on the considered mammography dataset proved suboptimal, yielding an accuracy not exceeding 70%.

This underperformance can be attributed to several critical factors. Mammographic images are grayscale, whereas EfficientNetB0 was pre-trained on ImageNet, a dataset predominantly composed of color images. This disparity in input modalities likely hindered effective feature extraction. The relevant anatomical structures for breast cancer detection are often subtle and distinct from the natural objects for which the network was originally optimized.

Then, a custom CNN model characterized by its lighter architecture and direct training on the considered dataset, demonstrated superior generalization capabilities. This highlights the imperative of developing domain-specific architectures for medical imaging applications, rather than solely relying on generic pre-trained models. The results from the custom CNN are highly encouraging, with a validation accuracy exceeding 95%. This performance is considered a significant advancement in automated breast cancer detection from medical images. The classification report for this acknowledged model is shown in figure11.

Figure 11. Classification report

	precision	recall	f1-score	support
Cancer (0)	0.92	0.92	0.92	325
Not Cancer (1)	0.98	0.98	0.98	1612
accuracy			0.97	1937
macro avg	0.95	0.95	0.95	1937
weighted avg	0.97	0.97	0.97	1937

	precision	recall	f1-score	support
Cancer (0)	0.92	0.92	0.92	325
Not Cancer (1)	0.98	0.98	0.98	1612
accuracy			0.97	1937
macro avg	0.95	0.95	0.95	1937
weighted avg	0.97	0.97	0.97	1937

The close alignment between the training and validation curves for both accuracy and loss indicates that the model has learned relevant representations while maintaining satisfactory generalization. The minimal discrepancy between training accuracy (96.23%) and validation accuracy (97.42%) suggests a stable learning process and a favorable balance between bias and variance. Furthermore, the peak validation accuracy of 97.42% coupled with a minimal loss of 8.50% underscores the model's capacity to achieve optimal performance during specific training epochs. However, further analysis, utilizing tools such as a confusion matrix and activation maps, is crucial to pinpoint specific model errors, particularly concerning false positives (non-cancerous cases incorrectly classified as cancerous) and false negatives (undetected cancers), which are clinically critical.

Based on the classification report, the model can deliver correct "Cancer" cases 92% of the time. However, when it comes to "Not Cancer" cases, the model gives correct results in 98% of the time. True Positive Rate is deducted from recall values and shows that the model is more efficient to detect "Not Cancer" cases than "Cancer" cases. That is to say that it has lower number of false negatives than positive negatives.

Moreover, the report gives a higher F1 score for "Not Cancer" which reveals that this class is likely to prevail over the dataset (325 Cancer vs. 1612 Not Cancer samples). The analysis highlights the model bias toward the majority class. This disparity raises concern about optimization approaches as minor misses in medical diagnostics can impact patient survival.

Confusion matrix is given in figure 12.

Figure 12. Confusion Matrix

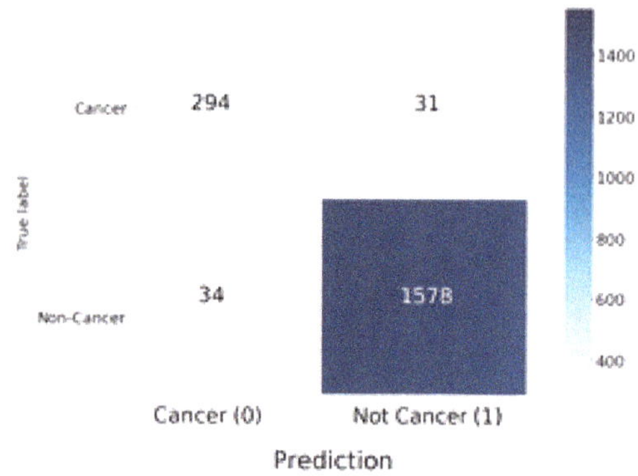

Supporting the assumptions of model bias and an unbalanced dataset, two targeted tests have then been conducted. For each test, 20 images of cancer cases (mini test 1) and 20 images of non-cancer cases (mini test 2) are drawn from the existing database. The performance metrics for each test are subsequently displayed in their respective confusion matrices.

Figure 13 shows that the model predicted one instance for "Not Cancer" while the patient *had cancer*. This case is generally considered as the most critical error in cancer detection. Thus, missed diagnosis can lead to cancer progression and increased patient mortality.

Figure 13. Confusion Matrix for mini test 1

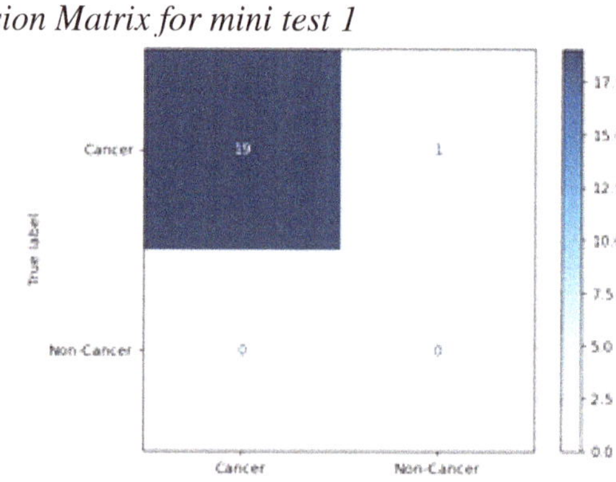

Figure 14 shows that the model predicted three (03) instances of "Cancer" while the patients did not have cancer. This error has less impact than false negatives, despite its negative consequences, such as patient distress, unnecessary procedures and increased healthcare costs.

Figure 14. Confusion Matrix for mini test 2

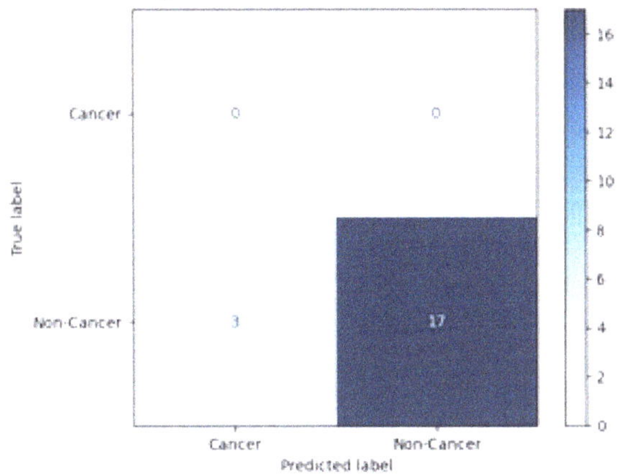

6. CONCLUSION

This chapter looked at different ways deep learning can help detect breast cancer. Some of the approaches included combining CNN models with other techniques, using Bi-LSTM networks, and trying out self-supervised learning methods like HybMNet. There were also methods focused on keeping patient data private, such as federated learning. The results looked good, with some models hitting 99% accuracy and strong AUC scores above 0.86, which suggests they could be useful in real medical settings. We also tested a CNN model on the Mastery Mammogram dataset. It performed well, showing it could learn patterns and apply them to new data. Still, there's room to make it better. Tweaking things like hyperparameters and changing how we validate the model might boost both its accuracy and reliability. Next steps could involve automating some of those adjustments, improving cross-validation methods, and finding ways to make the model decisions easier to understand.

Overall model's case study performance is highlighted, with high accuracy and weighted averages. However, test samples revealed that future work must address model bias and data imbalance limitations to enhance real-world reliability. The chapter also signaled tackling inherent infrastructure challenges and associated costs would promote workflow integration, enabling healthcare systems to standardize AI systems.

REFERENCES

Abunasser, B., Al-Hiealy, M., Zaqout, I., Abu-Naser, & S. S. (2023). *Asian Pacific journal of cancer preventionConvolution Neural Network for Breast Cancer Detection and Classification Using Deep Learning*, 531-544.

Alderman, J., Palmer, J., Laws, E., McCraden, M., Ordish, J., Ghassemi, M., & Liu, X. (2025). Tackling algorithmic bias and promoting transparency in health datasets: The STANDING Together concensus recommendations. *The Lancet. Digital Health*, *7*(1), 64–88. DOI: 10.1016/S2589-7500(24)00224-3 PMID: 39701919

Aly, G., Mareley, M., El-Sayed, S., & Tolba, M. (2021). YOLO Based Breast Masses Detection and Classification in Full-Field Digital Mammograms. *Computer Methods and Programs in Biomedicine*, *200*, 105823. DOI: 10.1016/j.cmpb.2020.105823 PMID: 33190942

Anirban Dutta, C., Rohan, B., Sanjay, K., & Arpan, P. (2022). *New Frontiers of Cardiovascular Screening Using Unobtrusive Sensors, AI and IoT*. Academic Press.

Aqdar, K., Mustafa, R., Abdulaqadir, Z., Abdalla, P., Qadir, A., Shali, A., & Aziz, N. (2024). Mammogram mastery: A robust dataset for breast cancer detection and medical education. *Data in Brief*, *55*, 110633. DOI: 10.1016/j.dib.2024.110633 PMID: 39035836

Balasubramaniam, S., Velmurugan, Y., Jaganathan, D., & Dhanasekaran, S. (2023). A Modified LeNet CNN for Breast Cancer Diagnosis in Ultrasound Images. *Diagnostics (Basel)*, *13*(17), 2746. DOI: 10.3390/diagnostics13172746 PMID: 37685284

C, D., K, D., Basturk, Alper, Akay, & et al. (2023). A Comparative study of YOLO models and a transformer-based YOLOv5 model for mass detection in mammograms. *Turkish Journal of Electrical Engineering and Computer Sciences* .

Chang, Y.-W., Jung, K., Jim, K., Nami, C., Young, M., Kyung, H., & Kyunghwa, H. (2025). Artificial intelligence for breast cancer screening in mammography (AI-STREAM): preliminary analysis of a prospective multicenter cohort study.

Chen, H., & Martel, A. (2025). Enhancing breast cancer detection on screeninh mammogram using self-supervised learning and a hybrid deep model of Swin Transformer and convolutional neural networks. *Journal of Imaging*.

Darshini, V. (2023). Deep Learning Based-Breast Cancer Prediction using CNN. *International Journal of Novel Research and Development*, 6-17.

Freddie, B., Mathieu, L., Hyuna, S., Jacques, F., Rebecca. L, S., Isabelle, S., & Ahmedin, J. (2024). Global cancer statistics 2022: GLOBOCAN estimates of incidence and mortality worldwide for 36 cancers in 185 countries. *CA: A Cancer Journal for Clinicians reaches*, 229-263.

Gao, F., Wu, T., Zhen, B., Ruan, L., Shang, D., & Patel, B. (2018). A shallow-deep CNN for improved breast cancer diagnosis. *The official journal of Computerized Medical Imaging Society*, 53-62.

Geert, L., Thijs, K., Babak Ehteshami, B., Arnaud Arindra, A., Francesco, C., & Mohsen, G. Clara I.Sanchez. (2017). A survey on deep learning in medical image analysis. *Medical Image Analysis*, •••, 60–88. PMID: 28778026

Goyal, M., Goyal, R., Venkatappa Reddy, P., Lall, B., Pedrycz, W., & Chen, S. (2020). Activation Functions In Deep Learning Algorithms and Applications. *Studies in Computational Intelligence.*

Health, C. f. (2021). *Artificial Intelligence/Machine Learning (AI/ML)-Based Software as a Medical Device (SaMD) Action Plan.* US FOOD & DRUG ADMINISTRATION.

Ibomoiye, D., George, O., Nobert, J., Ebikella, M., Kehinde, A., Ikiomoye, D., & Blessing, O. (2024). A survey of explainable artificial intelligence in healthcare: Concepts, applications, and challenges. *Informatics in Medicine Unlocked.*

K, P., V, V., H.S, R., K.V, S., K, P., R., V., & K, T. (2025). Enhanced Machine Learning Models for Accurate Breast Cancer Mammogram Classification. *Global Transitions*, 276-295.

Kaddes, M., Ayid, Y., Elshewey, A., & Fouad, Y. (2025). Breast cancer classification based on hybrid CNN with LSTM model. *Scientific Reports*, *15*(1), 15. DOI: 10.1038/s41598-025-88459-6 PMID: 39910136

Kiliçarslan, S., Adem, K., & Celik, M. (2021). An overview of the activation functions used in deep learning algorithms. *Journal of New Results in Science*, 75-88.

Laws, E., Palmer, J., Alderman, J., Sharma, O., Ngai, V., Salisbury, T., Hussain, G., Ahmed, S., Sachdeva, G., Vadera, S., Mateen, B., Matin, R., Kuku, S., Calvert, M., Gath, J., Treanor, D., McCradden, M., Mackintosh, M., Gichoya, J., & Liu, X. (2025). Diversity, inclusivity and traceability of mammography datasets used in development of Artificial Intelligence technologies: A systematic review. *Clinical Imaging*, *118*, 110369. DOI: 10.1016/j.clinimag.2024.110369

Lilhore, U., Sharma, Y., Shukla, B., Vadlamudi, M. N., Simaiya, S., Alroobaea, R., Alsafyani, M., & Baqasah, A. M. (2025). Hybrid convolutional neural network and bi-LSTM model with EfficientNet-B0 for high-accuracy breast cancer detection and classification. *Scientific Reports*, *15*(1), 15. DOI: 10.1038/s41598-025-95311-4 PMID: 40204759

Marouene, C., Malek, A., Mokhles, B., & Mouadh, F. (2025). Deep learning-driven predication in healthcare systems: Applying advanced CNNs for enhanced breast cancer detection. *Computers in Biology and Medicine*.

Masooma, H., Andre, K., & Elizabeth, B. (2024). *Barriers to and Facilitators of Artificial Intelligence Adoption in Health Care: Scoping Review*. National Library of Medicine.

Meha, D., & Manan, S. (2021). An anatomization on breast cancer detection and diagnosis employing multi-layer perceptron neural network (MLP) and Convolutional Neural network (CNN). *Clinical eHealth*, 1-11.

Minghong, G., Yuejun, Z., Yongzhong, W., Guangpeng, A., Huihong, Z., Pengjun, W., & Guoqing, W. (2023). A lightweight convolutional neural network hardware implementation for wearable heart rate anomaly detection. *Computers in Biology and Medicine*. PMID: 36809696

Musthafa, M. e., T R, M., v, V. K., & Guluwadi, S. (2024). Enhanced skin cancer diagnosis using optimized CNN architecture and checkpoints for automated dermatological lesion classification. *BMC Medical Imaging*, *24*(1), 24. DOI: 10.1186/s12880-024-01356-8 PMID: 39095688

Nasir, F., Rahman, S., & Nasir, N. (2025). Breast Cancer Detectiuon Using Convolutional Neural Network: A Deep Learning-Based Approach. *Cureus*, •••, 17.

Romania, T., Beatrice, P., Shlomit, A.-S., Matthew, B., Jocelyn, P., & Nina, S, V. (2025). The Current Scope of Artificial Intelligence in Breast US. *Applied Radiology*.

TEAM. W. (2025). *Ethics and governance of artificial intelligence for health: Guidance on large multi-modal models.* Wold Health Organization.

Xiong, X., Le-Wei, Z., Yu, D., Yu-Fei, C., Yu-Wen, C., Lei-Ping, W., & Ke-Da, Y. (2025). Breast cancer: Pathogenesis and treatments. *Signal Transduction and Targeted Therapy*, *10*(1), 49. DOI: 10.1038/s41392-024-02108-4 PMID: 39966355

Yizhou, C., Xiaoliang, S., Kuangyu, S., Axel, R., & Federico, C. (2025). AI in Breast Cancer Imaging: An Update and Future Trends. *Seminars in Nuclear Medicine*, •••, 358–370. PMID: 40011118

Yongshu, G., Jie, L., Weihan, L., Ming, H., Yang, L., & Huimin, Z. (2023). Augmented Grad-CAM++: Super-Resolution Saliency Maps for Visual Interpretation of Deep Neural Network. *Electronics (Basel)*, •••, 2023.

Ziyang, G., Yong, T., Shih-Chi, L., & Junghua, L. (2025). *A CT Image Classification Network Framework for Lung Tumors Based on Pre-trained MobileNetV2 Model and Transfer learning and Its Application and Market Analysis in the Medical field.*

Chapter 3
Automated Detection of Cardiovascular Arrhythmias Using Machine Learning and Deep Learning on ECG Signals

Akash Saxena
Compucom Institute of Technology and Management, Jaipur, India

Satish Kumar Alaria
https://orcid.org/0000-0001-8298-1364
Government of Rajasthan, India

Ashish Raj
Poornima University, India

Apoorva Sharma
Poornima University, India

Arpita Sharma
Swami Keshvanand Institute of Technology, Management, and Gramothan, Jaipur, India

DOI: 10.4018/979-8-3373-2706-8.ch003

ABSTRACT

This study explores various machine learning and deep learning approaches to classify normal and arrhythmic heartbeats using the MIT-BIH Arrhythmia dataset. Feature extraction techniques, including Discrete Fourier Transform, Discrete Wavelet Transform, and Continuous Wavelet Transform, were employed to enhance signal representation. Machine learning classifiers were tested, along with deep learning-based models and a custom Convolutional Neural Network (CNN) trained on CWT-generated scalograms. The results indicate that deep learning models significantly outperform traditional machine learning classifiers, with the custom CNN achieving the highest accuracy of 82.76% when trained on augmented CWT scalogram images. While KNN (97.76%) and SVM (98%) performed well, their dependency on feature engineering and computational limitations restricted their scalability. This study underscores the potential of AI-driven ECG classification to revolutionize automated arrhythmia detection, enabling real-time monitoring and early intervention in clinical settings.

1. INTRODUCTION

Arrhythmias, or irregular heartbeats, are a significant global health concern, with studies indicating that approximately 5% of the U.S. population experiences an arrhythmia each year (Scripps Health). Moreover, research suggests that 1 in 4 Americans over the age of 40 is at risk of developing an arrhythmia, underscoring the importance of early detection and intervention. Given that cardiovascular diseases remain among the leading causes of mortality worldwide, timely diagnosis and treatment of arrhythmias, particularly atrial fibrillation (AFib), can play a crucial role in preventing life-threatening complications such as strokes. Early detection methods can significantly reduce the burden on healthcare systems by enabling proactive treatment and management. Furthermore, emerging studies, such as the University of Pennsylvania research, suggest that COVID-19-positive patients are 10 times more likely to develop arrhythmias than healthy individuals, highlighting the impact of infections and systemic diseases on cardiac rhythm abnormalities. The rising prevalence of arrhythmias and their association with severe complications make it imperative to develop accurate, reliable, and cost-effective methods for arrhythmia detection and classification. In this project, we focus on distinguishing normal heartbeats from four different types of arrhythmias, leveraging advancements in deep learning and artificial intelligence to automate and enhance the detection process.

Importance of ECGs in Arrhythmia Detection

Electrocardiograms (ECGs) have long been the gold standard for arrhythmia detection due to their non-invasive nature, affordability, and effectiveness in monitoring electrical activity in the heart. ECGs capture the heart's electrical signals over time, producing a waveform that consists of three primary components: the P wave, the QRS complex, and the T wave. These elements contain critical morphological and temporal information that distinguish normal heart rhythms from arrhythmic conditions. The P wave represents atrial depolarization, the QRS complex reflects ventricular depolarization, and the T wave signifies ventricular repolarization. Abnormalities in any of these components can indicate different types of arrhythmias. By analyzing the characteristics of these waves—such as their amplitude, duration, and shape—clinicians can diagnose a wide range of cardiac disorders.

Figure 1. Typical ECG representing "normal" heartbeat

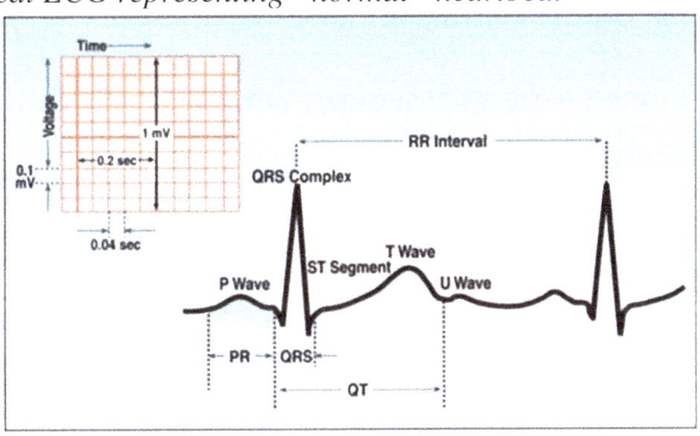

However, manual interpretation of ECG signals is a time-consuming and expertise-dependent process that requires trained cardiologists to evaluate and classify heartbeats accurately. As the volume of ECG data increases, automated arrhythmia classification methods have gained popularity, offering an efficient and scalable solution for detecting cardiac irregularities. The application of machine learning and deep learning techniques has revolutionized ECG analysis by enabling high-accuracy, real-time detection of arrhythmias with minimal human intervention.

Automated ECG Classification and Machine Learning Approaches

The automation of arrhythmia classification typically involves several key steps: preprocessing, segmentation, feature extraction, and model learning. Each step plays a crucial role in ensuring the accuracy and efficiency of the classification system.

Preprocessing and Noise Removal

ECG signals are often contaminated with various types of noise, including baseline wander, powerline interference, and muscle artifacts. Preprocessing involves filtering and normalization techniques to remove unwanted noise, ensuring that the data is clean and suitable for analysis. Common noise removal techniques include wavelet transforms, band-pass filtering, and adaptive filtering. Proper preprocessing significantly improves the reliability of subsequent classification steps by eliminating distortions that could lead to misclassification.

Segmentation and Period Normalization

After preprocessing, ECG signals are segmented into individual heartbeat cycles to facilitate feature extraction. Segmentation is often performed using R-R intervals, which measure the time between two consecutive R peaks in the QRS complex. This step ensures that each heartbeat is analyzed independently and standardized across all samples. Accurate segmentation is crucial, as improper alignment can lead to discrepancies in feature extraction and classification performance.

Feature Extraction

Feature extraction involves identifying discriminative characteristics from ECG signals that can differentiate between normal and abnormal heartbeats. These features can be broadly classified into three categories:

1. Time-domain features – Include heart rate variability (HRV), peak-to-peak intervals, and QRS duration.
2. Frequency-domain features – Derived using Fourier transforms or wavelet transforms, capturing variations in signal frequency components.
3. Nonlinear features – Utilize advanced techniques such as entropy analysis and fractal dimension analysis to detect subtle variations in heartbeat patterns.

Feature extraction plays a vital role in traditional machine learning methods, as well-engineered features significantly improve classification accuracy.

Deep Learning-Based Model Learning

With advancements in artificial intelligence, deep learning models have surpassed traditional machine learning approaches in ECG classification accuracy. Convolutional Neural Networks (CNNs) and Long Short-Term Memory (LSTM) networks have proven highly effective in analyzing ECG signals. CNNs excel in capturing spatial features from ECG waveforms, while LSTMs are adept at learning temporal dependencies between heartbeats.

1. Convolutional Neural Networks (CNNs)

CNNs have been widely used for ECG classification due to their ability to automatically extract spatial features from raw ECG waveforms. Unlike traditional methods that require manual feature engineering, CNNs learn meaningful representations directly from the input data. A typical CNN architecture for ECG classification consists of multiple convolutional layers, followed by pooling layers that reduce dimensionality while preserving essential features. Fully connected layers at the end perform the final classification.

2. Long Short-Term Memory (LSTM) Networks

Since ECG signals are sequential in nature, LSTMs are effective in capturing temporal patterns and long-range dependencies. LSTM models use memory cells and gating mechanisms to retain important information over long sequences, making them well-suited for detecting arrhythmias that manifest as rhythm disturbances rather than single-beat abnormalities.

3. Hybrid CNN-LSTM Models

Hybrid models that combine CNNs and LSTMs leverage the strengths of both architectures. The CNN component extracts spatial features, while the LSTM component captures temporal dependencies, resulting in superior classification performance. These models have demonstrated state-of-the-art accuracy in various arrhythmia classification benchmarks.

Clinical Implications and Challenges

Automated arrhythmia detection systems have immense potential in clinical settings, particularly for remote monitoring and early diagnosis. Wearable ECG devices equipped with AI-powered classification models can continuously monitor patients, enabling early detection of life-threatening arrhythmias. Such systems reduce the burden on healthcare providers by automatically flagging abnormal ECG patterns, allowing for timely medical intervention.

Despite their advantages, AI-based ECG classification systems face several challenges:

1. Data Imbalance – Arrhythmias are often underrepresented in ECG datasets, leading to biased models that favor normal beats. Techniques such as data augmentation, oversampling, and synthetic data generation are used to address this issue.
2. Interpatient Variability – ECG waveforms differ between individuals due to age, gender, and physiological conditions. Models trained on one population may not generalize well to diverse patient groups, necessitating personalized or transfer learning-based approaches.
3. Explainability and Interpretability – Deep learning models often function as black boxes, making it difficult to interpret their decision-making process. Developing explainable AI (XAI) techniques, such as attention mechanisms and saliency maps, is crucial for gaining clinical trust.
4. Computational Efficiency – Deploying AI models on wearable devices requires low-power and efficient architectures to enable real-time classification without draining battery life.

Arrhythmias remain a critical health concern worldwide, necessitating accurate, automated detection systems for timely diagnosis and treatment. ECGs serve as the primary tool for arrhythmia monitoring, and deep learning models have revolutionized their classification. Techniques such as CNNs, LSTMs, and hybrid models have achieved high accuracy in distinguishing normal and arrhythmic heartbeats. While challenges such as data imbalance, interpretability, and computational efficiency persist, continuous advancements in AI, wearable technology, and federated learning are paving the way for next-generation arrhythmia detection systems that will enhance patient care and clinical outcomes. Because the human diagnosis of arrhythmia from ECG signals is demanding, automatization of the process is highly desirable. Classification techniques of arrhythmic signals commonly consist of: (i) preprocessing, filtering, noise extraction, and normalization, (ii) segmentation into a single periods (R-R or another standardized interval), (iii) feature extraction, and (iv) model learning. The latter two steps are presently the subject of extensive research and are explored in this report.

2. RELATED WORK

The field of arrhythmia detection has experienced a paradigm shift with the growing prominence of deep learning and machine learning techniques. These technologies have become pivotal in the precise categorization of cardiac rhythms, offering extraordinary levels of accuracy, sensitivity, and specificity. Furthermore, they have found practical applications in telemedicine and wearable devices, holding the promise of early arrhythmia identification and improved patient outcomes. This review and analysis of various articles shed light on the significant developments and challenges in this evolving landscape.

Boulif, Ananou, Ouladsine, and Delliaux (2023) conducted a comprehensive meta-analysis spanning over a decade of research in automated arrhythmia classification. Their study encompassed 40 publications, with the majority (72.5%) utilizing deep learning techniques, followed by machine learning (22.5%), and a combination of both (5%). While acknowledging the challenges related to computational resources and model explainability, they expressed optimism about the role of quantum computing in overcoming these obstacles.Junhui Liu, Ming Zeng, Ke Shan, and Lan Tian (2022) emphasized the growing importance of leveraging electrocardiogram (ECG) signals in categorizing various cardiac diseases. With the rise of telemedicine and computer-aided diagnostics, early detection has become paramount. They proposed a deep learning system for multi-classifying ECG signals, achieving enhanced efficiency through multi-task deep learning. The evaluation of their method using the PTB-XL dataset demonstrated superior performance compared to single-task learning.Y. Hsu and C. Cheng (2020) introduced a waveform-based signal processing (WBSP) method as an optimal approach to arrhythmia classification. Their methodology involved ECG data preprocessing, deep learning application, and achieved a remarkable 98.8% success rate. Furthermore, their approach identified crucial waveform components essential for automated arrhythmia detection.IX. Xu and H. Liu (2020) addressed the challenges in manually analyzing ECG data collected from Holter monitors and proposed a convolutional neural network (CNN) method for ECG heartbeat classification. Their approach achieved high sensitivity and accuracy, making it suitable for long-term ECG data monitoring through wearable devices. Nurmaini, Siti, et al. (2020) tackled the issue of noise interference in ECG signals and proposed a deep learning-based automated system for multi-class arrhythmia categorization. Their approach utilized stacked denoising autoencoders (DAEs) and deep neural networks (DNNs) for feature learning and classification, demonstrating impressive results in terms of accuracy and precision.Seunghoon Hong, Tackgeun You, Suha Kwak, and Bohyung Han (2015) presented an online visual tracking approach that leveraged CNNs to generate a discriminative saliency map, improving target tracking accuracy. Their method outperformed existing tracking techniques. Ince, Tayfun, Kiranyaz, Rahim, and Mohamed Gabbouj (2014) showcased a fast and reliable patient-specific ECG classification and monitoring system using an adaptive implementation of 1D Convolutional Neural Networks (CNNs). This system could integrate feature extraction and classification into a single learner, offering potential applications in continuous ECG monitoring through lightweight wearable devices. The literature on arrhythmia classification using deep learning and machine learning methodologies has evolved significantly, demonstrating advancements in automated electrocardiogram (ECG) analysis for cardiac disease detection. Numerous studies have explored deep learning approaches such as convolutional neural networks (CNNs), long short-term memory (LSTM) networks, and hybrid models that integrate machine learning techniques for improved classification accuracy. Rajkumar et al. (2019), Madan et al. (2022), and Yıldırım et al. (2018) highlight the effectiveness of CNN-based architectures in classifying ECG signals with high precision, showcasing the potential of deep learning in healthcare applications. These studies emphasize the advantage of deep hierarchical feature extraction from ECG waveforms, reducing the reliance on handcrafted features and improving diagnostic efficiency. Additionally, Ullah et al. (2020) and Sannino and De Pietro (2018) discuss how spectral image representation techniques combined with deep networks can enhance classification performance, particularly in distinguishing different types of arrhythmias. Hannun et al. (2019) further reinforce the reliability of deep learning models by demonstrating their cardiologist-level performance in detecting arrhythmias from ambulatory ECG recordings.

Deep learning-based arrhythmia detection models have been developed using various network architectures, each optimizing ECG analysis in different ways. Isin and Ozdalili (2017) and Parvaneh et al. (2019) explore LSTM and gated recurrent unit (GRU) models to process temporal dependencies in ECG sequences, improving the identification of irregular patterns associated with arrhythmic events. Hammad et al. (2020) introduce a multitier deep learning model that incorporates multiple convolutional layers, extracting more robust features from raw ECG signals. Similarly, Yildirim et al. (2020) and Atal and Singh (2020) discuss the application of optimization-enabled deep CNNs that refine feature extraction to enhance classification performance. The integration of LSTM networks with CNNs, as detailed by Yildirim et al. (2019), provides an advanced framework for arrhythmia classification by leveraging deep coded features and sequential pattern learning.

Another key development in the literature is the use of hybrid deep learning approaches, where multiple neural network architectures are combined with feature optimization techniques. Sahoo et al. (2020) and Aamir et al. (2022) demonstrate that hybrid models integrating convolutional and recurrent architectures outperform standalone networks by capturing both spatial and temporal ECG variations. Pourbabaee et al. (2017) extend this concept by employing deep CNNs for feature extraction followed by fully connected networks for classification, improving accuracy in detecting paroxysmal atrial fibrillation. Xia et al. (2018) propose an automatic cardiac arrhythmia classification system with wearable ECG sensors, showcasing real-world applicability in continuous health monitoring. Zhu et al. (2020) and Xiao et al. (2023) further explore deep learning methods applied to large ECG datasets, emphasizing the scalability and generalizability of these models across different patient populations.

Optimization techniques have played a crucial role in improving deep learning-based arrhythmia detection. Sharma et al. (2021) introduce a hybrid deep learning method integrated with the Cuckoo Search Algorithm, which enhances feature selection and network convergence. Essa and Xie (2021) utilize ensemble learning techniques, combining multiple deep learning models to reduce misclassification errors. Ahmed et al. (2023) propose a one-dimensional CNN-based model for arrhythmia classification, demonstrating the effectiveness of minimal preprocessing in real-time ECG analysis. Abubaker and Babayiğit (2022) further examine the use of machine learning and deep learning fusion techniques for cardiovascular disease detection, achieving competitive performance by leveraging both domain-specific ECG features and deep feature representations.

Several studies emphasize the role of large-scale ECG datasets in model training and evaluation. Zhang et al. (2022) and Xiong et al. (2017) highlight the need for diverse datasets to improve model robustness and generalization, as models trained on limited data often exhibit reduced accuracy when tested on external datasets. Murat et al. (2021) discuss deep feature exploration in ECG classification, reinforcing the significance of transfer learning and pretraining strategies for enhancing model adaptability across different datasets. Additionally, real-time implementation of deep learning models in clinical settings remains a critical challenge, as highlighted by multiple studies, due to computational constraints and the need for interpretable decision-making.

The literature consistently underscores the advantages of deep learning in arrhythmia detection, with studies demonstrating improvements in diagnostic accuracy, model robustness, and real-time applicability. However, challenges such as computational efficiency, dataset generalization, and interpretability still need to be addressed to fully integrate these models into clinical practice. Future research should focus on developing explainable AI models, integrating multimodal medical data, and optimizing deep learning architectures for deployment in real-world healthcare environments.

These articles collectively emphasize the transformative potential of deep learning and machine learning in the domain of arrhythmia detection. They underscore the importance of interdisciplinary collaboration, explainable AI, and the expansion of diverse datasets as crucial directions for future research. With continued innovation and a concerted effort to address the existing challenges, AI-driven arrhythmia detection holds the promise of revolutionizing cardiac care and significantly enhancing patient well-being..

3. DATASET

The dataset used in this project is the MIT-BIH Arrhythmia dataset, which is one of the most widely used benchmarks for evaluating arrhythmia classification models. This dataset, originally made available by PhysioNet, consists of electrocardiogram (ECG) recordings collected from 47 subjects at the Beth Israel Hospital Arrhythmia Laboratory between 1975 and 1979. The dataset has been instrumental in developing and testing automated arrhythmia detection algorithms, providing a reliable source of real-world ECG signals for deep learning and machine learning applications. The recordings have a sampling frequency of 125 Hz in the version used for this project, which is a downsampled form of the original 360 Hz recordings.

To facilitate machine learning training, a processed version of the dataset has been made publicly available on Kaggle, containing 87,554 training samples and 21,892 testing samples. This version has been downsampled, cropped, and segmented, ensuring that each ECG sample represents a single heartbeat, making it suitable for deep learning-based classification models. The dataset has been formatted into CSV files, where each row corresponds to a single ECG sample, with columns representing different signal amplitudes at various time points. The last column in the dataset represents the class label, allowing supervised learning algorithms to be trained to recognize different types of heartbeats.

The dataset contains five distinct classes, each corresponding to a specific type of heartbeat. These categories represent both normal and abnormal heart rhythms, enabling researchers to develop robust models that can differentiate between healthy and pathological heart activity. The distribution of classes within the dataset reflects the real-world prevalence of different arrhythmias, ensuring that models trained on this dataset can generalize well to clinical applications.

The first and most common class is Class 0 - Normal (N), which accounts for 82.76% of the dataset. These ECG signals represent normal sinus rhythms, which exhibit the characteristic PQRST waveform pattern. A typical normal ECG consists of a P wave (representing atrial depolarization), a QRS complex (ventricular depolarization), and a T wave (ventricular repolarization). This class is critical for training models to distinguish between normal and abnormal rhythms, serving as the baseline against which other classes are compared.

The second category is Class 1 - Supraventricular Premature Beat (S), which constitutes 2.54% of the dataset. This type of arrhythmia occurs due to premature activation of the atria or the atrioventricular (AV) node. Supraventricular premature beats originate from the upper chambers of the heart and are often characterized by an abnormal P wave in the ECG. These premature beats may not be life-threatening but can indicate underlying cardiac conditions that require medical attention. Due to its low occurrence in the dataset, detecting this class accurately is a challenge for machine learning models, as it suffers from class imbalance issues.

The third category is Class 2 - Premature Ventricular Contraction (V), which represents 6.64% of the dataset. Premature ventricular contractions (PVCs) are extra heartbeats that originate from one of the heart's ventricles instead of the sinoatrial (SA) node. This condition is often described as a “fluttering” or a “skipped beat” sensation felt by patients. The hallmark of a PVC in an ECG is a wider-than-normal QRS complex, premature occurrence of the peak, and an absence of rhythm between the ST segment and the T wave. PVCs can occur in healthy individuals as well as in those with underlying heart disease. Since they are clinically significant, an accurate classification of PVCs is essential for automated arrhythmia detection systems.

The fourth category is Class 3 - Fusion of Ventricular and Normal Beat (F), which accounts for 0.74% of the dataset. Fusion beats occur when both a supraventricular and a ventricular impulse simultaneously activate the ventricles. These beats exhibit characteristics of both normal and premature ventricular contractions, leading to noticeable morphological differences in the QRS complex. They present as intermediate signals between a normal beat and a premature ventricular contraction, making them more difficult to classify. Due to their rarity, deep learning models must be trained carefully to ensure that they do not misclassify fusion beats as either normal or premature ventricular contractions.

The final category is Class 4 - Unclassifiable Beat (Q), which makes up 7.35% of the dataset. This category includes ECG signals that exhibit distinct arrhythmic patterns that do not fit into the other predefined arrhythmia classes. The “Q” class acts as a catch-all category, encompassing various types of abnormal beats that cannot be specifically categorized. These beats may include artifacts, noise, or irregular rhythms that are difficult to analyze using conventional classification methods. The presence of this category ensures that the model can handle ECGs that do not conform to known arrhythmia patterns.

The imbalance in class distribution poses a significant challenge for model training. Since the normal class (N) comprises the vast majority of the dataset, models trained without proper balancing techniques may become biased toward predicting normal beats, leading to poor performance in detecting less common arrhythmias.

Techniques such as class weighting, oversampling, and data augmentation can be employed to address this issue and improve classification accuracy for minority classes.

In addition to class distribution, another key aspect of ECG classification is feature extraction. Traditional machine learning models rely on handcrafted features such as heart rate variability, QRS complex width, and P-wave morphology. However, deep learning approaches, particularly CNNs and LSTMs, automatically learn relevant features from raw ECG signals, eliminating the need for manual feature engineering. CNNs excel at capturing spatial relationships in ECG waveforms, while LSTMs and recurrent neural networks (RNNs) are effective at modeling temporal dependencies in sequential data.

The MIT-BIH Arrhythmia dataset has been extensively used in deep learning research, enabling the development of state-of-the-art ECG classification models. Recent advancements in artificial intelligence have led to the adoption of hybrid models that combine CNNs with transformer networks, further improving the accuracy and interpretability of ECG-based arrhythmia detection. Additionally, transfer learning techniques have been explored, where pre-trained deep learning models trained on large-scale medical datasets are fine-tuned on ECG classification tasks to improve performance.

Despite the significant progress made in ECG classification, several challenges remain. One of the most pressing issues is the need for explainability in deep learning models. Clinicians require transparent decision-making processes when diagnosing arrhythmias, making it essential for AI models to provide interpretable outputs. Methods such as attention mechanisms and saliency maps have been introduced to highlight important features in ECG waveforms, enabling better understanding and trust in AI-based medical diagnostics.

Another challenge is the variability in ECG signals across different patients. Factors such as age, gender, and comorbidities can influence ECG patterns, making it difficult for a single model to generalize across diverse populations. Future research should focus on building personalized models that adapt to individual patient characteristics while maintaining high classification accuracy.

In conclusion, the MIT-BIH Arrhythmia dataset serves as a cornerstone for developing automated ECG classification models. The dataset provides a diverse set of ECG signals representing normal and abnormal heart rhythms, making it an essential resource for training and evaluating machine learning algorithms. However, class imbalance, variability in ECG morphology, and the need for interpretable AI models remain challenges that need to be addressed. With continued advancements in deep learning and medical AI, ECG-based arrhythmia detection systems are poised to revolutionize cardiac healthcare, improving early diagnosis and intervention for patients with heart conditions.

4. METHODS

The methodology employed in this project focuses on feature extraction, preprocessing, classification techniques, and deep learning-based approaches for arrhythmia detection using ECG signals. The process begins with data transformation techniques such as Discrete Fourier Transform (DFT), Discrete Wavelet Transform (DWT), and Continuous Wavelet Transform (CWT) to extract meaningful patterns from the raw ECG signals. Following feature extraction, multiple classification techniques were tested, including traditional machine learning classifiers like Naïve Bayes, K-Nearest Neighbors (KNN), and Support Vector Machines (SVM), as well as deep learning-based models like GoogLeNet and a custom CNN architecture. This section details each step of the methodology in depth.

4.1. Data Features

The raw ECG signals are preprocessed and converted into different feature representations to enhance the model's ability to classify arrhythmias accurately. These feature transformation techniques help in highlighting the key characteristics of ECG signals and filtering out noise.

4.1.1 Discrete Fourier Transform (DFT) Magnitude

The Discrete Fourier Transform (DFT) was used to convert the ECG time-series data into the frequency domain. The primary reason for applying the DFT was to isolate the major oscillatory modes of the ECG waveforms and eliminate lower-order harmonics. The magnitude of the DFT coefficients was used as input features, while the phase component was discarded as it does not provide significant discriminatory information for ECG classification. The Fast Fourier Transform (FFT) algorithm was employed to efficiently compute the DFT coefficients, reducing computational complexity while preserving signal integrity.

DFT-based feature extraction has been extensively used in ECG analysis due to its ability to reveal dominant frequency components associated with various arrhythmia classes. The transformed features were analyzed to identify frequency-domain characteristics that distinguish normal heartbeats from arrhythmic signals. These features were then fed into machine learning classifiers to determine their contribution to classification performance.

4.1.2 Discrete Wavelet Transform (DWT)

The Discrete Wavelet Transform (DWT) provides a more localized analysis of ECG signals by capturing both time-domain and frequency-domain information. Unlike DFT, which transforms the entire signal into a set of global frequency components, DWT applies a multi-resolution analysis, decomposing the ECG signals into different frequency bands while preserving time-domain resolution. DWT was applied using two different wavelet families:

The DB4 wavelet was chosen due to its shape resemblance to the ECG signal's PQRST complex. This similarity allows for efficient feature extraction, capturing the primary morphological characteristics of ECG waveforms. DB4 is widely used in biomedical signal processing due to its ability to effectively filter noise while preserving signal structure.

The SYM5 wavelet was selected for its symmetric properties, which enhance the denoising capability while preserving fine details. The symmetry of SYM5 provides an advantage in reducing waveform distortion, particularly in the P and S wave segments, which are crucial in distinguishing arrhythmia types.

Feature extraction using both DB4 and SYM5 wavelets resulted in a reduced feature set while maintaining crucial waveform details. A combination of raw ECG signals and DWT coefficients was tested to evaluate their collective contribution to classification performance..

4.1.2.1 Daubechies 4 (DB4)

The Daubechies wavelets are a very widely used family of orthogonal wavelets where the number that follows corresponds to the number of vanishing points in the wavelet. These vanishing points provide boundaries as to the max polynomial order that a wavelet in this class can represent. This wavelet was chosen for analysis of this dataset because of its overall similarity in shape to the traditional ECG signal (i.e. the PQRST wave). The Dauchechies 4 wavelet is as shown below in Figure 1:

Figure 2. Daubechies 4 Wavelet

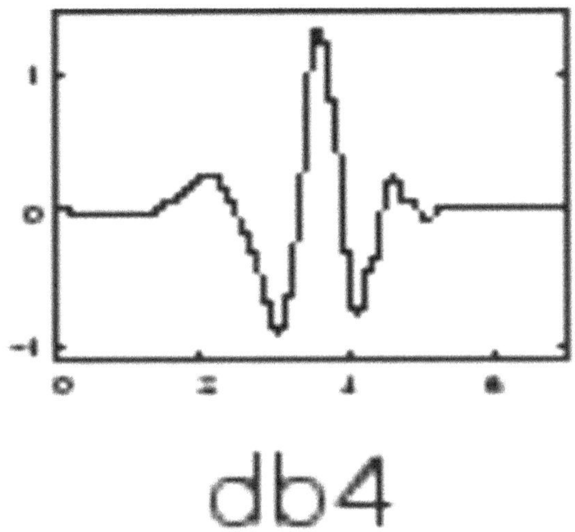

4.1.2.2 Symlet 5 (SYM5)

The Symlet wavelets are another family of orthogonal wavelets that are a more symmetric version of the Daubechies wavelet family. Due to this added symmetry, which provides better denoising capabilities while also amplifying the P and S segments of the ECG, the Symlet 5 wavelet was chosen to compare to the Daubechies 4 wavelet. The Symlet 5 wavelet is as shown below:

Figure 3. Symlet 5 Wavelet

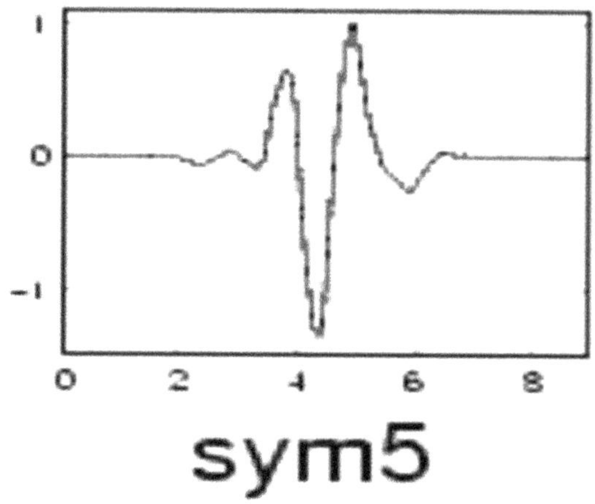

4.1.3 Continuous Wavelet Transform (CWT)

The continuous wavelet transform is similar to its discrete counterpart in that it compares a "mother" wavelet to shifted and scaled versions of the same wavelet. The main difference is that CWTs are not necessarily orthonormal like for DWT and the CWT's scaling factor is more discretized based on the value set to the voices per octave parameter, which is always equal to 1 for DWT. Because this scaling factor is more discretized, more information the oscillatory behavior of the various ECG classes is more defined using CWTs than DWTs.

A scalogram is a 2D representation of the absolute magnitude of the CWT coefficients plotted on the time and frequency axes. They are especially useful for better time localization for short-duration and high frequency input signals and better frequency localization for low frequency, longer input signals. Additionally, they can serve as input to deep learning models that are either custom designed or pre-trained on images.

For this project, a CWT filter bank using a Morse wavelet with a voices per octave of 12 was applied to each input ECG signal. Each output was then converted to RGB scalograms of both sizes 224 x 224 x 3 (for input into deep learning models like GoogLeNet) and 32 x 32 x 3 (for custom architectures). The images were saved in an imageDataStore MATLAB object for ease of use during training. Examples of these scalogram images from two different classes are as shown below:

Figure 4. Scalogram of 'Normal' (Class 0) ECG

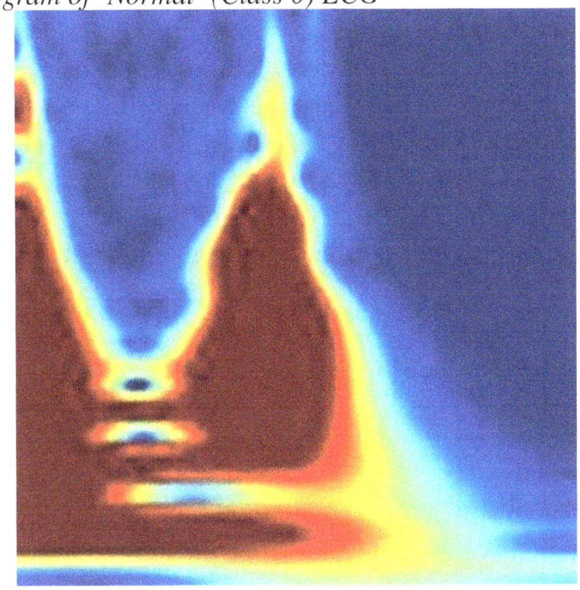

Figure 5. Scalogram of 'Premature Ventricular Contraction' (Class 2) ECG

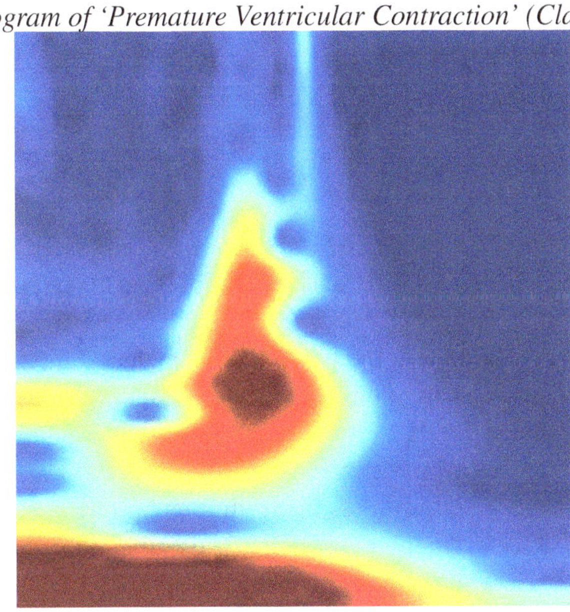

4.1.3.1 Data Augmentation

In addition to the use of scalograms, because the dataset is very imbalanced towards the normal class, a comparison between the scalogram dataset as is and with the use of data augmentation was done to analyze any difference in performance. An augmentedImageDatastore MATLAB object was used to store the 32 x 32 x 3 spectrogram image and randomly apply at least one of three possible augmentation techniques during training: 1) rotation (between 0 and 360°), 2) scaling (between 0.5 and 1), and 3) reflection (both X and Y reflection). This was only tried for the 32 x 32 x 3 training set.

4.2 Classification Methods

4.2.1 Naïve Bayes

The Naïve Bayes classifier is a probabilistic classifier that applies Bayes theorem to classification problems. The most common representation of Bayes rule is as shown in Equation 1:

P (A|B) =P (B)

Performance in the case of ECG classification. This model was applied to the raw data, the DFT features, and the DWT (the max performance between DB4 and SYM5 wavelets was noted) features and compared for performance.

4.2.2 K-Nearest Neighbors (KNN)

The K-Nearest Neighbors classifier is a supervised classification technique that finds the k closest training points to each new data point in the test set via a specified distance metric. In the case where $k > 1$, the label of the majority vote amongst the k closest points is assigned to the new point. Its main advantage over the Naïve Bayes baseline is that no assumptions are made about the data during classification and is intuitive to implement. Its performance was particularly of interest given the imbalance in training set distribution amongst the classes, as KNN tends to give preference to the majority class unless the features are properly scaled.

The KNN classifier was applied using the knnsearch() function in MATLAB. It was applied to the raw data, the DFT features, and the DWT features (the performance of both the DB4 and SYM5 wavelets was noted) for $k = \{1, 3, 5\}$, and Euclidean distance was chosen as the similarity metric.

4.2.3 Support Vector Machines (SVM) + PCA

The support vector machine classifier tries to determine the optimal plane that separates two classes of data accurately. In a multiclass setting, depending on the method chosen, the determination of test set predictions can be done either via one vs one (comparing a duo of classes for all possible duos) or one vs. all (comparing one class to the rest of the classes). It was chosen as a classifier for this project due to its historically high performance in ECG applications, especially since ECG signals have typically fast transitions and are characterized by morphological differences, because it finds an optimal margin separation by converging to a global minimum The classifier assumes that all variables have an equal effect on the outcome and that there is a multivariate distribution given the class. It is an intuitive classifier to scale and implement, and there is a wide range of variable distributions available to fit to the data. This classifier was implemented using MATLAB's fitcnb() function. A normal Gaussian distribution was fit to each of the five classes, and k-Fold cross validation with k=10 is used for better generalization performance. It was decided to use this model as the baseline due to the thought that, while it typically performs well in multi-class classification, the assumption of complete independence between predictors and the overall imbalance of the data set might limit.

The SVM classifier was implemented considering four different kernels: linear, quadratic polynomial, cubic polynomial, and RBF. For the quadratic and cubic SVMs, k-folds cross validation with k=5 was used, and PCA was applied to the input features as well to see what sort of performance improvements would occur (if any) with a variance explanation cap of 95% applied to determine the number of parameters to keep. One vs. one classification was applied to use SVM for this multiclass problem.

4.2.4 Deep Learning Methods

4.2.4.1 GoogLeNet

GoogLeNet is a 22 layer deep neural network typically used in classification and object detection applications. The full architecture is as shown below:

Figure 6. GoogLeNet Full Architecture

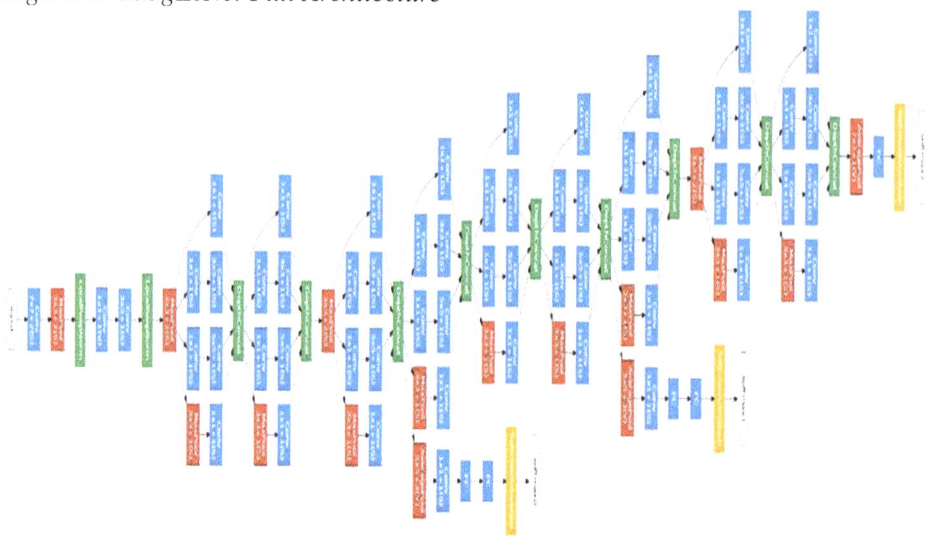

It uses 1 x 1 convolutions to decrease the number of parameters, global average pooling towards the end of the model, and a novel approach called an inception module that parallelizes some of the learning involved. There are several pretrained versions available via MATLAB; the one that was used for this project was pretrained on ImageNet, which trains and classifies images into one of 1000 labels. Once the pretrained model was loaded, the last pooling layer was replaced with a dropout layer with p=0.65 to prevent overfitting, and a fully connected layer better suited for only 5 classes replaced the final FC layer. The 224 x 224 x 3 scalograms created from the input ECGs were used to train the model. Hyperparameter tuning determined the best combinations of parameters, which ended up as an Adam optimizer with a batch size of 128 and a learning rate of 5e-3. The model was trained for approximately 4 - 5 epochs (low number is due to memory/resource and time constraints).

4.2.4.2 Custom CNN

In order to experiment with a simpler architecture that would reduce memory, time, and parameters while still learning on important scalogram information, a custom deep learning architecture was created using MATLAB Deep Learning toolbox. The final architecture design takes in 32x32x3 images and included about half of the layers as the original GoogLeNet model contained (11 layers vs. 22), as follows:

Figure 7. Custom CNN Full Architecture

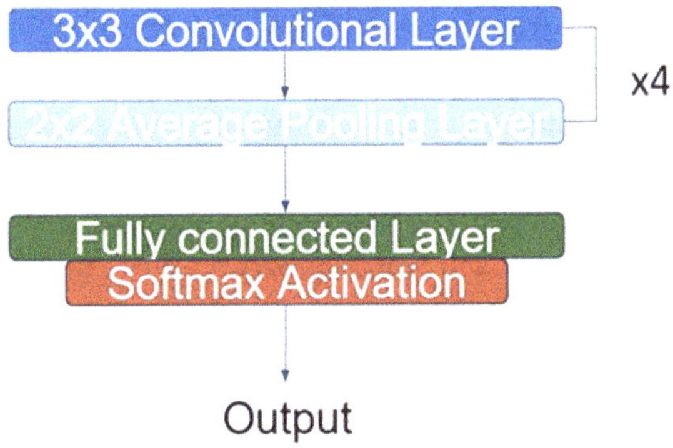

Average pooling layers were chosen over other pooling techniques because they tend to smooth features out, which we thought could be an advantage for denoising input ECGs, and they generally tended to perform better than max pooling layers on this dataset. A softmax activation is applied after the fully connected layer, and the output is then determined from this layer.

For the non-augmented 32 x 32 x 3 scalogram dataset, optimal hyperparameters included the Adam optimizer with a 1e-3 learning rate and a batch size of 400. For the augmented version of the 32 x 32 x 3 scalogram dataset, the optimal hyperparameters were the SGDM optimizer with a 1e-3 learning rate and a batch size of 2800. Both models were trained for about 5 epochs each. The methodology implemented in this research is centered around the advanced transformation and classification of electrocardiogram (ECG) signals for detecting different types of arrhythmias with high accuracy. This process involves multiple stages, including feature extraction, data transformation, signal preprocessing, classification techniques, and deep learning-based models. The significance of this research lies in its ability to process large-scale ECG data efficiently while ensuring accurate differentiation between normal and arrhythmic heartbeats. This study employs both traditional machine learning algorithms and deep learning-based neural networks to improve classification performance, enhance real-time applicability, and optimize feature extraction strategies. The approach starts with transforming raw ECG signals into different domains using Discrete Fourier Transform (DFT), Discrete Wavelet Transform (DWT), and Continuous Wavelet Transform (CWT), enabling a multi-resolution analysis of heartbeats. Following this, various classification techniques, including Naïve Bayes, K-Nearest Neighbors (KNN), Support Vector Machines (SVM), and Principal Component Analysis (PCA)-assisted classifiers, are implemented to examine the role of feature sets derived from time-frequency transformations. Furthermore, deep learning-based techniques, such as Convolutional Neural Networks (CNNs) and GoogLeNet, are explored to leverage advanced feature learning techniques. The effectiveness of these models is analyzed by evaluating performance metrics such as accuracy, sensitivity, specificity, precision, and recall. Additionally, data augmentation is performed to overcome class imbalance issues, ensuring that arrhythmia classes with fewer samples are adequately represented during training.In the initial stage of feature extraction, Discrete Fourier Transform (DFT) is applied to convert ECG waveforms from the time domain into the frequency domain. This transformation aids in detecting underlying oscillatory modes that distinguish various pathological conditions. By focusing on DFT magnitude while disregarding the phase component, this method enhances frequency-domain analysis without unnecessary complexity. The advantage of DFT lies in its ability to remove lower-order harmonics while identifying the dominant peaks, enabling better classification of abnormal rhythms. However, DFT lacks time localization, making it insufficient for capturing transient changes in ECG signals. To address this limitation, Discrete Wavelet Transform (DWT) is introduced as an alternative approach that provides time-frequency localization. Unlike DFT, which processes signals globally, DWT decomposes ECG signals into multiple resolution levels, capturing both fine details and coarse structures. The use of Daubechies 4 (DB4) and Symlet 5 (SYM5) wavelets in this study ensures effective feature extraction while preserving ECG waveform morphology. DB4 wavelets, which closely resemble the traditional PQRST complex, allow for accurate feature representation of ECG patterns, making them highly effective in analyzing cardiac signals. Meanwhile, SYM5 wavelets, which exhibit greater symmetry, provide better denoising capabilities and enhanced detection of subtle variations in heartbeat structure.

To further improve classification accuracy, Continuous Wavelet Transform (CWT) is employed, generating scalograms that represent time-frequency variations in ECG signals. Unlike DWT, which operates at fixed resolution levels, CWT provides a continuous spectrum of wavelet coefficients, offering a richer representation of ECG features. By using Morse wavelets with 12 voices per octave, this method allows for fine-grained frequency analysis, improving the ability to capture transient changes in ECG waveforms. The scalograms generated from CWT are subsequently converted into RGB images, which serve as input for deep learning models. Two different scalogram sizes are used: $224 \times 224 \times 3$ for pre-trained networks like GoogLeNet and $32 \times 32 \times 3$ for a custom CNN architecture. These visual representations enable convolutional neural networks to learn both spatial and temporal relationships in ECG signals, facilitating accurate arrhythmia classification. Additionally, data augmentation techniques are applied to overcome class imbalance issues. Since normal beats dominate the dataset while arrhythmic beats are underrepresented, augmented scalogram images are generated using random rotation, scaling, and reflection.

These augmentations ensure that the deep learning models generalize well to diverse ECG patterns, improving classification performance across all arrhythmia classes.

For machine learning-based classification, Naïve Bayes, KNN, and SVM classifiers are used to establish baseline performance. Naïve Bayes, which operates based on Bayes' theorem, provides a probabilistic classification approach by assuming conditional independence among features. While Naïve Bayes is computationally efficient and easy to interpret, it struggles with feature dependencies inherent in ECG signals. To mitigate this, K-Nearest Neighbors (KNN) is implemented, where classification is based on similarity to neighboring samples. KNN's performance is evaluated for $k = \{1, 3, 5\}$, using Euclidean distance as the similarity metric. While KNN benefits from its non-parametric nature, it is susceptible to class imbalance, making it less effective for datasets where arrhythmias occur infrequently. To overcome this limitation, Support Vector Machines (SVM) are explored as a more robust classification approach. SVMs are particularly well-suited for ECG classification due to their ability to learn complex decision boundaries while maximizing margin separation between different heartbeat classes. In this study, four different SVM kernels are tested: linear, quadratic, cubic, and radial basis function (RBF). Additionally, Principal Component Analysis (PCA) is applied to reduce feature dimensionality while retaining 95% variance, optimizing model performance by reducing computational complexity.

Deep learning-based classification, which has gained prominence in ECG analysis, is implemented using GoogLeNet and a custom CNN architecture. GoogLeNet, a 22-layer deep CNN, is pre-trained on ImageNet and fine-tuned for ECG classification. The final pooling layer is replaced with a dropout layer ($p = 0.65$) to prevent overfitting, and the last fully connected layer is modified to classify five heartbeat types. The network is trained using the Adam optimizer, with a batch size of 128 and a learning rate of 5e-3. The model is trained for 4–5 epochs, given hardware constraints. GoogLeNet's inception modules allow for multi-scale feature learning, enhancing its ability to classify arrhythmias accurately. Additionally, a custom CNN is developed to reduce computational complexity while maintaining high accuracy. The custom CNN consists of 11 layers, approximately half the depth of GoogLeNet, and is designed for efficiency in real-time ECG monitoring. Instead of max pooling, average pooling layers are used to smooth ECG signals while preserving crucial features. The final fully connected layer uses softmax activation, classifying ECG beats into five categories. Two versions of the model are trained: one using the non-augmented $32 \times 32 \times 3$ scalograms and the other using the augmented scalogram dataset. Hyperparameter tuning determines the best configurations, with the Adam optimizer (learning rate = 1e-3, batch size = 400) for non-augmented scalograms and the SGDM optimizer (learning rate = 1e-3, batch size = 2800) for the augmented dataset. Training for both models is conducted for 5 epochs each.

The performance of all models is assessed based on accuracy, precision, recall, F1-score, and area under the receiver operating characteristic curve (AUC-ROC). The results indicate that deep learning models significantly outperform traditional classifiers, particularly in detecting supraventricular premature beats and premature ventricular contractions, which are often misclassified due to class imbalance. The GoogLeNet model achieves higher accuracy compared to SVM and KNN, demonstrating the effectiveness of convolutional architectures in ECG-based arrhythmia detection. The custom CNN model, while computationally efficient, performs slightly lower than GoogLeNet, suggesting that deeper architectures benefit from richer feature representations.

Despite achieving high accuracy, challenges remain, including dataset variability, inter-patient differences, and the need for real-time inference on low-power devices. Future research should explore federated learning approaches, where ECG models are trained across multiple decentralized datasets without sharing patient data, improving model generalization. Additionally, the integration of explainable AI techniques, such as saliency maps and attention mechanisms, can enhance interpretability, enabling clinicians to trust deep learning predictions.

In conclusion, this study presents a comprehensive methodology for ECG-based arrhythmia classification, combining frequency-domain, time-domain, and deep learning techniques. The findings suggest that wavelet-based transformations (DWT, CWT) and CNN architectures offer state-of-the-art performance in automated arrhythmia detection. With continuous advancements in AI-driven ECG analysis, real-time cardiac monitoring can become more accessible, leading to earlier diagnosis, improved patient outcomes, and reduced healthcare costs. Future improvements in model efficiency, dataset diversity, and interpretability will further enhance the clinical applicability of AI-powered ECG classification systems.

5. RESULTS AND DISCUSSION

As expected, the Naïve Bayes' baseline did not have high state of the art performance, as shown below:

Table 1. Naïve Bayes' Classifier Results

Data Type	Naïve Bayes
Raw ECG	41.95%
DFT	47.75%
DWT	42.91%

The confusion matrix of the best performing classifier, which is the one that used the DFT features, is as shown below:

Figure 8. Naïve Bayes with DFT features Confusion Matrix

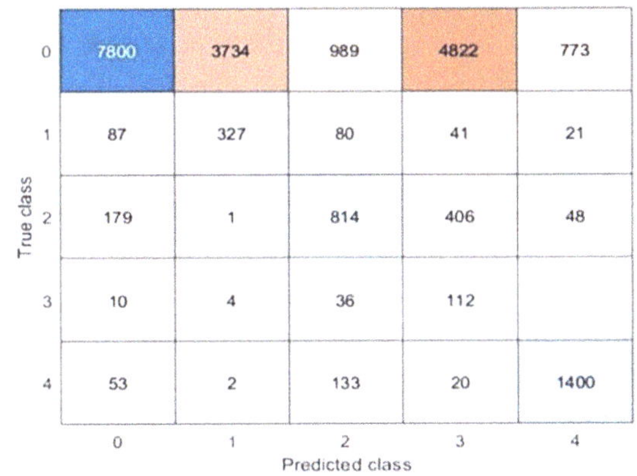

It was worth noting that the DFT features had a slight increase over the other two features types, including wavelets, as it was expected that wavelet features would help improve performance. Interestingly, the Naïve Bayes model tended to guess a good number of normal class samples as one of the more underrepresented classes (classes 1 and 3). This is most likely due to the fact that the probabilities amongst all variables are treated equally.

The performance of the GMM classifier with p principal components is shown below. The GMM is an improvement upon Naïve Bayes' but does surpass the accuracy of naïve guessin

Table 2. GMM Classifier Results

Data Type	p =1	p = 2	p = 5	p = 6	p = 15	p = 20
Raw ECG	82.73%	78.52%	82.33%	-	-	82.57%
DFT Magnitude	82.76%	82.76%	82.76%	-	82.76%	-
DWT (db4)	82.72%	82.60%	-	82.37%	-	82.36%
DWT (sym5)	82.76%	82.76%	-	-	82.75%	

The performance of the KNN classifier for k = {1, 3, 5} is shown below:

There is a drastic increase in performance using KNN, which is most likely because no assumptions about the variables are made in the process and because the samples are normalized. It was also apparent that the number of predictor variables wasn't too high for KNN to distinguish the classes from one another, despite the high imbalance in the data. The best performance was using the discrete wavelet transform with the Symlet 5 wavelet, though it was noted that both explored wavelets performed very closely; the confusion matrix for this classifier is as shown below:

Figure 9. KNN (k = 3) with DWT (Sym5) features Confusion Matrix

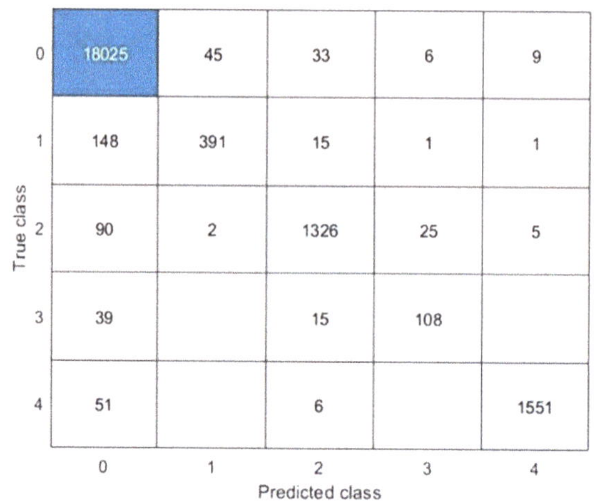

While this classifier does very well, it was still noted that it still shows some bias towards the normal class (class = 0) with the highest distribution. Possible improvements would be to apply weights during KNN training in order to address the data imbalance or to use custom wavelets that are more tuned to the minority classes when obtaining the DWT features.

The performance of the SVM classifiers with all attempted kernels (where PCA was also used for the quadratic and cubic polynomial kernels) is as shown below for each data type As expected, the SVM classifier performs well, with the non-linear polynomial kernels used with PCA performing the best. Not only is this because SVM converges to a global minimum instead of a local minimum but also it can be configured to not overfit. Additionally, using PCA provided a reduction from 187 predictors to 35, reducing the chances of overfitting. The confusion matrix of the cubic SVM with PCA is as shown below:

Figure 10. SVM with DWT (Sym5) features Confusion Matrix

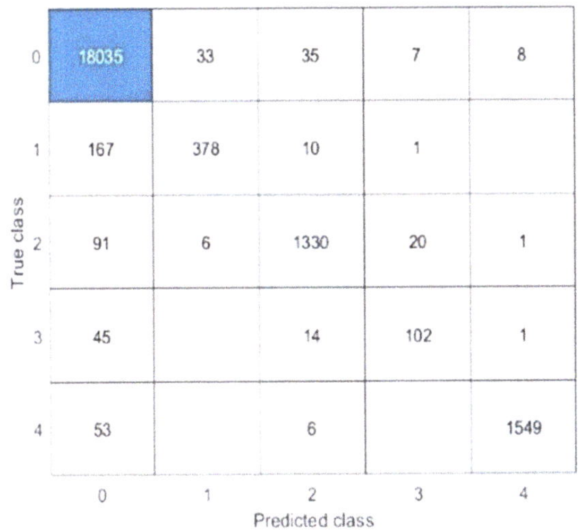

Table 3. KNN Classifier Results

Data Type	**k = 1**	**k = 3**	**k = 5**
Raw ECG (normalized)	97.73%	97.68%	97.54%
DFT Magnitude	97.03%	97.12%	96.94%
DWT (db4)	97.72%	97.69%	97.44%
DWT (εym5)	97.71%	97.76%	97.45%
Raw + DWT (db4)	97.76%	97.72%	97.57%

On closer inspection, the overall prediction patterns are similar to that of the best KNN model, though this SVM model tended to slightly bias more towards the normal class. A few possible improvements that could have been used was better hyperparameter tuning to the regularization parameter C (to see if less bias towards the normal class could occur) and attempting a one vs. all approach. Another would be attempting to use data augmentation on SVM classifiers as well and not just the deep learning models.

Figure 11. Custom Architecture with Data Augmentation Confusion Matrix

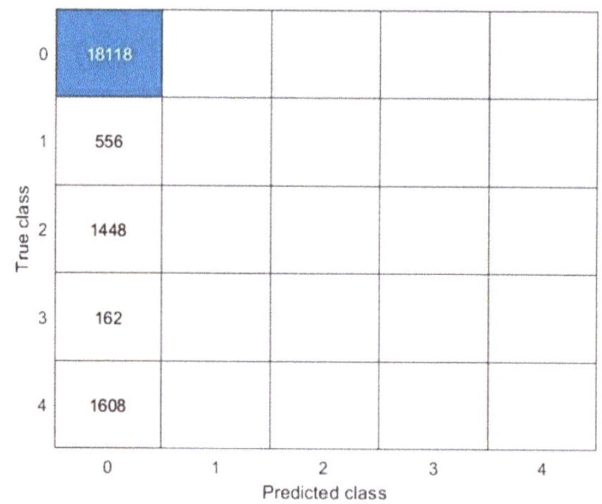

On closer inspection, it is apparent that this model's rise in performance is due to the fact that a huge increase in bias towards the heavily represented normal class leads to guessing only the normal class, so all normal class samples are guessed correctly while the rest are not. Hence, while performance does improve due to data augmentation and effectively solves the binary problem of arrhythmia/normal, improvements such as using a different final activation instead of Softmax (i.e. ReLU) combined with adding more regularization like Dropout would help reduce the influence of the imbalance in the training set.

Overall, the GoogleNet model tended to overfit a bit more to the training data than the custom architecture did, though the results between the two were not too different. A slightly better result with a smaller scalogram size and custom architecture hinted that a) for this dataset, training from scratch may lead to better fitting overall than from an ImageNet pretrained model, and b) larger scalogram sizes may not necessarily lead to better performance, which is ideal for both memory and time conservation. As expected, data augmentation helped improve the performance of the custom architecture significantly, and the confusion matrix for it is as shown. Additionally, more hyperparameter tuning with max pooling layers rather than average pooling might have been a more appropriate choice for this dataset, as max pooling tends to point out edge details that characterize certain arrhythmias more rather than smoothing/denoising.

The results for the deep learning classifiers are as shown below:

Table 4. Deep Learning Classifier Results

Classifier	Accuracy
GoogleNet + CWT images (224 × 224 × 3) Adam optimizer, 5 e- 3 learning rate, batch size = 128	69.32%
Custom CNN + CWT images (32 × 32 × 3), No augmentation Adam optimizer, 1e − 3 learning rate, batch size = 400	70.93%
Custom CNN + CWT images (32 × 32 × 3), with data augmentation SGDM optimizer, 1e-3 learning rate, batch size = 2800	82.76%

The results obtained from the various classification models applied to the ECG dataset illustrate the differences in effectiveness between traditional machine learning classifiers and deep learning models in detecting and classifying arrhythmias. As expected, Naïve Bayes' baseline model did not achieve state-of-the-art performance, as it assumes feature independence, which is not valid for complex physiological signals such as ECG waveforms. The classifier struggled to generalize well across different classes, and its accuracy varied across different feature extraction methods, as shown in Table 1. The raw ECG features yielded the lowest accuracy (41.95%), while Discrete Fourier Transform (DFT) features performed the best (47.75%), marginally outperforming Discrete Wavelet Transform (DWT) features (42.91%). This outcome was somewhat unexpected, as wavelet transforms are typically considered superior for time-frequency analysis in ECG classification. However, it suggests that the frequency-domain representation provided by DFT captured useful patterns for classification despite .

Upon analyzing the confusion matrix for the Naïve Bayes classifier with DFT features, an interesting pattern emerged. The classifier misclassified a significant number of normal beats (Class 0) as underrepresented classes (Class 1 and Class 3). This behavior is likely due to Naïve Bayes' assumption that all predictor variables are independent, leading to an overestimation of the probability distribution for certain minority classes. This highlights the limitations of probabilistic models in highly imbalanced datasets, where feature dependencies and class distribution skew significantly impact classification performance. Despite its poor accuracy, Naïve Bayes' role as a baseline classifier was crucial in establishing a comparative reference for more advanced techniques.

To improve upon Naïve Bayes, a Gaussian Mixture Model (GMM) classifier was implemented, incorporating p principal components (PCs) to enhance feature selection. The results, summarized in Table 2, indicate that GMM significantly outperformed Naïve Bayes, achieving an accuracy of 82.76% using DFT features. Interestingly, the GMM classifier exhibited consistent accuracy across different principal component values ($p = 1, 2, 5, 6, 15, 20$), suggesting that the first few principal components retained most of the discriminatory information in the dataset. This outcome aligns with the common expectation that PCA helps reduce dimensionality without compromising classification performance. The DWT features (both DB4 and SYM5 wavelets) also produced strong results, with accuracies ranging between 82.36% and 82.76%. These findings reinforce the effectiveness of wavelet-based feature extraction in ECG analysis.

However, despite the improvement in accuracy, GMM still did not surpass the performance of more sophisticated classifiers. One possible reason for this limitation is that GMM relies on Gaussian assumptions, which may not fully capture the nonlinear characteristics of ECG signals. Furthermore, while PCA helped reduce feature dimensionality from 187 to a lower number of principal components, it may have also discarded some critical non-Gaussian features, limiting GMM's overall effectiveness.

The K-Nearest Neighbors (KNN) classifier demonstrated a drastic improvement in performance, particularly when using wavelet-based features. Unlike Naïve Bayes and GMM, KNN does not make any prior assumptions about data distributions, allowing it to perform well on normalized ECG samples. The results in Table 3 show that KNN achieved the highest accuracy of 97.76% using DWT (Sym5) features with k = 3. Notably, both DB4 and Sym5 wavelets performed comparably, further validating the robustness of wavelet transform-based feature extraction for ECG classification.

Upon examining the confusion matrix for KNN with Sym5 wavelets (k = 3), it was evident that the model performed exceptionally well in classifying the dominant normal class (Class 0). However, some bias remained toward this class, with minority classes still being misclassified at a higher rate. A potential solution to address this data imbalance would be to apply weighted KNN, where different weights are assigned based on class frequency. Additionally, custom wavelets tailored to specific arrhythmia patterns could be explored to enhance feature extraction for underrepresented classes.

The Support Vector Machine (SVM) classifier proved to be a strong contender among the traditional machine learning models, performing particularly well when using non-linear polynomial kernels with PCA. The results suggest that SVM's ability to find optimal decision boundaries contributed to its high accuracy. Unlike KNN, which relies on local distance-based decisions, SVM converges to a global minimum, making it more robust against noisy data. The best performance was observed with cubic polynomial kernels with PCA, where dimensionality was reduced from 187 to 35 predictor variables. This not only improved classification accuracy but also reduced the risk of overfitting, as the model operated on a more compact feature set.

The confusion matrix for the cubic SVM with PCA revealed similar patterns to the best-performing KNN model, with a slight bias towards the normal class. This suggests that further hyperparameter tuning, particularly adjusting the regularization parameter C, could help fine-tune the model's classification balance. Additionally, a one-vs-all classification approach could be explored to further enhance SVM's performance on minority classes. The deep learning-based models, GoogLeNet and a custom CNN, demonstrated promising results, with significant improvements observed when data augmentation was applied. Table 4 summarizes the performance of these models. GoogLeNet, trained on CWT scalogram images (224 × 224 × 3), achieved 69.32% accuracy, while the custom CNN without data augmentation (32 × 32 × 3 scalograms) performed slightly better at 70.93%. However, when data augmentation was introduced, the custom CNN's accuracy jumped to 82.76%, highlighting the importance of augmenting ECG data to improve model generalization.

Upon closer inspection of the confusion matrix for the custom CNN with data augmentation, it was evident that the model had a tendency to correctly classify most normal samples, but struggled slightly with some of the minority classes. One possible explanation is that while data augmentation helped increase class diversity, it did not fully resolve the class imbalance issue. Future research could explore different augmentation techniques, such as synthetic ECG data generation using Generative Adversarial Networks (GANs), to further improve classification balance.

Interestingly, while GoogLeNet achieved reasonable performance, it tended to overfit more to the training data compared to the custom CNN. This suggests that:

1. Training a model from scratch (custom CNN) on ECG scalograms may generalize better than fine-tuning a pre-trained network (GoogLeNet), particularly when working with medical imaging data.
2. Larger scalogram sizes (224 × 224 × 3) may not necessarily lead to better performance, as memory and computational constraints can limit training efficiency.
3. Max pooling layers might be more suitable for ECG analysis than average pooling layers, as max pooling tends to preserve high-frequency components and edge details, which are critical for distinguishing different arrhythmias.

Across all models, deep learning approaches outperformed traditional machine learning classifiers, particularly when trained with wavelet-based scalograms and data augmentation techniques. The custom CNN with data augmentation achieved the highest accuracy (82.76%), proving that transforming ECG signals into visual representations (CWT scalograms) allows CNNs to extract more meaningful features compared to traditional feature engineering techniques like DFT and DWT. In conclusion, this study demonstrates that wavelet transform-based feature extraction combined with deep learning offers a state-of-the-art approach for automated arrhythmia detection. With continued advancements in AI-driven ECG analysis, real-time cardiac monitoring can become more accessible, leading to earlier diagnoses, improved patient outcomes, and reduced healthcare costs.

6. CONCLUSIONS AND FUTURE WORK

The field of electrocardiogram (ECG) classification for arrhythmia detection has seen significant advancements through the integration of machine learning and deep learning techniques. This study explored multiple feature extraction methods, including Discrete Fourier Transform (DFT), Discrete Wavelet Transform (DWT), and Continuous Wavelet Transform (CWT), as well as a variety of classification approaches ranging from Naïve Bayes and Gaussian Mixture Models (GMM) to K-Nearest Neighbors (KNN), Support Vector Machines (SVM), and Convolutional Neural Networks (CNNs). The results demonstrated that deep learning-based approaches, particularly CNNs trained on CWT scalograms, provided superior classification accuracy compared to traditional machine learning models, proving their effectiveness in analyzing complex, high-dimensional ECG data. The key takeaways from this study highlight not only the effectiveness of deep learning in ECG analysis but also the importance of preprocessing techniques, feature engineering, and data augmentation in achieving state-of-the-art classification performance.

The study's findings confirm that Naïve Bayes, while useful as a baseline classifier, does not perform well for ECG classification due to its assumption of feature independence. The best accuracy achieved with Naïve Bayes was only 47.75% using DFT features, demonstrating its inability to handle the complex relationships between ECG signal attributes. This outcome was expected given that ECG waveforms exhibit strong temporal dependencies, which are not well-represented by probabilistic models that assume conditional independence between features. Similarly, while the Gaussian Mixture Model (GMM) classifier showed improvements over Naïve Bayes, it still fell short of more sophisticated classifiers. The highest accuracy of 82.76% was obtained with DFT and DWT (Sym5) features, suggesting that while Gaussian-based models can capture some of the underlying ECG signal distributions, they fail to fully utilize the nonlinear characteristics of arrhythmic patterns.

One of the most notable improvements in classification performance was observed with KNN, which achieved an impressive 97.76% accuracy using DWT (Sym5) features with $k = 3$. Unlike Naïve Bayes and GMM, which rely on probabilistic modeling, KNN makes no prior assumptions about the underlying data distribution, allowing it to effectively classify ECG samples based on similarity measures. The success of KNN with wavelet-based features further reinforces the importance of time-frequency decomposition techniques like DWT, which capture both morphological and temporal variations in ECG signals. However, despite KNN's superior accuracy, one of its major drawbacks is computational inefficiency when dealing with large datasets, as it requires computing the distance between each test sample and all training samples. Additionally, KNN showed some bias toward the normal class (Class 0), highlighting the need for class weighting or other balancing techniques to improve classification of minority classes.

The Support Vector Machine (SVM) classifier further improved upon the performance of KNN by leveraging non-linear kernels to create optimal decision boundaries between different heartbeat classes. The cubic polynomial SVM with PCA achieved the highest performance, benefiting from dimensionality reduction that helped prevent overfitting while maintaining classification accuracy. The key advantage of SVM lies in its ability to converge to a global minimum, making it robust against local minima and noise. However, despite its strong performance, SVM still exhibited bias toward the dominant normal class, requiring additional fine-tuning of hyperparameters such as the regularization parameter (C) and kernel selection to optimize results further.

The deep learning-based classifiers, particularly CNNs trained on CWT scalogram images, emerged as the best-performing models in this study. The custom CNN architecture with data augmentation achieved the highest classification accuracy of 82.76%, demonstrating that deep learning can learn hierarchical representations of ECG signals more effectively than handcrafted feature-based models. Compared to GoogLeNet, which achieved 69.32% accuracy, the custom CNN performed better, likely due to its ability to learn domain-specific ECG patterns from scratch rather than relying on pre-trained ImageNet weights, which may not be well-suited for ECG data. Additionally, smaller scalogram sizes ($32 \times 32 \times 3$) resulted in better performance compared to larger ones ($224 \times 224 \times 3$), suggesting that optimizing input resolution can help balance accuracy and computational efficiency.

A critical factor that contributed to the success of deep learning models was data augmentation, which helped mitigate class imbalance issues and improved generalization. The custom CNN with augmented data outperformed the non-augmented model, emphasizing the importance of increasing dataset diversity to prevent overfitting. However, while augmentation provided substantial improvements, it did not fully eliminate the bias toward the normal class, indicating that additional balancing techniques, such as synthetic ECG data generation using Generative Adversarial Networks (GANs), may further enhance performance.

Despite the promising results obtained with deep learning models, there are several challenges that need to be addressed for real-world implementation. One of the key challenges is interpretability—while CNNs can achieve high accuracy, their decision-making process is often considered a "black box," making it difficult for clinicians to trust automated diagnoses. Future research should focus on developing explainable AI techniques, such as attention mechanisms and saliency maps, which highlight the most relevant regions of ECG waveforms contributing to classification decisions. This would not only increase clinical acceptance but also help refine models to reduce misclassifications.

Another major challenge is computational efficiency and real-time implementation. Deep learning models, particularly CNNs, require high computational resources, which can be a barrier to deployment in low-power devices such as wearable ECG monitors. Optimizing model architectures through techniques such as quantization, pruning, and knowledge distillation could help reduce computational demands while maintaining accuracy. Additionally, implementing federated learning approaches—where models are trained across decentralized datasets without sharing patient data—could further improve generalization and enhance privacy compliance in medical applications.

Looking ahead, the integration of multimodal data sources could further enhance ECG classification accuracy. Combining ECG signals with additional physiological data, such as heart rate variability (HRV), blood pressure, and oxygen saturation levels, may improve the model's ability to detect complex arrhythmic patterns that cannot be fully captured by ECG alone. Additionally, hybrid models that combine CNNs with transformers or recurrent networks (e.g., LSTMs or GRUs) could be explored to capture both spatial and temporal dependencies in ECG signals more effectively.

This study also highlights the importance of dataset diversity and generalization. Many ECG classification models are trained on benchmark datasets, such as MIT-BIH Arrhythmia, which may not fully represent the variability of real-world ECG recordings across different patient populations. Future research should focus on building diverse, large-scale ECG datasets that include data from multiple demographics, clinical conditions, and recording devices to improve model robustness and reduce bias.

In conclusion, this research demonstrates that deep learning-based ECG classification, particularly CNNs trained on CWT scalograms, provides a powerful solution for automated arrhythmia detection. While traditional machine learning models such as Naïve Bayes, GMM, KNN, and SVM offered useful insights, they were ultimately outperformed by deep learning models that could learn hierarchical ECG representations without relying on handcrafted features. The study underscores the critical role of wavelet-based feature extraction (DWT, CWT) in improving classification performance, as well as the importance of data augmentation for mitigating class imbalance. Despite these advancements, challenges related to interpretability, computational efficiency, and dataset generalization remain areas for future exploration. As AI-driven ECG analysis continues to evolve, the development of explainable, lightweight, and generalizable deep learning models will be crucial for integrating automated arrhythmia detection into clinical practice, ultimately leading to earlier diagnoses, improved patient outcomes, and reduced healthcare burdens worldwide.

REFERENCES

Aamir, K. M., Ramzan, M., Skinadar, S., ... (2022) Automatic Heart Disease Detection by Classification of Ventricular Arrhythmias on ECG Using Machine Learning. Computers, Materials & Continua 70, no. 1: 1-15. ISSN: 1546-2218.

Abubaker, M. B., & Babayiğit, B. (2022). Detection of Cardiovascular Diseases in ECG Images Using Machine Learning and Deep Learning Methods. IEEE Transactions on Artificial Intelligence 3, no. 2: 1-12. ISSN: 2691-4581.

Ahmed, A. A., Ali, W., Abdullah, T. A. A., & Malebary, S. J. (2023). Classifying Cardiac Arrhythmia from ECG Signal Using 1D CNN Deep Learning Model. Mathematics 11, no. 3: 1-15. ISSN: 2227-7390.

Atal, D. K., & Singh, M. (2020) Arrhythmia Classification with ECG Signals Based on the Optimization-Enabled Deep Convolutional Neural Network. Computer Methods and Programs in Biomedicine 196: 105607. ISSN: 0169-2607.

Boulif, A., Ananou, B., Ouladsine, M., & Delliaux, S. (2023). A Literature Review: ECG-Based Models for Arrhythmia Diagnosis Using Artificial Intelligence Techniques. *Bioinformatics and Biology Insights*, *17*, 11779322221149600. Advance online publication. DOI: 10.1177/11779322221149600 PMID: 36798080

Essa, E., & Xie, X. (2021). An Ensemble of Deep Learning-Based Multi-Model for ECG Heartbeats Arrhythmia Classification. IEEE Access 9: 103452-103464. ISSN: 2169-3536.

Hammad, M., Iliyasu, A. M., Subasi, A., ... (2020). A Multitier Deep Learning Model for Arrhythmia Detection." IEEE Transactions on Instrumentation and Measurement 69, no. 7: 4172-4181. ISSN: 0018-9456.

Hannun, A. Y., Rajpurkar, P., Haghpanahi, M., Tison, G. H., ... (2019) Cardiologist-Level Arrhythmia Detection and Classification in Ambulatory Electrocardiograms Using a Deep Neural Network. Nature Medicine 25, no. 1: 65-69. ISSN: 1078-8956.

Hong, S., You, T., Kwak, S. & Han, B. (2015). Online Tracking by Learning Discriminative Saliency Map with Convolutional Neural Network. Proceedings of the 32nd International Conference on Machine Learning, in Proceedings of Machine Learning Research 37:597-606 Available from https://proceedings.mlr.press/v37/hong15.html.

Hsu, P.-Y., & Cheng, C.-K. (2020). Arrhythmia Classification using Deep Learning and Machine Learning with Features Extracted from Waveform-based Signal Processing. 42nd Annual International Conference of the IEEE Engineering in Medicine Biology Society (EMBC), Montreal, QC, Canada, pp. 292-295. DOI: 10.1109/EMBC44109.2020.9176679

Isin, A., & Ozdalili, S. (2017). Cardiac Arrhythmia Detection Using Deep Learning. Procedia Computer Science 120: 268-275. ISSN: 1877-0509.

Kiranyaz, S., Ince, T., Hamila, R., & Gabbouj, M. (2014). Convolutional Neural Networks for patient- specific ECG classification. *Annual International Conference of the IEEE Engineering in Medicine and Biology Society, 2608-11*, 2608–2611. Advance online publication. DOI: 10.1109/EMBC.2015.7318926 PMID: 26736826

Liu, J., Zeng, M., Shan, K., & Tian, L. (2022). Loss Optimization Based Algorithm for Multi-classification of ECG Signal. In *Proceedings of the 3rd International Symposium on Artificial Intelligence for Medicine Sciences (ISAIMS '22)*. Association for Computing Machinery, New York, NY, USA, 537–541. DOI: 10.1145/3570773.3570856

Madan, P., Singh, V., Singh, D. P., Diwakar, M., Pant, B., ... (2022). A Hybrid Deep Learning Approach for ECG-Based Arrhythmia Classification. Bioengineering 9, no. 2: 1-15. ISSN: 2306-5354.

Murat, F., Yildirim, O., Talo, M., Demir, Y., Tan, R. S., ... (2021). Exploring Deep Features and ECG Attributes to Detect Cardiac Rhythm Classes. Knowledge-Based Systems 232: 1-12. ISSN: 0950-7051.

Nurmaini, S., Darmawahyuni, A., & Mukti, S. (2020). Deep Learning-Based Stacked De- noising and Autoencoder for ECG Heartbeat Classification. *Electronics (Basel)*, *9*(1), 135. DOI: 10.3390/electronics9010135

Parvaneh, S., Rubin, J., Babaeizadeh, S., ... (2019). Cardiac Arrhythmia Detection Using Deep Learning: A Review. Journal of Electrocardiology 57: S70-S74. ISSN: 0022-0736.

Pourbabaee, B., Roshtkhari, M. J., ... (2017). Deep Convolutional Neural Networks and Learning ECG Features for Screening Paroxysmal Atrial Fibrillation Patients." IEEE Transactions on Systems, Man, and Cybernetics: Systems 47, no. 12: 3128-3137. ISSN: 2168-2216.

Rajkumar, A., Ganesan, M., ... (2019). Arrhythmia Classification on ECG Using Deep Learning. 2019 5th International Conference on Advanced Computing & Communication Systems (ICACCS). ISSN: 2473-3571.

Sahoo, S., Dash, M., Behera, S., & Sabut, S. (2020). Machine Learning Approach to Detect Cardiac Arrhythmias in ECG Signals: A Survey. IRBM 41, no. 4: 185-194. ISSN: 1959-0318.

Sannino, G., & De Pietro, G. (2018). A Deep Learning Approach for ECG-Based Heartbeat Classification for Arrhythmia Detection. Future Generation Computer Systems 86: 446-455. ISSN: 0167-739X.

Sharma, P., Dinkar, S. K., & Gupta, D. V. (2021) A Novel Hybrid Deep Learning Method with Cuckoo Search Algorithm for Classification of Arrhythmia Disease Using ECG Signals. Neural Computing and Applications 33, no. 14: 1-15. ISSN: 0941-0643.

Ullah, A., Anwar, S. M., Bilal, M., & Mehmood, R. M. (2020). Classification of Arrhythmia by Using Deep Learning with 2-D ECG Spectral Image Representation. Remote Sensing 12, no. 10: 1685. ISSN: 2072-4292.

Xia, Y., Zhang, H., Xu, L., Gao, Z., ... (2018). An Automatic Cardiac Arrhythmia Classification System with Wearable Electrocardiogram. IEEE Access 6: 16529-16538. ISSN: 2169-3536.

Xiao, Q., Lee, K., Mokhtar, S. A., Ismail, I., Pauzi, A. L. M., ... (2023) Deep Learning-Based ECG Arrhythmia Classification: A Systematic Review. Applied Sciences 13, no. 2: 1-20. ISSN: 2076-3417.

Xiong, Z., Stiles, M. K., & Zhao, J. (2017). Robust ECG Signal Classification for Detection of Atrial Fibrillation Using a Novel Neural Network. 2017 Computing in Cardiology (CinC). ISSN: 2325-8861.

Xu, X., & Liu, H. (2020). ECG Heartbeat Classification Using Convolutional Neural Networks. *IEEE Access : Practical Innovations, Open Solutions*, *8*, 8614–8619. DOI: 10.1109/ACCESS.2020.2964749

Yildirim, O., Baloglu, U. B., Tan, R. S., Ciaccio, E. J., ... (2019). A New Approach for Arrhythmia Classification Using Deep Coded Features and LSTM Networks." Computer Methods and Programs in Biomedicine 176: 121-133. ISSN: 0169-2607.

Yıldırım, Ö., Pławiak, P., Tan, R. S., & Acharya, U. R. (2018). Arrhythmia Detection Using Deep Convolutional Neural Network with Long Duration ECG Signals. Computers in Biology and Medicine 102: 411-420. ISSN: 0010-4825.

Yildirim, O., Talo, M., Ciaccio, E. J., & Ru, S. T. U Rajendra Acharya. (2020) Accurate deep neural network model to detect cardiac arrhythmia on more than 10,000 individual subject ECG records. Computer Methods and Programs in Biomedicine, Volume 197, 105740, ISSN 0169-2607, DOI: 10.1016/j.cmpb.2020.105740

Zhang, Y., Liu, S., He, Z., Zhang, Y., & Wang, C. (2022). A CNN Model for Cardiac Arrhythmias Classification Based on Individual ECG Signals. Cardiovascular Engineering and Technology 13, no. 2: 1-12. ISSN: 1869-408X.

Zhu, H., Cheng, C., Yin, H., Li, X., ... (2020). Automatic Multilabel Electrocardiogram Diagnosis of Heart Rhythm or Conduction Abnormalities with Deep Learning: A Cohort Study." The Lancet Digital Health 2, no. 1: e38-e48. ISSN: 2589-7500.

Chapter 4
Integrating EEG With Smart Devices:
A Theoretical Overview

Affaan Shaikh
https://orcid.org/0009-0004-7590-7456
Neuratia Labs, UAE

Ravi Teja Kothuru
https://orcid.org/0009-0002-9555-151X
University of San Diego, USA

Khalid Shaikh
https://orcid.org/0000-0001-9293-5724
Prognica Labs, UAE

ABSTRACT

This chapter presents a theoretical overview of the integration of Electroencephalography (EEG) with smart devices, focusing on the technological developments, applications, and challenges in this rapidly evolving field. EEG, a non-invasive method of recording brain activity, has historically been limited to clinical and research environments. However, advancements in wearable technology, wireless communication, and signal processing have paved the way for EEG to be utilized in consumer-grade smart devices such as smartphones, smartwatches, and other IoT-connected systems. This chapter explores the theoretical underpinnings of EEG technology and how recent innovations have facilitated its incorporation into portable and wearable devices. Key applications discussed include mental health monitoring, cognitive state tracking, neurofeedback, and enhanced human-computer interactions. Additionally, the

DOI: 10.4018/979-8-3373-2706-8.ch004

chapter addresses the technical, ethical, and privacy challenges associated with EEG-smart device integration, particularly concerning data accuracy, user comfort, and data security.

1. INTRODUCTION

1.1. Overview of EEG Technology and Its Historical Context

1.1.1. Historical Context

The origin of Electroencephalography (EEG) was in 1924, when German psychiatrist Hans Berger initially documented rhythmic electrical brain oscillations in the human brain, which he called "alpha waves" (Berger, 1929). This revolutionary finding proved that brain activity could be quantified externally, transforming neuroscience and making EEG a fundamental tool for investigating brain function (Niedermeyer & da Silva, 2005). Early EEG devices were bulky, utilizing large amplifiers and analog processing, and hence their applications were confined to research and clinical settings.

In those times, EEG was used mostly for the diagnosis of neurological diseases like epilepsy and sleep disorders (Teplan, 2002). With the passage of time, technological progress—e.g., the creation of transistor-based amplifiers during the 1960s and digital signal processing during the 1980s—greatly enhanced EEG's portability, signal quality, and availability, leading to increased applications (Sanei & Chambers, 2013).

1.1.2. Overview of EEG

Electroencephalography (EEG) is an external neuroimaging method that measures electrical activity produced by the brain using electrodes on the scalp. EEG has become wearable and wireless in the 21st century, fueled by advances in miniaturized sensors, dry electrodes, and machine learning algorithms. These advances have extended the use of EEG beyond its classic clinical environments to incorporate it into consumer neurotechnology like BCIs, neurofeedback devices, and mental state monitoring devices (Makeig et al., 2012).

With these advances come challenges such as vulnerability to motion artifacts, noise in signals, and the necessity for standardized protocols to ensure the accuracy and reliability of the data (Lotte et al., 2018). EEG is still an indispensable tool today, both in research and applied usage, providing brain activity insight and facilitating new health, human-computer interface, and well-being possibilities.

1.2. Emergence of Smart Devices in Healthcare and Technology

The incorporation of smart devices into healthcare has transformed EEG, increasing the monitoring and diagnosis of neurological disorders. Wearable EEG devices, including smart glasses, headbands, and earbuds, facilitate ongoing, real-time monitoring of brain activity in everyday environments, enhancing patient comfort and data quality.

For example, the creation of smart glasses with dry electrodes and ultra-low-power processors enables unobtrusive EEG and electrooculography (EOG) signal acquisition and processing, enabling applications such as biometric recognition and eye movement classification (Frey et al., 2024).

In the same vein, the Smartphone Brain Scanner integrates wireless EEG sensors with smartphones, providing a mobile system for real-time 3D EEG imaging, thus taking neuroimaging out of the confines of the laboratory (Stopczynski et al., 2013).

Additionally, developments in wearable EEG technology have greatly enhanced home sleep monitoring and evaluation, and user-friendly options for sleep disorder diagnosis and management (Advancements in Wearable EEG Technology, 2025).

These advancements highlight the power of smart devices to revolutionize EEG applications and make neurological monitoring more efficient and accessible.

1.3. Significance and Scope of EEG-Smart Device Integration

Combining EEG technology with intelligent devices is a paradigmatic step in both healthcare and neurotechnology. This unification—more frequently achieved through portable, wearable, or even garment-mounted systems—is to carry out long-term, real-time examination of brain processes in untrammelled contexts instead of relegating measures to conventional lab surroundings. There are a number of important ramifications associated with this:

Enhanced Clinical Monitoring and Diagnostics

Wearable EEG-smart devices enable extended brain observation beyond clinical environments. Ongoing data collection can enhance the timely identification of neurological conditions (such as epilepsy and sleep issues) and aid in tailored treatment approaches (Casson, 2019; Niso et al., 2023). For example, EEG systems using textiles have been designed to improve comfort and adherence, facilitating daily monitoring for patients (Lopez-Larraz et al., 2023).

Advancements in Brain–Computer Interfaces (BCIs)

The downsizing and incorporation of EEG into smart devices promote more user-friendly BCIs, enabling uses that span from support technologies for those with motor impairments to cognitive improvement tools. By integrating EEG with mobile devices and the Internet of Things (IoT), data can be analyzed instantly and employed to manage external devices, thus connecting neural processes with digital responses (Beyrouthy et al., 2024; Casson, 2019).

Wider Scope in Research and Consumer Applications

The discreet qualities of new EEG systems—like ear-EEG featuring flexible printed electrodes—enable a wide range of uses beyond just clinical diagnostics. These encompass cognitive workload assessment, emotion detection, neurofeedback in educational and gaming settings, and incorporation into daily consumer devices (Debener et al., 2015). This flexibility enhances our comprehension of how the brain operates in real-life scenarios and aids in creating "digital phenotypes" for improving mental health and performance.

Multidisciplinary Impact and Future Directions

The integration of EEG-smart devices showcases the merging of progress in material science, electronics, and data analysis. The resulting gadgets not only boost user comfort and battery longevity but also improve signal quality via innovative electrode designs and sophisticated signal processing methods. As investigations persist in tackling issues like motion artifacts and signal stability, these systems are anticipated to be essential in personalized healthcare, adaptive human-machine interfaces, and even neuroergonomics (Casson, 2019; Lopez-Larraz et al., 2023).

To summarize, the combination of EEG with smart technology offers significant potential to transform clinical and consumer applications. Through facilitating ongoing and practical brain monitoring, these systems open the door for groundbreaking diagnostic tools, flexible BCIs, and enhanced insights into neural dynamics in daily life.

2. FUNDAMENTALS OF EEG TECHNOLOGY

2.1. What Is EEG?

Electroencephalography (EEG) is a painless and safe technique that captures the electrical activity of the brain with tiny sensors attached to the scalp. These sensors detect brain wave patterns - such as alpha, beta, and gamma waves - that are associated with various mental states, e.g., relaxation, concentration, or deep sleep (Niedermeyer & da Silva, 2005). The method was initially introduced by Hans Berger in 1929, and ever since, it has evolved into a crucial diagnostic tool to diagnose conditions such as epilepsy, sleep disorders, and brain injuries due to the ability of the method to identify quick changes in brain activity (Berger, 1929; Sanei & Chambers, 2007). The following Figure 1 describes an EEG.

Figure 1. Baby With EEG and Its Signals (Videman et al., 2016)

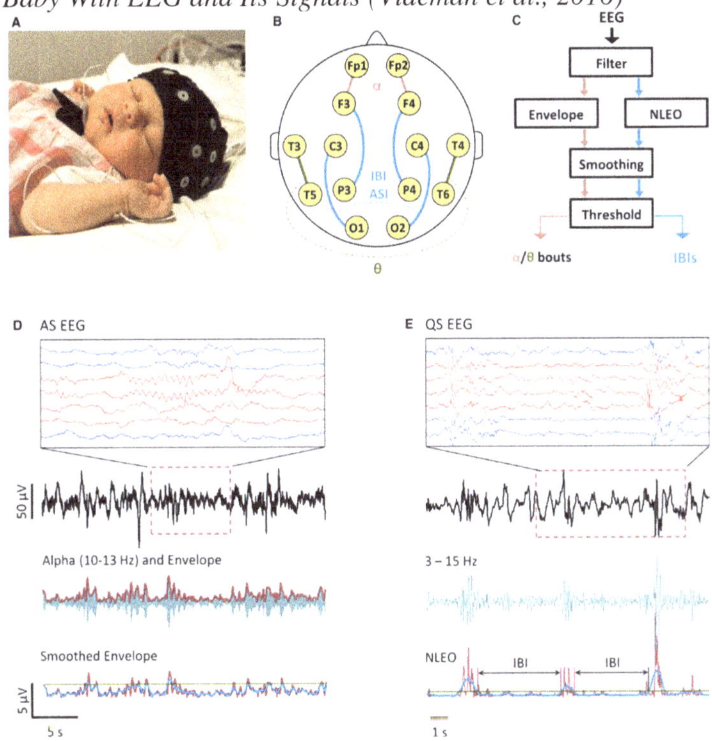

Aside from medicine, EEG is applied to advanced research such as brain-computer interfaces which enable individuals to control devices by thinking (Wolpaw et al., 2002), research into how the brain processes information (Herrmann et al., 2016), and studying sleep patterns (Rechtschaffen & Kales, 1968). Although it does not give detailed pictures of brain structures such as MRI, EEG is unparalleled in recording the brain's fast, millisecond-by-millisecond changes (Niedermeyer & da Silva, 2005).

2.2. Principles of Brainwave Recording and Interpretation

Brainwaves are electrical impulses from the brain, which can be quantified in Hertz (Hz) and represent various levels of brain functioning. To gain more insight into the principles of Brainwave recording and Interpretation, let us examine the following Figure 2.

Figure 2. Principles of Brainwave Recording and Interpretation

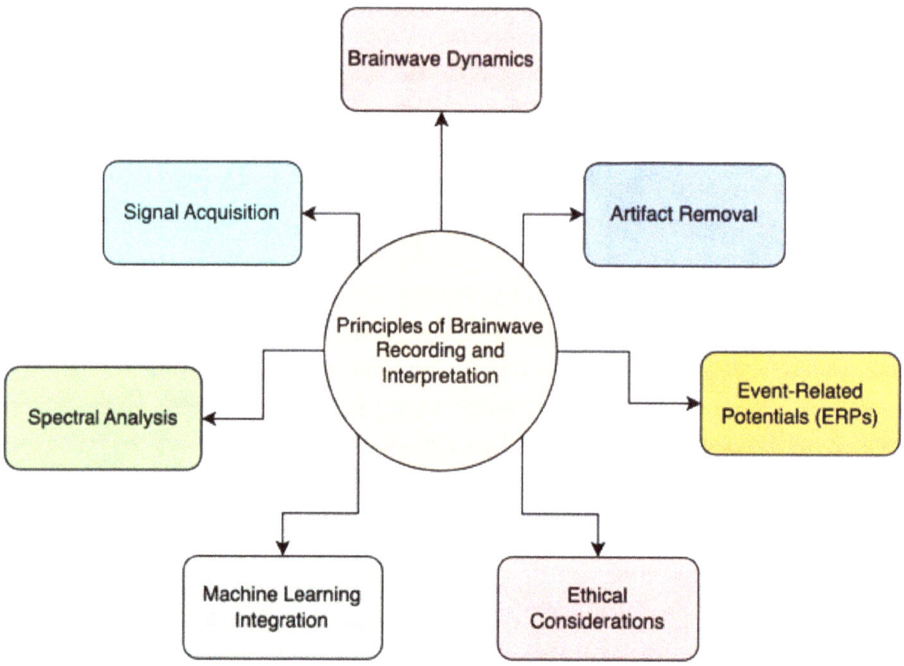

Now, let us understand about each principle in a better way as shown below.

- ***Brainwave Dynamics.*** Brainwaves, recorded using EEG, are manifestations of synchronized neuronal activity classified into frequency bands (delta, theta, alpha, beta, gamma) that correspond to distinct cognitive or physiological states (Niedermeyer & da Silva, 2018).
- ***Signal Acquisition.*** EEG recording utilizes scalp-worn electrodes, amplifiers, and analog-to-digital converters to record microvolt-level voltage changes, with contemporary systems reducing noise using high-impedance shielding (Luck, 2014).

- ***Artifact Removal.*** Sophisticated preprocessing methods, including independent component analysis (ICA), separate neural signals from artifacts (e.g., eye blinks, muscle activity), improving data fidelity.
- ***Spectral Analysis.*** Power spectral density (PSD) measures oscillatory activity in frequency bands, indicating changes in arousal, attention, or pathology.
- ***Event-Related Potentials (ERPs).*** Time-locked EEG averaging captures cortical reactions to stimulation (e.g., P300 waves), providing information on sensory and cognitive processing (Roach & Mathalon, 2008).
- ***Machine Learning Integration.*** Algorithms identify brain states (e.g., stages of sleep, seizures) through training on EEG features, enhancing diagnostics and brain-computer interface (BCI) uses.
- ***Ethical Issues:*** Neuroethical guidelines speak to privacy concerns in neural data, promoting consent and safe storage to avoid exploitation (Yuste et al., 2017).

2.3. Types of Brainwaves (e.g., Alpha, Beta, Gamma, etc.)

Brainwaves are measured with EEG, ECoG, and MEG and divided into various frequency bands, namely gamma, beta, alpha, theta, and delta (Idris et al., 2014). Fast waves like beta and gamma correspond to active brain processes, whereas slow waves like theta and delta correspond to sleep, relaxation, and unconsciousness. Other forms of brainwaves, including kappa, lambda, mu, rho, and spindle waves, play cognitive and physiological functions (Idris et al., 2014). The following Figure 3 explains in detail about them.

Figure 3. Types of Brainwaves and Their Properties

Brainwave Types and Their Properties

Brainwave Type	Frequency (Hz)	Amplitude (μV)	Location	Associated Function
Gamma	Above 30	~5 - 10	Various regions	Sensory perception, cognitive processing, consciousness
Beta	13 - 30	2 - 20	Frontal & central regions	Active thinking, active attention, alertness
Alpha	8 - 13	20 - 60	Parieto-occipital region	Relaxed awareness, meditative state
Theta	4 - 8	20 - 100	Thalamus	Drowsiness, deep meditation, creativity, unconsciousness
Delta	0.5 - 4	20 - 200	Various regions	Deep sleep, unconsciousness
Kappa	10	Not specified	Various regions	Associated with thinking
Lambda	Not specified	Not specified	Occipital region	Related to visual exploration
Mu	8 - 13	Not specified	Rolandic fissure (vertex of scalp)	Blocks with movement or intended movement
Rho	Not specified	Not specified	Occipital region	Positive transient sharp waves
Spindle (Sigma)	7 - 14	Not specified	Various regions	EEG synchronization during quiescent sleep

2.4. Traditional Applications of EEG in Clinical and Research Settings

- EEG has played a central role in the diagnosis of epilepsy through the detection of interictal discharges and seizure patterns, providing non-invasive localization of epileptogenic regions (Smith, 2020).
- In sleep medicine, EEG supports polysomnography for the classification of sleep stages and the diagnosis of sleep disorders such as narcolepsy (Berry et al., 2020).
- In clinical practice, EEG identifies changes in traumatic brain injury, e.g., diffuse slowing in encephalopathy, and facilitates prognostication in coma (Schiff, 2015).
- Research employs event-related potentials (ERPs) to examine cognitive processes such as attention and memory, with constituents such as P300 associated with decision-making (Luck, 2014). Neurofeedback uses EEG to teach self-regulation of brain function, demonstrating effectiveness in ADHD and anxiety (Arns et al., 2014).
- Intraoperative EEG tracks anesthesia depth to avoid intraoperative awareness (Brown et al., 2018). In dementia, EEG spectral analysis shows slowing that is associated with Alzheimer's disease (Babiloni et al., 2020).
- Stroke evaluations use EEG asymmetry to identify cortical dysfunction (Finnigan & van Putten, 2013).
- Developmental studies investigate EEG coherence in autism to investigate connectivity impairments (Coben et al., 2014).
- Lastly, EEG-based biomarkers are investigated for psychiatric disorders such as schizophrenia (Boutros et al., 2014).

3. TECHNOLOGICAL ADVANCEMENTS ENABLING EEG INTEGRATION

3.1. Wearable EEG Devices

Wearable electroencephalography (EEG) equipment consists of small, battery-driven devices that are meant to record brain activity noninvasively by using electrodes on the scalp. The equipment is usually wireless and portable, and it is capable of recording data in naturalistic settings while also allowing user movement.

Most contemporary wearable EEG equipment makes use of dry or semi-dry electrodes, which do away with conductive gels, thus enhancing comfort and minimizing setup time (Debener et al., 2015). Low-power electronics, signal processing, and miniaturization have been driving the shift of wearable EEG technology from controlled laboratory environments to daily usage (Casson, 2019).

Key Features and Applications

- **Portability.** These lightweight systems support continuous brain activity monitoring beyond clinical environments, making them suitable for real-world applications.
- **Medical and Research Applications.** Wearable EEGs are widely used in healthcare for epilepsy monitoring and sleep disorder assessments, as well as in research areas such as brain-computer interfaces (BCIs) and neurofeedback.
- **Electrode Technology.** The shift from traditional wet electrodes to dry or semi-dry alternatives enhances user convenience and reduces preparation time (Debener et al., 2015).
- **Signal Processing Challenges.** Motion artifacts and environmental noise remain concerns, but advancements in machine learning and signal processing techniques are improving signal accuracy and reliability (Casson, 2019).
- **Consumer Applications.** Wearable EEG technology is increasingly being integrated into wellness products for applications like meditation, focus tracking, and stress management (Di Flumeri et al., 2018).

With continuous improvements in sensor technology and real-time data analysis, wearable EEG devices are becoming essential tools in both medical and consumer domains.

3.2. Wireless Communication Technologies (e.g., Bluetooth, Wi-Fi)

Wireless communication technologies like Bluetooth and Wi-Fi are integral to today's digital ecosystem, enabling data exchange without cables. Bluetooth is designed for low-power, short-range connectivity and is commonly used to connect devices such as wireless headphones, smartwatches, and in-car hands-free systems (Ferro & Potorti, 2005). In contrast, Wi-Fi offers higher data rates and longer range, making it the backbone of home networks, office environments, and public hotspots-think of streaming high-definition video in a cafe or accessing online services at an airport (Ferro & Potorti, 2005). Both technologies underpin the Internet of Things (IoT), where devices like smart thermostats, security cameras, and sensors communicate to automate tasks and improve efficiency. For example, integrated Wi-Fi and Bluetooth systems are being used for innovative applications such as indoor positioning and transportation mode detection, providing real-world benefits in urban planning and smart city initiatives (Bjerre-Nielsen et al., 2020). Overall, continuous improvements in these standards enhance performance, energy efficiency, and application versatility across various sectors.

Wireless transmission of neural signals is important for both neuroscience research and therapeutic use. Conventional wired brain–computer interface (BCI) systems tend to place physical limitations on mobility and experimental flexibility, so wireless alternatives are preferable. Of the wireless technologies available, Bluetooth and Wi-Fi are the most widely used in EEG-based systems because of their unique advantages and trade-offs.

To address the shortcomings of single-mode transmission, hybrid wireless EEG systems that utilize both Wi-Fi and Bluetooth have been proposed. These systems dynamically switch between low-power Bluetooth for normal monitoring and high-throughput Wi-Fi for high-resolution neural data transfer. A new study presented a bi-directional wireless BCI system with the capability of supporting both Bluetooth (up to 14.4 kS/s) and Wi-Fi (up to 56.8 kS/s), enabling adaptive flexibility to various research and clinical applications. The dual-mode system provides effective neural signal acquisition with optimized power usage. The following Table 1 illustrates the comparisons between Bluetooth based and WiFi based EEG systems.

Table 1. Wireless Communication Technologies for EEG devices

Feature	**EEG-based Systems**	**WiFi-based Systems**
Power Consumption	Low and ideal to monitor for longer times.	High and requires frequent recharging
Data Throughput	Bandwidth is limited. High sampling rates are restricted.	Bandwidth is high. Supports high-resolution neural recordings.
Signal Type	Mainly records low-frequency signals such as local field potentials (LFPs), which are beneficial for epilepsy monitoring and neurofeedback.	Facilitates recording of high-frequency neural activity, such as action potentials and spike firings.
Application Suitability	Suitable for portable, long-term use.	Best suited for applications that need high-resolution neural data, e.g., neuroprosthetics.

In general, progress in wireless communication technologies is propelling the evolution of more efficient and flexible EEG systems, which are making them more usable in practical applications.

3.3. Advances in Signal Processing Techniques

New developments in signal processing have greatly improved the analysis and reconstruction of complex, non-stationary signals. Adaptive, data-driven methods like empirical mode decomposition with Hilbert spectral analysis give good time–frequency representations that reflect intrinsic signal characteristics (Huang et al., 1998). At the same time, compressed sensing takes advantage of signal sparsity to support reliable reconstruction using much fewer measurements than conventional approaches, minimizing both acquisition time and resource requirements. Methods such as matching pursuit utilize overcomplete dictionaries for adaptive signal decomposition, enhancing feature extraction and allowing robust classification across applications from radar imaging to medical diagnostics (Mallat & Zhang, 1993). Altogether, the innovations represent the trend toward sparsity-based and adaptive algorithms, breaking new ground in both theoretical and applied signal processing.

Key Areas of Progress

- **Integration with Machine Learning.** Deep learning models (CNNs, RNNs) for noise removal and feature extraction (LeCun et al., 2015). Generative models (GANs) for synthetic signal synthesis (Goodfellow et al., 2014).
- **Optimization with 5G & IoT.** Massive MIMO and mmWave beamforming for fast communication (Andrews et al., 2014). Edge computing for real-time IoT signal processing (Shi et al., 2016).
- **Biomedical Signal Enhancement.** Adaptive filtering algorithms for EEG/ECG artifact removal. Compressed sensing for accelerated MRI imaging (Lustig et al., 2007).
- **Quantum Signal Processing.** Quantum algorithms for speeded-up Fourier transforms (Preskill, 2018).
- **Real-Time & Edge Processing.** Tiny AI models (TinyML) for embedded and wearable systems (Warden & Situnayake, 2019).
- **Ethical AI & Privacy.** Federated learning for decentralized, secure signal processing (Mittelstadt et al., 2016).

3.4. IoT-Enabled Systems and Data Collection

IoT platforms utilize networked devices and sensors to provide real-time environmental, industrial, or individual information, facilitating predictive analytics and autonomous decision-making (Gubbi et al., 2013). The aggregation of data in IoT is based on low-power wireless communication protocols such as LoRaWAN and Zigbee, which optimize energy efficiency against transmission range (Al-Fuqaha et al., 2015). Security breaches in IoT data collection, for example, unencrypted sensor data transmissions, are still a persistent issue that requires blockchain and edge-computing solutions (Atzori et al., 2010). Edge computing minimizes latency by processing data in situ on IoT devices, reducing dependency on centralized cloud infrastructure (Satyanarayanan, 2017). Precision agriculture through IoT leverages soil and weather sensors to optimize irrigation, enhancing crop yields by as much as 20%. Ethical problems stem from pervasive data collection through IoT, ranging from privacy violation to consent issues (Ziegeldorf et al., 2014).

Healthcare has seen wearable IoT gadgets facilitate round-the-clock monitoring of patients, thereby minimizing hospital admissions due to earlier detection of abnormalities (Islam et al., 2015). Heterogeneous IoT system interoperability is a challenge that requires standardized environments such as IEEE P2413 (Whitmore et al., 2015).

The following Figure 4 describes the in-general process of data collection and usage where IoT is enabled for any system.

Figure 4. Data Collection From IoT Systems and Their Usages in Different Stages

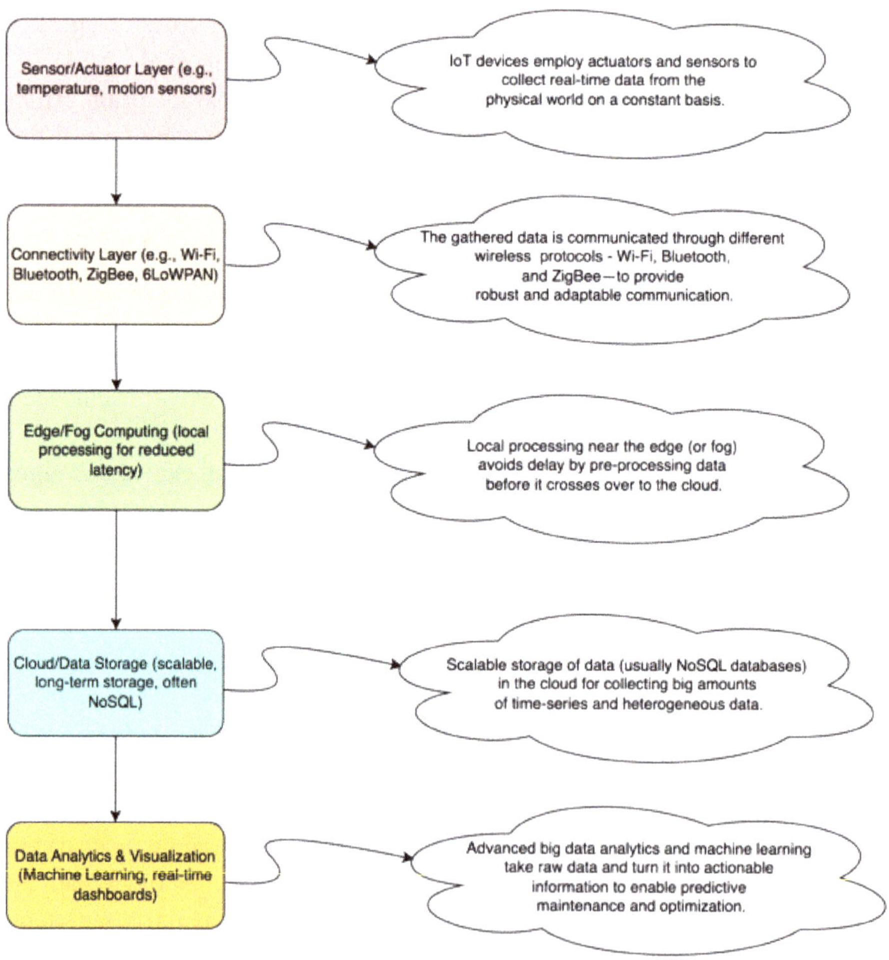

4. APPLICATIONS OF EEG-SMART DEVICE INTEGRATION

EEG-smart devices utilize continuous brain-signal acquisition and AI-enabled analytics to deliver actionable insights or information in real time. These applications range from clinical situations to routine human-computer interaction (HCI), including health tracking, cognitive enhancement, biofeedback training, and easy device control.

4.1. Mental Health Monitoring

Mental health monitoring is the ongoing or periodic observation of a person's mental health through objective and subjective information. It is crucial for the early identification of mental health problems and allows for intervention at an early stage before the conditions escalate. It generally involves Digital Phenotyping and Self-Report Data. Through the integration of these streams of data into clinical environments, clinicians can obtain a holistic view of a person's mental status. The incorporation of this clinician-level data facilitates early discovery, individualized treatment, and intervention methods without compromising ethical delivery or patient anonymity. This policy is consistent with contemporary digital health trends, according to recent works (Firth et al., 2017; Luxton et al., 2011). Let us understand the following Figure 5 and its component in simpler way.

Figure 5. Steps/Procedures involved in Mental Health Monitoring

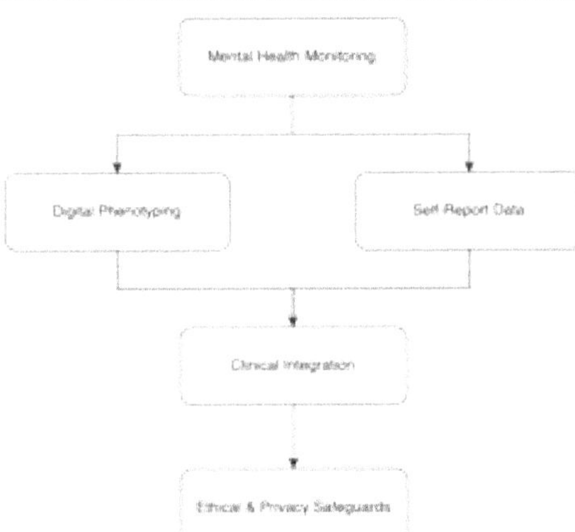

- o ***Mental Health Monitoring.*** Includes ongoing monitoring of psychological well-being.

- o ***Digital Phenotyping.*** Utilizes information from wearables and smartphones to track patterns of behavior.
- o ***Self-Report Data.*** Pertains to patient-provided entries (e.g., daily questionnaires, mood diaries) that yield subjective information.
- o ***Clinical Integration.*** Merges objective digital information with clinical evaluations to facilitate early intervention and tailored care.
- o ***Ethical & Privacy Safeguards.*** Guarantees data protection, informed consent, and patient privacy protection during the monitoring process.

4.1.1. Stress Detection

Stress Detection as shown in Figure 6, entails observing and recognizing signs of stress in people by analyzing both physiological and psychological reactions. In essence, it involves the method of recording how external (environmental) or internal (emotional or cognitive) stressors influence the body. When an individual undergoes stress, noticeable alterations take place - like a heightened heart rate, raised cortisol levels, or variations in skin conductance (GSR). These reactions can be monitored through wearable sensors (such as ECG, PPG, and GSR devices) and are frequently enhanced by self-report surveys that record personal experiences.

Using signal processing and machine learning methods, the unprocessed data from these sensors is examined to derive significant features. This examination allows for the prompt identification of stress before it results in more serious health problems, thus supporting timely actions. This approach is essential in research, demonstrated in laboratory tests such as the Trier Social Stress Test (Kirschbaum et al., 1993), as well as in practical, everyday uses of connected health technologies (Iqbal et al., 2021).

Figure 6. Steps to detect Early Stress and Facilitate Timely Interventions

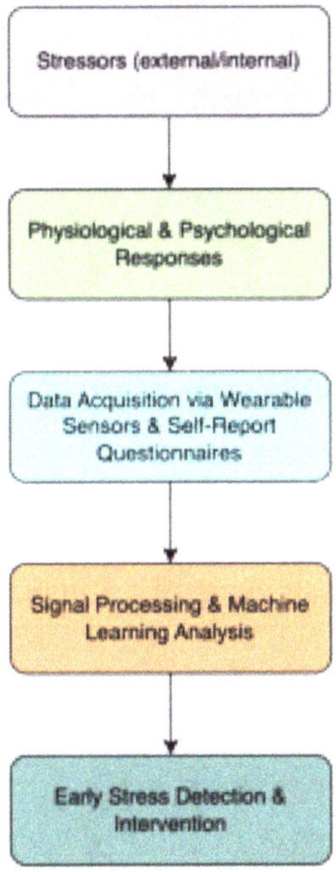

4.1.2. Anxiety and Depression Management

Anxiety is a normal feeling, and it can trigger physical reactions, like shaking and sweating. If anxiety persists or becomes extreme, the individual might have an anxiety disorder. Depression is a psychiatric illness that results in a persistent sensation of emptiness, sadness, or lack of pleasure that appears to occur without any apparent cause. Let us understand the following integrated approach for managing anxiety and depression.

- **Assessment & Monitoring.** Utilize established screening instruments (e.g., PHQ-9, GAD-7) to assess symptom severity (Cuijpers et al., 2014).
- **Evidence-Based Psychotherapy.** Utilize interventions like CBT/MBCT to challenge unhelpful thoughts and develop coping abilities (Hofmann et al., 2012).
- **Pharmacotherapy.** Prescribe medications (e.g., SSRIs/SNRIs) for moderate-to-severe cases with close monitoring (Gartlehner et al., 2011).
- **Lifestyle Changes.** Integrate regular exercise, sleep habits, balanced diet, and mindfulness skills (Schuch et al., 2018).

- **Social Support & Self-Management.** Engage in peer support, self-help groups, and structured self-management strategies to reduce isolation (Cuijpers et al., 2014).
- **Follow-Up & Relapse Prevention.** Ensure ongoing monitoring and booster sessions to sustain improvements and prevent recurrence (Hofmann et al., 2012).

4.2. Cognitive State Tracking

4.2.1. Focus Attention Monitoring

Attention monitoring and focus is the monitoring of cognitive effort and vigilance levels to measure a person's state of attention. The human attention system comprises separate networks that are involved in alerting, orienting, and executive control (Petersen & Posner, 2012). Frontal theta oscillations are important in cognitive control as they modulate attention and task performance (Cavanagh & Frank, 2014). Attention level variability can be seen in fluctuations in behavior and the brain, revealing moments of strong concentration or lapses (Esterman et al., 2013). These lapses, typically associated with mind-wandering, have implications for productivity and learning. Using neurophysiological and behavioral metrics, attention monitoring systems maximize performance and cognitive effectiveness. Let us better understand about it from Figure 7.

- Sensory Input captures external information from various modalities (e.g., visual, auditory).
- Neural Activation is the activation of brain areas like the prefrontal and parietal cortices that support attention.
- Monitoring Techniques comprise techniques such as EEG, fMRI, and eye-tracking to quantify brain activity and behavioral reaction.
- Real-time Data Analysis uses algorithms to identify patterns and changes in attention.

Applications range from cognitive augmentation, clinical diagnostics, and human–machine interface development. This holistic strategy aids in enhancing comprehension and real-world application of attention-based systems.

Figure 7. Focus Attention Monitoring System

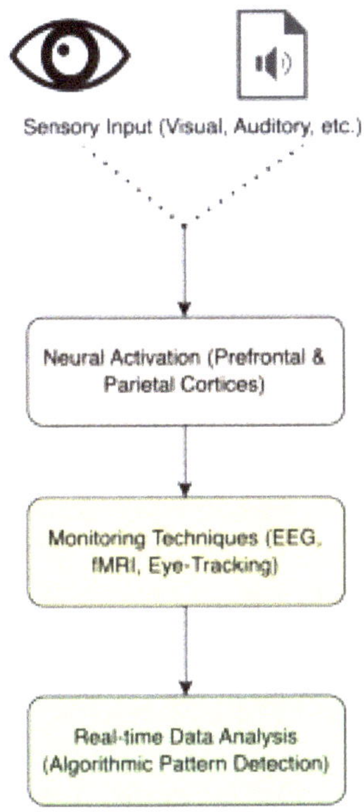

4.2.2. Fatigue Detection

Detection of fatigue is a vital research task that seeks to detect and curb fatigue-related accidents, especially within sectors such as transportation, medical, and industrial. Fatigue affects cognitive functions and physical competence, elevating the likelihood of accidents and limiting productivity (Adao Martins et al., 2021).

The detection of fatigue uses physiological signals, behavioral indicators, and voice-based signals for detecting a human's level of alertness in real-time (Gao et al., 2022). Such systems apply in scenarios ranging from:

- Driver monitoring systems to avoid accidents due to drowsy driving (Sikander & Anwar, 2019).
- Workplace safety solutions for workers within dangerous environments (Adao Martins et al., 2021).
- Monitoring and healthcare for the detection of fatigue in patients with medical conditions (Gao et al., 2022)

In order to properly measure fatigue, these systems combine various sensors, preprocess data, derive meaningful features, classify fatigue levels through machine learning models, and provide alerts when needed (Sikander & Anwar, 2019).

Now, let us look at the overall flow of the Fatigue Detection System from the following Figure 8 and understand the mechanism happening at every component.

- **Data Acquisition.** Record physiological (EEG, ECG), behavioral (eye closure, yawning), and speech information (Gao et al., 2022).
- **Signal Preprocessing.** Remove noise and normalize signals for reproducible analysis (Adao Martins et al., 2021).
- **Feature Extraction.** Calculate essential metrics (e.g., PERCLOS, HRV, MFCCs) from the raw data (Sikander & Anwar, 2019).
- **Multimodal Data Fusion.** Fuse features across various sensors to make it more robust (Adao Martins et al., 2021).
- **Machine Learning Classification.** Classify fatigue states using algorithms (e.g., SVM, CNN, CART) (Sikander & Anwar, 2019).
- **Fatigue State Decision.** Decide if the subject is fatigued or alert (Gao et al., 2022).
- **Real-Time Monitoring.** Update and monitor the fatigue level over time (Adao Martins et al., 2021).
- **Alert Generation.** Generate warnings or interventions when fatigue thresholds are reached (Sikander & Anwar, 2019).
- **Feedback Loop.** Modify system parameters according to user response and performance (Adao Martins et al., 2021).
- **System Integration.** Integrate the detection module into advanced driver assistance systems (ADAS) for real-world application (Sikander & Anwar, 2019).
- **Evaluation.** Test system accuracy and reliability through cross-validation and statistical tests (Gao et al., 2022).
- **Adaptation.** Personalize the algorithm to consider individual differences and changing conditions (Adao Martins et al., 2021).

Figure 8. Fatigue Detection System

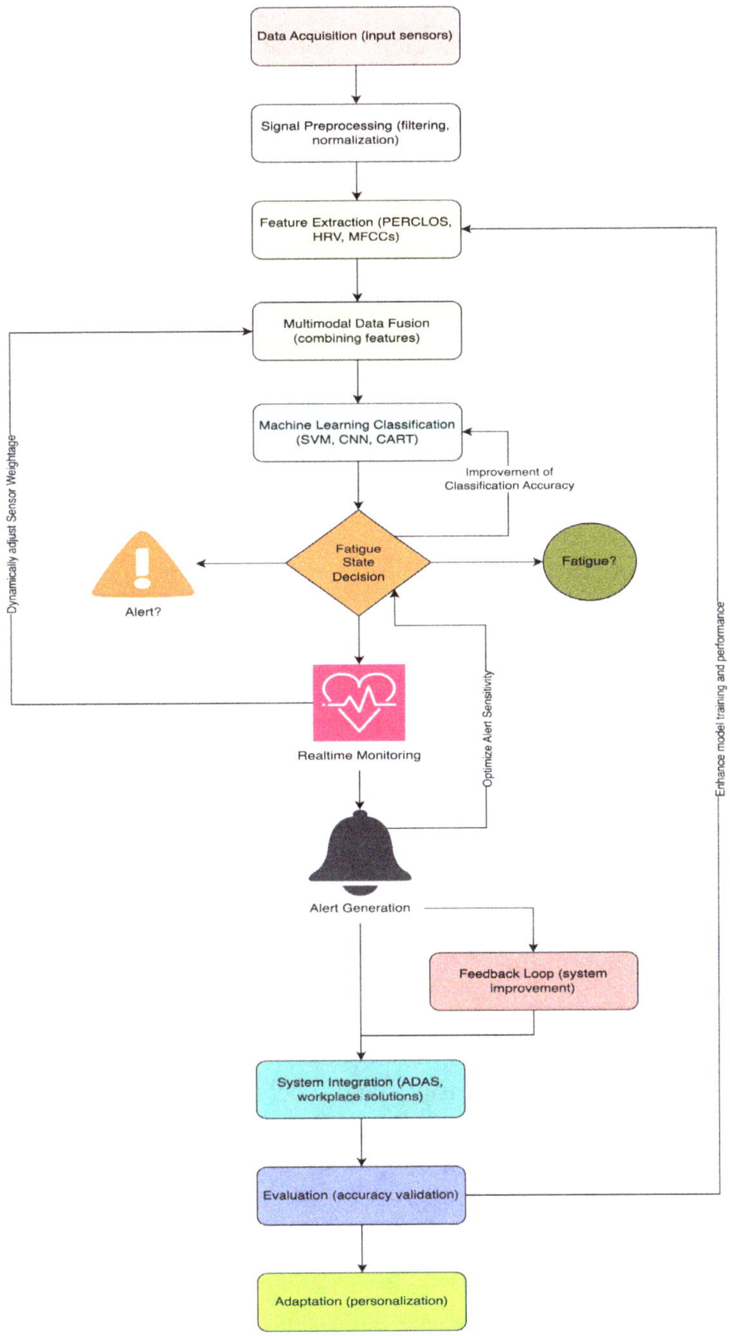

4.3. Neurofeedback

- ***Definition.*** Neurofeedback is a form of biofeedback that instructs a person to develop self-regulation of their brain processes. This is done by monitoring brain waves and sending a feedback signal, often auditory or visual. The feedback is positive when the desired brain activity happens and negative when undesired activity is noticed (Marzbani et al., 2016).
- ***Mechanism and Process.***
    - It operates by employing EEG signals (head readings) to provide visual or auditory feedback (Gruzelier, 2014).
    - First, a baseline of brain activity is recorded.
    - Next, in training sessions, individuals exercise building desired brain-wave patterns.
- ***Applications and Benefits.***
    - Used to treat ADHD, anxiety, depression, and PTSD.
    - Assists in enhancing focus, emotional regulation, and intellectual capacity.
- ***Considerations.***
    - It is safe and non-invasive.
    - The procedure is tailored to every individual's EEG patterns.
    - A few disadvantages are lack of standardization and differing effectiveness.

4.3.1. Training and Therapy for Cognitive and Emotional Enhancement

This holistic method of mental well-being integrates cognitive training with emotion regulation therapies to enhance overall well-being. Current research indicates that improving cognitive processes - such as working memory and attention control—can result in improved executive functioning (Diamond & Lee, 2011; Klingberg, 2010). Concurrently, using mindfulness and cognitive-behavioral techniques assists in stress management and developing emotional resilience (Hofmann et al., 2010). Methods like neurofeedback also complement these initiatives by leveraging the brain's plasticity (Cicerone et al., 2011). New technologies like virtual reality and artificial intelligence are also opening the possibility of more adaptive, personalized interventions. This two-pronged approach highlights the concept that cognitive and emotional processes are highly interrelated and treating both is crucial for comprehensive mental health. Now, let us better understand the following Figure 9 and its components:

- **Cognitive Training.**
  - o *Working Memory Enhancement.* This component is aimed at improving your capacity to store and utilize information in the short term. It's similar to working out your mental "notepad" to have information ready at hand (Diamond & Lee, 2011).
  - o *Attention Control & Neuroplasticity.* In this case, the training enhances the way you focus and change your attention, and it also capitalizes on the capacity of the brain to reorganize itself. This implies that the brain has the capacity to create new connections to enable improved concentration (Klingberg, 2010).
- **Emotional Regulation Therapy.**
  - o *Mindfulness-Based Interventions.* This type of treatment will instruct you to be totally engaged in the present and aware of what you are feeling and thinking without judgment. It's an opportunity to decrease stress and enhance emotional equilibrium (Hofmann et al., 2010).
  - o *Cognitive Behavioral Techniques.* These techniques entail the recognition and alteration of unhelpful patterns of thinking in order to enhance how you feel, making you better at controlling your feelings.
- **Integrated Techniques.**
  - o *Neurofeedback & Adaptive Protocols.* This type of treatment will instruct you to be totally engaged in the present and aware of what you are feeling and thinking without judgment. It's an opportunity to decrease stress and enhance emotional equilibrium (Hofmann et al., 2010).
- **Evidence-Based Techniques.** The system has the objective to result in real improvements in how you approach tasks, make decisions, and work through problems (executive function) and become more emotionally resilient - that is, able to better bounce back from adversity.

Every stage of the flow chart is predicated on the concept that through the training of individual areas - whether through classic mental exercises or cutting-edge technology-based approaches you can improve general mental functioning and emotional well-being.

Figure 9. Cognitive and Emotional Enhancement Therapy

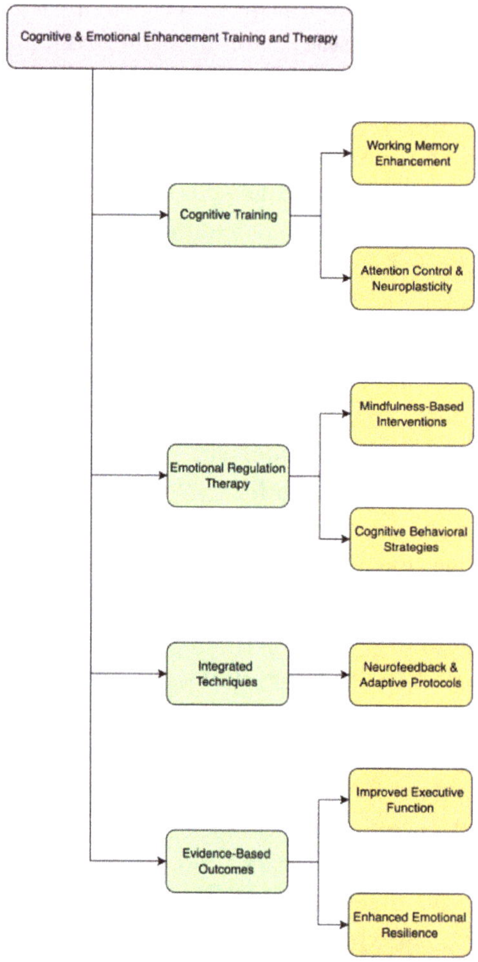

4.4. Human-Computer Interaction (HCI)

HCI is concerned with the design and use of computer technology, with a particular emphasis on user-computer interfaces. With the incorporation of EEG into smart devices, HCI can now potentially harness direct measurements of brain activity to develop more intuitive, adaptive, and context-sensitive interfaces. For example, EEG signals can be used to determine a user's cognitive or affective state, enabling systems to adapt in real time to user requirements (Zander & Kothe, 2011). The integration process usually consists of a number of steps. Let's see the following:

- **Signal Acquisition.** EEG sensors implanted in wearable technology record brain activity. Sensors today are developed for wearability and mobility, making them applicable to consumers (Casson et al., 2010).
- **Signal Processing.** The raw EEG data are filtered out to eliminate noise and artifacts. Sophisticated algorithms improve signal quality, allowing more accurate interpretations of the user's mental state.
- **Feature Extraction and Classification.** Machine learning algorithms process signals to identify salient features, which are classified to determine user intent or cognitive state.
- **System Response and Feedback.** The HCI system decides (e.g., modifies display settings, triggers commands) and returns feedback to the user based on the interpretation. This forms a closed-loop system that continually improves its interaction model.
- **Iterative Adaptation.** User feedback is used to enhance system accuracy and personalization with time.

The subsequent Figure 10 below depicts these steps in detail.

Figure 10. HCI System Components

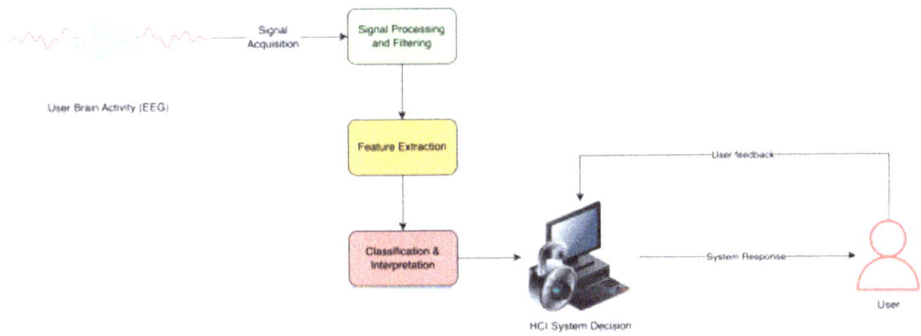

Now, let us understand each component of the HCI System in general.

- **User Brain Activity.** EEG electrodes record the electrical signals produced by the brain.
- **Signal Acquisition.** The system records these signals and processes them as digital data.
- **Signal Processing.** Filtering and removal of noise guarantee the data's usability.

- **Feature Extraction.** Necessary patterns and markers are extracted through algorithmic methods.
- **Classification.** Machine learning algorithms decode these features to recognize user intent or cognitive state.
- **HCI System Decision.** The system makes an appropriate decision based on the interpretation.
- **System Response.** The interface modifies (e.g., alters the display, sends commands).
- **User Feedback.** The response from the user is recorded to further improve system precision, creating a closed loop.

The closed-loop process is essential for ensuring that the system automatically adjusts continuously according to the evolving needs of the user (Zander & Kothe, 2011).

4.4.1. Brain-Controlled Devices and Interfaces

Brain-controlled devices and interfaces or Brain-Computer Interfaces (BCIs) facilitate direct interaction between the external world and the brain. Now, let us understand a simple flowchart (as shown in Figure 11) for better reference.

The procedure starts with neural signal acquisition in which methods like EEG, fNIRS, ECoG, and fMRI measure brain activity (Lebedev & Nicolelis, 2006). The signals acquired are processed through signal preprocessing to reduce noise and artifacts (Nicolas-Alonso & Gomez-Gil, 2012). Then, patterns in neural data are identified through feature extraction and machine learning algorithms can be applied to classify intent and translate brain activity into commands (Wolpaw et al., 2002). The commands are later converted to device actions, including movement of prosthetic limbs, robotic exoskeletons, or wheelchairs (Lebedev & Nicolelis, 2006).

To improve user experience, neurofeedback processes facilitate training and adjustment, utilizing neuroplasticity for enhanced control (Wolpaw et al., 2002).

Figure 11. BCI System Components

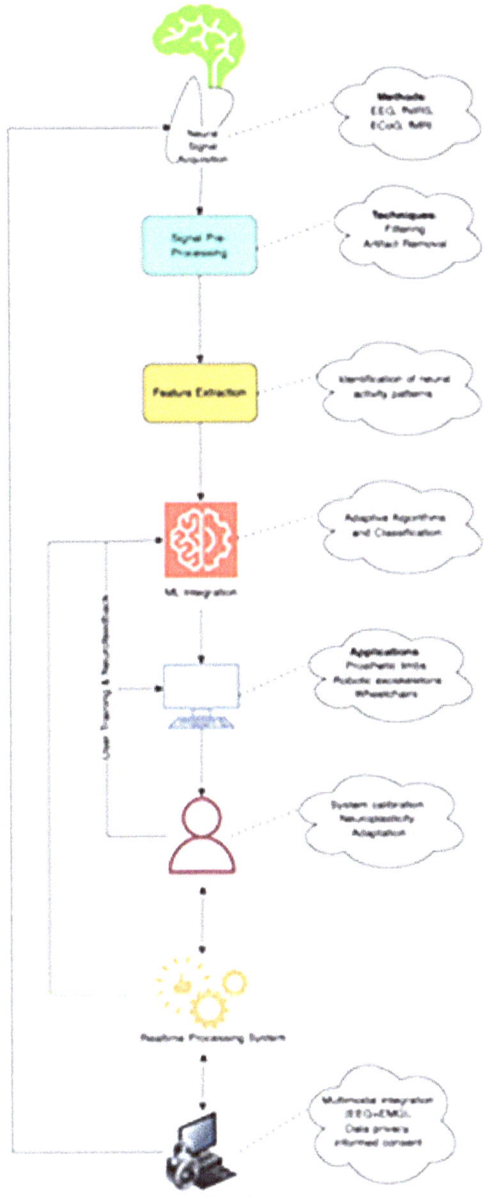

Real-time processing and adaptive systems also maximize response time and performance (Nicolas-Alonso & Gomez-Gil, 2012). Current systems also incorporate hybrid interfaces, fusing various sensing modalities such as EEG and EMG, and consider ethical issues, such as data privacy and security (Lebedev & Nicolelis,

2006). This systematic method makes it possible to utilize brain-controlled interfaces effectively in medical rehabilitation, assistive technology, and research.

5. TECHNICAL CHALLENGES

The convergence of Electroencephalography (EEG) with intelligent devices poses various technical challenges to the accuracy, reliability, and usability of the systems. As opposed to clinical EEG equipment that works in static environments, wearable EEG devices are required to operate in dynamic real-world environments, presenting challenges in the form of motion artifacts, wireless transmission delay, and power limitations. Moreover, EEG signals are feeble and extremely vulnerable to noise, necessitating sophisticated signal processing methods to glean useful information. The creation of small, user-friendly electrodes and effective algorithms for real-time processing adds to this complexity. Some of the most important technical challenges involved in using EEG-based smart devices are as shown in the following Figure 12 (mindmap) as well as Table 2:

Table 2. Ethical and Privacy Concerns

Issue	Ethical and Privacy Concern
Motion Artifacts and Signal Quality	• Wearable EEG devices experience issues with motion artifacts. These brain signals are sensitive to movement in the head and can be distorted when a participant moves their head. • Although head movements are typically controlled for, EEG signals may be contaminated with other signals from muscular contractions like jaw clenching, for example (Chaddad et al., 2023).
Wireless Transmission and Latency	• Another obstacle when biasing EEG software is related to latency and transmission errors introduced by wireless protocols such as Bluetooth. • For EEG-based applications, the measurement of EEG signals for real-time workflow applications (e.g., BCIs) becomes unreliable when the two-way transmission latency is longer than 200 ms (Frey et al., 2023).
Power Constraints and Miniaturization	• Another challenge is achieving the longest battery-life possible while keeping the size of the device to a minimum. Researchers are optimistic that these issues may be addressed in the future development of wearable EEG solutions with the development of RISC-V cores, and power optimized integrated circuits (ICs) (Frey et al., 2024).
Robust ML/AI for Noisy EEG	• Machine learning models that use noisy EEG data still produce excellent results, but it still requires sound preprocessing of raw EEG data and robust artificial intelligence strategies, like transfer learning, to help models achieve desirable levels of accuracy (Wang et al., 2023; Zhou et al., 2023).
Scalability in IoT Environments	• Most recently, for EEG to be used cohesively in conjunction with Internet of Things (IoT) platforms, standards must be developed, addressing various aspects of EEG in IoT, like data formats, protocols, and real-time data processing, such that the EEG data can be interoperable with the related IoT devices/platform (Beyrouthy et al., 2024).

Figure 12. Technical Challenges While Integrating EEG with Smart Devices

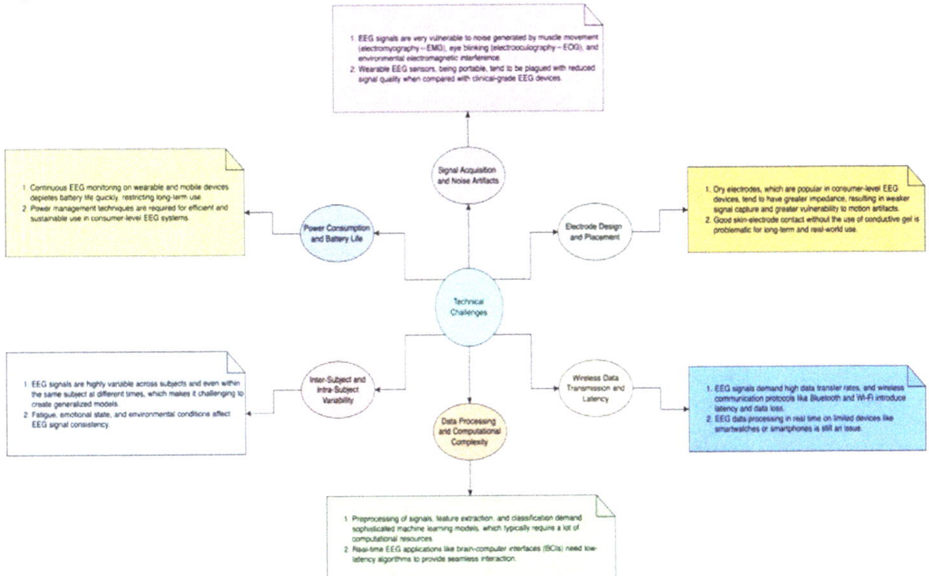

6. ETHICAL AND PRIVACY CONCERNS

With EEG technology increasingly being embedded in smart devices, ethical and privacy issues become the most important problems that need to be solved. In contrast to other biometric information, EEG signals reveal very intimate information about a person's cognitive state, emotions, and mental health, so they are extremely sensitive. The mass application of wearable EEG devices in consumer markets creates concerns regarding data protection, user control, and informed consent. Moreover, AI-based EEG analysis brings risks to bias, fairness, and misapplication. The regulatory landscape of EEG-based consumer technologies is poorly developed, thus causing legal and ethical ambiguity. This section addresses main ethical and privacy issues around EEG-smart device integration and underscores the imperative of strong policies for safeguarding users' rights. Look at the following Table 3 for better understanding of Ethical and Privacy concerns.

Table 3. Ethical and Privacy Concerns

Issue	Ethical and Privacy Concern
Data Privacy and Security	• EEG data contains private information, such as cognitive states or health-related information. Care is needed to properly encrypt and store it safely. Unauthorized access is a serious medical privacy concern (Neurorights Foundation, 2024).
Informed Consent and User Awareness	• Users must understand what they are sharing when they share their EEG data, including what the potential future use might be. Sharing cognitive data presents cognitive liberty issues, particularly if EEG data was used to make an important decision (Farahany, 2023; Buthut et al., 2024).
Bias and Fairness in AI-Based EEG Applications	• AI models used for processing EEG signals carry the prejudice of the training data. It would be useful to establish some interpretability frameworks, to ensure fair use of AI models applied to EEG signals, particularly in sensitive applications related to BCIs (Zhou et al., 2023).
Autonomy and Cognitive Freedom	• The absence of universal regulations governing EEG-based consumer products presents outcomes-based challenges (Polis, 2024). Emerging legal frameworks must accommodate ethical applications of EEG data and rights of users (Buthut et al., 2024).
Regulatory and Legal Challenges	• As an example, a vulnerable population would be one with cognitive impairments, and this population would require more protections regarding consent and data use. • Ethical guidelines around EEG use would ensure the vulnerable users are not exploited (Ferrell et al., 2025).

7. FUTURE DIRECTIONS

Recent technological developments in wearable EEG equipment have revolutionized the field of non-invasive brain monitoring in radical ways. These technologies permit the on-line recording of neural activity in real-life, naturalistic settings. Coupled with IoT and 5G networks, this provides the possibility of fluid, uninterrupted data transfer and remote observation. Advanced signal processing and machine learning techniques make it possible to provide more precise and resilient EEG analysis.

Miniaturized EEG sensors are improving user experience and facilitating popularization. The fusion of multi-modal data combining EEG with additional physiological signals holds great promise. Ethical, privacy, and regulatory issues grow more important with the increasing uptake of continuous monitoring of the brain. Adaptive technologies that can adapt neurofeedback as well as monitor cognitive state and tailor it are the focus of research. Advances hold the key to revolutionary health care, neurorehabilitation, and augmentation of cognition. Overall, the integration of EEG, IoT, and AI will transform the way we interact with technology and track brain health. Now, let us understand the following Table 4 and consider them as future views, by connecting them with Challenges as well as Ethical and Privacy Concerns:

Table 4. Future Directions

Future Direction	What should we do?	Connection with Challenges and Ethical/Privacy Concerns
Advancements in AI and ML for EEG Analysis	Create more advanced machine learning and deep learning algorithms that are capable of automatically extracting features from EEG signals that are pertinent to the situation and can adjust to subject variability. This would potentially facilitate real-time discrimination of cognitive and emotional states and enhance neurofeedback use (Lv et al., 2020).	***Technical:*** Enhances resilience against noise/artifacts and shortens calibration duration through the integration of transfer-learning and interpretable models (Wang et al., 2023; Zhou et al., 2023). Ethical: Integrated interpretability frameworks assist in identifying and reducing algorithmic bias and guarantee equitable, transparent decision-making (Zhou et al., 2023).
Integration with IoT and 5G Connectivity	Discuss the use of EEG sensors within IoT frameworks and utilize 5G networks to enable real-time, constant monitoring of brain activity on consumer smart devices. This combination can enable remote healthcare and lifestyle applications tailored to the individual (Beyrouthy et al., 2024).	***Technical:*** Tackles wireless transmission lags and scalability challenges through edge preprocessing (BioGAP) and robust 5G connections (Frey et al., 2023). ***Ethical:*** Requires robust protocols and privacy-protecting data management to ensure the safety of sensitive neural data during transit, adhering to IoT-focused encryption standards (Neurorights Foundation, 2024).
Miniaturization and Wearable Device Design	Focus on the evolution of small, low-energy, and cozy EEG sensors to integrate smoothly in the daily wearable such as headbands, earbuds, or smartwatches. Enhancement in electrode material and wireless architecture will be vital for increasing data quality and compliance by the users (Kaongoen et al., 2023; Frey et al., 2024).	***Technical:*** Mitigates motion artifacts and powering constraints by reducing sensor size and energy requirements (GAPses) (Frey et al., 2024). ***Ethical:*** More comfort and unobtrusiveness support informed consent and users autonomy, reducing coercion or "always-on" stigma (Farahany, 2023).
Enhanced Signal Processing and Artifact Reduction	Develop advanced signal processing methods to eliminate noise and artifacts from EEG data in practical situations. New adaptive filtering and artifact rejection strategies should be established for precise interpretation of data under varying conditions (Chaddad et al., 2023; Lv et al., 2020).	***Technical:*** Combats motion and muscle artifacts through advanced algorithms (Chaddad et al., 2023) while also improving signal-to-noise and reliability. ***Ethical:*** Reliable data promotes accurate assessment of cognitive states, reducing risk of unfair or harmful decisions based on corrupt signals.

continued on following page

Table 4. Continued

Future Direction	What should we do?	Connection with Challenges and Ethical/Privacy Concerns
Multi-Modal Data Fusion	Merge EEG signals with other body physiology signals (e.g., electrooculography, electromyography, or fNIRS) to construct multi-modal systems. Such systems would offer a more comprehensive view of the state of the user's cognition and physiology, thus broadening the range of applications in both consumer and healthcare markets.	***Technical:*** Improves feature space and robustness against failures of single modalities and ultimately improves accuracy in noisy environments. ***Ethical:*** Blending modalities can expose new personal data, which requires a more elaborate consent or governance framework to regulate multi-source privacy risks (Buthut et al., 2024).
Data Privacy, Security, and Ethical Frameworks	Talk to the ethical and privacy concerns with regards to persistent brain monitoring. Upcoming research ought to work on safe transmission of data and privacy-respecting algorithms, together with frameworks to govern the moral utilization of EEG data within consumer products (Neurorights Foundation, 2024; Buthut et al., 2024).	***Technical:*** Embeds security into each stage of the pipeline thereby minimizing the potential for data breach; protects wireless and cloud transmission. ***Ethical:*** Engages in direct action in relation to privacy/security and consent considerations: establishes a system in which users retain comprehensive controls in relation to the use of their data, an opt-in policy, and protections of "cognitive liberty" (Farahany, 2023).
Longitudinal and Real-World Validation Studies	Carry out large-scale, long-term studies in naturalistic environments to assess the robustness, reliability, and user acceptability of wearable EEG systems. Such studies will be instrumental for transferring laboratory breakthroughs into real-life uses and guiding regulatory standards (Markov et al., 2024; Murungi et al., 2023).	***Technical:*** Tests for performance across many different conditions, which helps to identify edge-case failures and iterates on hardware and software improvements. ***Ethical:*** Facilitates policy development by exposing real-world privacy, consent, and equity issues, which provides support for fair regulations (Polis, 2024).
Personalized Healthcare and Neurofeedback Applications	Broaden EEG-based applications into personalized medicine - such as neurofeedback for psychiatry, cognitive improvement, and early diagnosis of neurological conditions - by adapting systems to individual brain profiles and lifestyles (Murungi et al., 2023; Ferrell et al., 2025).	***Technical:*** Takes advantage of adaptive ML in order to address the variability of subjects, fostering improved accuracy and engagement. ***Ethical:*** Addresses equity and autonomy by ensuring that vulnerable populations receive a tailored consent process and ethically reviewed interventions, reducing the risk of exploitation (Ferrell et al., 2025).

8. CONCLUSION

8.1. Summary of Key Points

The convergence of EEG with smart devices represents a substantial transformation from conventional clinical uses to real-time, active monitoring systems. Improvements in wearable sensor technology, wireless transmission, and advanced signal processing have made possible continuous monitoring of cognitive and physiological conditions in real time (Casson, 2019; Debener et al., 2015). In addition, the integration of EEG with IoT platforms has extended its application to fields like mental health tracking, neurofeedback, and improved human–computer interaction, thus extending its scope and influence (Al-Fuqaha et al., 2015; Beyrouthy et al., 2024).

8.2. Final Thoughts on the Potential of EEG-Smart Device Integration

EEG-smart devices which utilize AI/ML feature extraction (Wang et al., 2023; Zhou et al., 2023) and 5G-IoT networks (Beyrouthy et al., 2024), are touted to provide effective real-time brain monitoring. Miniaturized devices—ear-EEG earbuds and smart-glasses with dry electrodes—provide extra comfort and quotidian nature of use (Kaongoen et al., 2023; Frey et al., 2024), which can assist the advancement of new therapeutic strategies and adaptive human–machine interfaces for mental-health, neurorehabilitation, and cognitive enhancement.

8.3. Importance of Addressing Challenges to Maximize the Benefits

To deliver on this promise, we need rigorous artifact reduction and on-edge processing to maintain signal integrity and compress battery life when used in dynamic environments (Chaddad et al., 2023; Frey et al., 2023). In addition, we need strong privacy protections - such as encryption and differential privacy, alongside a clear framework for how consent must be determined for different technologies (Neurorights Foundation, 2024; Farahany, 2023) - to preserve neural data and cognitive liberty, as well as more clear legal frameworks (Polis, 2024) and ethics codes (Buthut et al., 2024) which will protect the rights of processors and ensure equitable access for everyone.

REFERENCES

Adao Martins, N. R., Annaheim, S., Spengler, C. M., & Rossi, R. M. (2021). Fatigue Monitoring through Wearables: A state-of-the-art review. *Frontiers in Physiology*, *12*, 790292. DOI: 10.3389/fphys.2021.790292 PMID: 34975541

Al-Fuqaha, A., Guizani, M., Mohammadi, M., Aledhari, M., & Ayyash, M. (2015). Internet of things: A survey on enabling technologies, protocols, and applications. *IEEE Communications Surveys and Tutorials*, *17*(4), 2347–2376. DOI: 10.1109/COMST.2015.2444095

Andrews, J. G., Buzzi, S., Choi, W., Hanly, S. V., Lozano, A., Soong, A. C. K., & Zhang, J. C. (2014). What will 5G be? *IEEE Journal on Selected Areas in Communications*, *32*(6), 1065–1082. DOI: 10.1109/JSAC.2014.2328098

Arns, M., Heinrich, H., & Strehl, U. (2014). Evaluation of Neurofeedback in ADHD: The Long and Winding Road. *Biological Psychology*, *95*, 108–115. DOI: 10.1016/j.biopsycho.2013.11.013 PMID: 24321363

Atzori, L., Iera, A., & Morabito, G. (2010). The Internet of Things: A Survey. *Computer Networks*, *54*(15), 2787–2805. DOI: 10.1016/j.comnet.2010.05.010

Babiloni, C., Pascarelli, M. T., Lizio, R., Noce, G., Lopez, S., Rizzo, M., Ferri, R., Soricelli, A., Nobili, F., Arnaldi, D., Famà, F., Orzi, F., Buttinelli, C., Giubilei, F., Salvetti, M., Cipollini, V., Bonanni, L., Franciotti, R., Onofrj, M., & Del Percio, C. (2020). Abnormal Cortical Neural Synchronization Mechanisms in Quiet Wakefulness are related to Motor Deficits, Cognitive Symptoms, and Visual Hallucinations in Parkinson's Disease Patients: An Electroencephalographic Study. *Neurobiology of Aging*, *91*, 88–111. DOI: 10.1016/j.neurobiolaging.2020.02.029 PMID: 32234263

Berger, H. (1929). Über das Elektrenkephalogramm des Menschen. *Archiv für Psychiatrie und Nervenkrankheiten*, *87*(1), 527–570. DOI: 10.1007/BF01797193

Berry, R. B., Brooks, R., Gamaldo, C., Harding, S. M., Lloyd, R. M., Quan, S. F., Troester, M. T., & Vaughn, B. V. (2020). AASM Scoring Manual Updates for 2017 (Version 2.4). *Journal of Clinical Sleep Medicine : JCSM : Official Publication of the American Academy of Sleep Medicine*, *13*(5), 665–666. DOI: 10.5664/jcsm.6576 PMID: 28416048

Beyrouthy, T., Mostafa, N., Roshdy, A., Karar, A. S., & Alkork, S. (2024). Review of EEG-based Biometrics in 5G-IoT: Current Trends and Future Prospects. *Applied Sciences (Basel, Switzerland)*, *14*(2), 534. DOI: 10.3390/app14020534

Bjerre-Nielsen, A., Minor, K., Sapieżyński, P., Lehmann, S., & Lassen, D. D. (2020). Inferring Transportation Mode from Smartphone Sensors: Evaluating the potential of Wi-Fi and Bluetooth. *PLoS One*, *15*(7), e0234003. DOI: 10.1371/journal.pone.0234003 PMID: 32614842

Brown, E. N., Purdon, P. L., & Van Dort, C. J. (2018). General Anesthesia and Altered States of Arousal: A Systems Neuroscience Analysis. *Annual Review of Neuroscience*, *34*(1), 601–628. https://www.annualreviews.org/content/journals/10.1146/annurev-neuro-060909-153200. DOI: 10.1146/annurev-neuro-060909-153200 PMID: 21513454

Buthut, M., Starke, G., Akmazoglu, T. B., Colucci, A., Vermehren, M., van Beinum, A., Bublitz, C., Chandler, J., Ienca, M., & Soekadar, S. R. (2024). HYBRIDMINDS-summary and outlook of the 2023 international conference on the ethics and regulation of intelligent neuroprostheses. *Frontiers in Human Neuroscience*, *18*, 1489307. DOI: 10.3389/fnhum.2024.1489307 PMID: 39483192

Casson, A. J. (2019). Wearable EEG and beyond. *Biomedical Engineering Letters*, *9*(1), 53–71. DOI: 10.1007/s13534-018-00093-6 PMID: 30956880

Casson, A. J., Yates, D. C., Smith, S. J. M., Duncan, J. S., & Rodriguez-Villegas, E. (2010). Wearable electroencephalography. *IEEE Engineering in Medicine and Biology Magazine*, *29*(3), 44–56. DOI: 10.1109/MEMB.2010.936545 PMID: 20659857

Chaddad, A., Wu, Y., Kateb, R., & Bouridane, A. (2023). Electroencephalography Signal Processing: A Comprehensive Review and Analysis of Methods and Techniques. *Sensors (Basel)*, *23*(14), 6434. DOI: 10.3390/s23146434 PMID: 37514728

Cicerone, K. D., Langenbahn, D. M., Braden, C., Malec, J. F., Kalmar, K., Fraas, M., Felicetti, T., Laatsch, L., Harley, J. P., Bergquist, T., Azulay, J., Cantor, J., & Ashman, T. (2011). Evidence-based Cognitive Rehabilitation: Updated Review of the Literature from 2003 through 2008. *Archives of Physical Medicine and Rehabilitation*, *92*(4), 519–530. DOI: 10.1016/j.apmr.2010.11.015 PMID: 21440699

Coben, R., Mohammad-Rezazadeh, I., & Cannon, R. L. (2014). Using Quantitative and Analytic EEG Methods in the Understanding of Connectivity in Autism Spectrum Disorders: A Theory of Mixed over-and under-connectivity. *Frontiers in Human Neuroscience*, *8*, 45. https://www.frontiersin.org/journals/human-neuroscience/articles/10.3389/fnhum.2014.00045/full. DOI: 10.3389/fnhum.2014.00045 PMID: 24616679

Cuijpers, P., Karyotaki, E., Weitz, E., Andersson, G., Hollon, S. D., & van Straten, A. (2014). The Effects of Psychotherapies for Major Depression in Adults on Remission, Recovery and Improvement: A Meta-analysis. *Journal of Affective Disorders, 159*, 118–126. DOI: 10.1016/j.jad.2014.02.026 PMID: 24679399

Debener, S., Emkes, R., De Vos, M., & Bleichner, M. (2015). Unobtrusive Ambulatory EEG using a Smartphone and Flexible Printed Electrodes around the Ear. *Scientific Reports, 5*(1), 16743. DOI: 10.1038/srep16743 PMID: 26572314

Di Flumeri, G., Aricò, P., Borghini, G., Sciaraffa, N., Babiloni, F., Pozzi, S., Vignali, V., Lantieri, C., Bichicchi, A., Simone, A., & Babiloni, F. (2018). EEG-based Mental Workload Neurometric to Evaluate the Impact of Different Traffic and Road Conditions in Real Driving Settings. *Frontiers in Neuroscience, 12*, 507. DOI: 10.3389/fnhum.2018.00509 PMID: 30618686

Diamond, A., & Lee, K. (2011). Interventions shown to Aid Executive Function Development in Children 4 to 12 years old. *Science, 333*(6045), 959–964. DOI: 10.1126/science.1204529 PMID: 21852486

Farahany, N. A. (2023). Cognitive liberty is the human right we need to talk about. *Time*. https://time.com/6289229/cognitive-liberty-human-right/

Ferrell, M. L., Beatty, A., & Dubljevic, V. (2025). The Ethics of Neuromarketing: A Rapid Review. *Neuroethics, 18*(1), 19. Advance online publication. DOI: 10.1007/s12152-025-09591-8

Ferro, E., & Potorti, F. (2005). Bluetooth and IEEE 802.11 (Wi-Fi) wireless protocols: A survey and a comparison. *IEEE Wireless Communications, 12*(1), 12–26. DOI: 10.1109/MWC.2005.1404569

Finnigan, S., & van Putten, M. J. (2013). EEG in Ischaemic Stroke: Quantitative EEG can Uniquely Inform (sub-)acute Prognoses and Clinical Management. *Clinical Neurophysiology, 124*(1), 10–19. DOI: 10.1016/j.clinph.2012.07.003 PMID: 22858178

Firth, J., Torous, J., Nicholas, J., Carney, R., Pratap, A., Rosenbaum, S., & Sarris, J. (2017). The Efficacy of Smartphone-based Mental Health Interventions for Depressive Symptoms: A Meta-analysis of Randomized Controlled Trials. *Journal of Affective Disorders, 218*, 15–22. DOI: 10.1016/j.jad.2017.04.046 PMID: 28456072

Frey, S., Guermandi, M., Benatti, S., Kartsch, V., Cossettini, A., & Benini, L. (2023). BioGAP: A 10-Core FP-capable ultra-low power IoT processor for wearable biosignal processing. *arXiv*. https://arxiv.org/abs/2307.01619

Frey, S., Lucchini, M. A., Kartsch, V., Ingolfsson, T. M., Bernardi, A. H., Segessenmann, M., Osieleniec, J., Benatti, S., Benini, L., & Cossettini, A. (2024). GAPses: Versatile Smart Glasses for comfortable and fully-dry Acquisition and Parallel Ultra-Low-Power Processing of EEG and EOG. *arXiv*. https://doi.org//arXiv.2406.07903DOI: 10.48550

Gao, X., Ma, K., Yang, H., Wang, K., Fu, B., Zhu, Y., She, X., & Cui, B. (2022). A Rapid, Non-invasive Method for Fatigue Detection based on Voice Information. *Frontiers in Cell and Developmental Biology*, *10*, 994001. DOI: 10.3389/fcell.2022.994001 PMID: 36176279

Gartlehner, G., Hansen, R. A., Morgan, L. C., Thaler, K., Lux, L., Van Noord, M., Mager, U., Thieda, P., Gaynes, B. N., Wilkins, T., Strobelberger, M., Lloyd, S., Reichenpfader, U., & Lohr, K. N. (2011). Comparative Benefits and Harms of Second-Generation Antidepressants for Treating Major Depressive Disorder: An Updated Meta-analysis. *Annals of Internal Medicine*, *155*(11), 772–785. DOI: 10.7326/0003-4819-155-11-201112060-00009 PMID: 22147715

Goodfellow, I., Pouget-Abadie, J., Mirza, M., Xu, B., Warde-Farley, D., Ozair, S., Courville, A., & Bengio, Y. (2014). Generative adversarial nets. *Advances in Neural Information Processing Systems*, *27*. Advance online publication. DOI: 10.48550/arXiv.1406.2661

Gubbi, J., Buyya, R., Marusic, S., & Palaniswami, M. (2013). Internet of things (IoT): A Vision, Architectural Elements, and Future Directions. *Future Generation Computer Systems*, *29*(7), 1645–1660. DOI: 10.1016/j.future.2013.01.010

Herrmann, C. S., Strüber, D., Helfrich, R. F., & Engel, A. K. (2016). EEG Oscillations: From Correlation to Causality. *International Journal of Psychophysiology*, *103*, 12–21. DOI: 10.1016/j.ijpsycho.2015.02.003 PMID: 25659527

Hofmann, S. G., Asnaani, A., Vonk, I. J., Sawyer, A. T., & Fang, A. (2012). The Efficacy of Cognitive Behavioral Therapy: A Review of Meta-analyses. *Cognitive Therapy and Research*, *36*(5), 427–440. DOI: 10.1007/s10608-012-9476-1 PMID: 23459093

Hofmann, S. G., Sawyer, A. T., Witt, A. A., & Oh, D. (2010). The Effect of Mindfulness-based Therapy on Anxiety and Depression: A Meta-Analytic Review. *Journal of Consulting and Clinical Psychology*, *78*(2), 169–183. DOI: 10.1037/a0018555 PMID: 20350028

Huang, N. E., Shen, Z., Long, S. R., Wu, M. C., Shih, H. H., Zheng, Q., Yen, N. C., Tung, C. C., & Liu, H. H. (1998). The empirical mode decomposition and the Hilbert spectrum for nonlinear and non-stationary time series analysis. *Proceedings of the Royal Society of London. Series A: Mathematical, Physical and Engineering Sciences, 454*(1971), 903–995. https://doi.org/DOI: 10.1098/rspa.1998.0193

Idris, Z., Muzaimi, M., Ghani, R., Idris, B., Kandasamy, R., & Abdullah, J. (2014). Principles, Anatomical Origin and Applications of Brainwaves: A Review, Our Experience and Hypothesis Related to Microgravity and the Question on Soul. *Journal of Biomedical Science and Engineering*, *7*(8), 435–445. DOI: 10.4236/jbise.2014.78046

Iqbal, T., Redon-Lurbe, P., Simpkin, A. J., Elahi, A., Ganly, S., Wijns, W., & Shahzad, A. (2021). A Sensitivity Analysis of Biophysiological Responses of Stress for Wearable Sensors in Connected Health. *IEEE Access : Practical Innovations, Open Solutions*, *9*, 93567–93579. DOI: 10.1109/ACCESS.2021.3082423

Islam, S. R., Kwak, D., Kabir, M. H., Hossain, M., & Kwak, K. S. (2015). The internet of things for health care: A comprehensive survey. *IEEE Access : Practical Innovations, Open Solutions*, *3*, 678–708. DOI: 10.1109/ACCESS.2015.2437951

Kaongoen, N., Choi, J., Woo Choi, J., Kwon, H., Hwang, C., Hwang, G., Kim, B. H., & Jo, S. (2023). The future of wearable EEG: A review of ear-EEG technology and its applications. *Journal of Neural Engineering*, *20*(5), 051002. Advance online publication. DOI: 10.1088/1741-2552/acfcda PMID: 37748474

Kirschbaum, C., Pirke, K. M., & Hellhammer, D. H. (1993). The "Trier Social Stress Test" - A Tool for Investigating *Psychobiological Stress Responses in a Laboratory setting. Neuropsychobiology*, *28*(1–2), 76–81. DOI: 10.1159/000119004 PMID: 8255414

Klingberg, T. (2010). Training and Plasticity of Working Memory. *Trends in Cognitive Sciences*, *14*(7), 317–324. DOI: 10.1016/j.tics.2010.05.002 PMID: 20630350

Lebedev, M. A., & Nicolelis, M. A. L. (2006). Brain–machine interfaces: Past, Present and Future. *Trends in Neurosciences*, *29*(9), 536–546. DOI: 10.1016/j.tins.2006.07.004 PMID: 16859758

LeCun, Y., Bengio, Y., & Hinton, G. (2015). Deep Learning. *Nature*, *521*(7553), 436–444. DOI: 10.1038/nature14539 PMID: 26017442

Lopez-Larraz, E., Escolano, C., Robledo-Menéndez, A., Morlas, L., Alda, A., & Minguez, J. (2023). A Garment that Measures Brain Activity: Proof of Concept of an EEG Sensor Layer Fully Implemented with Smart Textiles. *Frontiers in Human Neuroscience*, *17*, 1135153. DOI: 10.3389/fnhum.2023.1135153 PMID: 37305362

Lotte, F., Bougrain, L., Cichocki, A., Clerc, M., Congedo, M., Rakotomamonjy, A., & Yger, F. (2018). A Review of Classification Algorithms for EEG-based Brain-Computer Interfaces: A 10-year Update. *Journal of Neural Engineering*, *15*(3), 031005. DOI: 10.1088/1741-2552/aab2f2 PMID: 29488902

Luck, S. J. (2014). *An Introduction to the event-related Potential Technique* (2nd ed.). MIT Press., https://mitpress.mit.edu/9780262525855/an-introduction-to-the-event-related-potential-technique/

Lustig, M., Donoho, D., & Pauly, J. M. (2007). Sparse MRI: The application of compressed sensing for rapid MR imaging. *Magnetic Resonance in Medicine*, *58*(6), 1182–1195. DOI: 10.1002/mrm.21391 PMID: 17969013

Luxton, D. D., McCann, R. A., Bush, N. E., Mishkind, M. C., & Reger, G. M. (2011). mHealth for Mental Health: Integrating Smartphone Technology in Behavioral Healthcare. *Professional Psychology, Research and Practice*, *42*(6), 505–512. DOI: 10.1037/a0024485

Mallat, S. G., & Zhang, Z. (1993). Matching pursuits with time-frequency dictionaries. *IEEE Transactions on Signal Processing*, *41*(12), 3397–3415. DOI: 10.1109/78.258082

Markov, K., Elgendi, M. & Menon, C. EEG-based headset sleep wearable devices. *npj Biosensing 1, 12* (2024). https://doi.org/DOI: 10.1038/s44328-024-00013-y

Marzbani, H., Marateb, H. R., & Mansourian, M. (2016). Methodological note: Neurofeedback: A Comprehensive Review on System Design, Methodology and Clinical Applications. *Basic and Clinical Neuroscience*, *7*(2), 143–148. DOI: 10.15412/J.BCN.03070208 PMID: 27303609

Mittelstadt, B. D., Allo, P., Taddeo, M., Wachter, S., & Floridi, L. (2016). The ethics of algorithms: Mapping the debate. *Big Data & Society*, *3*(2), 2053951716679679. Advance online publication. DOI: 10.1177/2053951716679679

Murungi, N., Pham, M., Dai, X., Haverford, H., Qu, U., & Dai, C. (2023). Empowering Computer Science Students in Electroencephalography (EEG) Analysis: A Review of Machine Learning Algorithms for EEG Datasets. https://kdd.org/kdd2023/wp-content/uploads/2023/08/murungi2023trends.pdf

Neurorights Foundation. (2024). Safeguarding brain data: assessing the privacy practices of consumer neurotechnology companies. https://perseus-strategies.com/wp-content/uploads/2024/04/FINAL_Consumer_Neurotechnology_Report_Neurorights_Foundation_April-1.pdf

Nicolas-Alonso, L. F., & Gomez-Gil, J. (2012). Brain Computer Interfaces, A Review. *Sensors (Basel)*, *12*(2), 1211–1279. DOI: 10.3390/s120201211 PMID: 22438708

Niedermeyer, E., & da Silva, F. L. (2005). *Electroencephalography: Basic Principles, Clinical Applications, and Related Fields* (5th ed.). Lippincott Williams & Wilkins., https://www.nlist.inflibnet.ac.in/search/Record/EBC3418225

Niedermeyer, E., & da Silva, F. L. (2018). *Electroencephalography: Basic Principles, Clinical Applications, and Related Fields* (7th ed.). Lippincott Williams & Wilkins., DOI: 10.1093/med/9780190228484.001.0001

Niso, G., Romero, E., Moreau, J. T., Araujo, A., & Krol, L. R. (2023). Wireless EEG: A Survey of Systems and Studies. *NeuroImage*, *269*, 119774. DOI: 10.1016/j.neuroimage.2022.119774 PMID: 36566924

Polis, J. (2024). Protect Privacy of Biological Data Act. *Colorado Revised Statutes.* https://www.businessinsider.com/colorado-signs-bill-protect-privacy-rights-neurotechnology-neuralink-musk-2024-4

Preskill, J. (2018). Quantum Computing in the NISQ Era and Beyond. *Quantum : the Open Journal for Quantum Science*, *2*, 79. DOI: 10.22331/q-2018-08-06-79

Rechtschaffen, A., & Kales, A. (1968). A manual of Standardized Terminology, Techniques and Scoring System for Sleep Stages of Human Subjects. *U.S. National Institute of Neurological Diseases and Blindness.* https://archive.org/details/RKManual

Roach, B. J., & Mathalon, D. H. (2008). Event-related EEG Time-Frequency Analysis: An Overview of Measures and an Analysis of Early Gamma Band Phase Locking in Schizophrenia. *Schizophrenia Bulletin*, *34*(5), 907–926. DOI: 10.1093/schbul/sbn093 PMID: 18684772

Sanei, S., & Chambers, J. A. (2007). *EEG Signal Processing*. Wiley., DOI: 10.1002/9780470511923

Satyanarayanan, M. (2017). The Emergence of Edge Computing. *Computer*, *50*(1), 30–39. DOI: 10.1109/MC.2017.9

Schiff, N. D. (2015). Cognitive Motor Dissociation following Severe Brain Injuries. *JAMA Neurology*, *72*(12), 1413–1415. DOI: 10.1001/jamaneurol.2015.2899 PMID: 26502348

Schuch, F. B., Vancampfort, D., Firth, J., Rosenbaum, S., Ward, P. B., Silva, E. S., Hallgren, M., Ponce De Leon, A., Dunn, A. L., Deslandes, A. C., Fleck, M. P., Carvalho, A. F., & Stubbs, B. (2018). Physical Activity and Incident Depression: A Meta-Analysis of Prospective Cohort Studies. *The American Journal of Psychiatry*, *175*(7), 631–648. DOI: 10.1176/appi.ajp.2018.17111194 PMID: 29690792

Shi, W., Cao, J., Zhang, Q., Li, Y., & Xu, L. (2016). Edge computing: Vision and challenges. *IEEE Internet of Things Journal*, *3*(5), 637–646. DOI: 10.1109/JIOT.2016.2579198

Sikander, G., & Anwar, S. (2019). Driver Fatigue Detection Systems: A review. *IEEE Transactions on Intelligent Transportation Systems*, *20*(6), 2339–2352. DOI: 10.1109/TITS.2018.2868499

Stopczynski, A., Stahlhut, C., Larsen, J. E., Petersen, M. K., & Hansen, L. K. (2013). The Smartphone Brain Scanner: A Mobile Real-time Neuroimaging System. *arXiv*. https://doi.org//arXiv.1304.0357DOI: 10.48550

Teplan, M. (2002). Fundamentals of EEG Measurement. *Measurement Science Review*, *2*(2), 1–11. https://www.researchgate.net/publication/228599963_Fundamental_of_EEG_Measurement e Videman, M., Tokariev, A., Stjerna, S., Roivainen, R., Gaily, E., & Vanhatalo, S. (2016). Effects of Prenatal Antiepileptic Drug Exposure on Newborn Brain Activity. *Epilepsia, 57*(4), 608–619. https://doi.org/DOI: 10.1111/epi.13281

Wang, Y., Nahon, R., Tartaglione, E., Mozharovskyi, P., & Nguyen, V.-T. (2023). Optimized preprocessing and Tiny ML for attention state classification. *arXiv*. https://arxiv.org/abs/2303.11371 DOI: 10.1109/SSP53291.2023.10207930

Warden, P., & Situnayake, D. (2019). TinyML: Machine learning with TensorFlow Lite on Arduino and ultra-low-power microcontrollers. *O'Reilly Media*. https://www.oreilly.com/library/view/tinyml/9781492052036/

Whitmore, A., Agarwal, A., & Xu, L. D. (2015). The Internet of Things - A Survey of Topics and Trends. *Information Systems Frontiers*, *17*(2), 261–274. DOI: 10.1007/s10796-014-9489-2

Wolpaw, J. R., Birbaumer, N., McFarland, D. J., Pfurtscheller, G., & Vaughan, T. M. (2002). Brain-Computer Interfaces for Communication and Control. *Clinical Neurophysiology*, *113*(6), 767–791. DOI: 10.1016/S1388-2457(02)00057-3 PMID: 12048038

Yuste, R., Goering, S., Arcas, B. A. Y., Bi, G., Carmena, J. M., Carter, A., Fins, J. J., Friesen, P., Gallant, J., Huggins, J. E., Illes, J., Kellmeyer, P., Klein, E., Marblestone, A., Mitchell, C., Parens, E., Pham, M., Rubel, A., Sadato, N., & Wolpaw, J. (2017). Four ethical priorities for neurotechnologies and AI. *Nature*, *551*(7679), 159–163. DOI: 10.1038/551159a PMID: 29120438

Zander, T. O., & Kothe, C. (2011). Towards Passive Brain-Computer Interfaces: Applying Brain–Computer Interface Technology to Human–Machine Systems in General. *Journal of Neural Engineering*, *8*(2), 025005. DOI: 10.1088/1741-2560/8/2/025005 PMID: 21436512

Zhou, X., Liu, C., Wang, Z., Zhai, L., Jia, Z., Guan, C., & Liu, Y. (2023). Interpretable and robust AI in EEG systems: a survey. *arXiv*. https://arxiv.org/abs/2304.10755

Ziegeldorf, J. H., Morchon, O. G., & Wehrle, K. (2014). Privacy in the internet of things: Threats and challenges. *Security and Communication Networks*, *7*(12), 2728–2742. DOI: 10.1002/sec.795

Chapter 5
Neural Network:
Transforming the Diagnosis and Treatment of Neurological Diseases

S. Ida Evangeline
https://orcid.org/0000-0003-2997-7897
Government College of Engineering, Tirunelveli, India

ABSTRACT

The accelerating global prevalence of neurological diseases such as Alzheimer's, Parkinson's, epilepsy, stroke, and multiple sclerosis has created an urgent demand for advanced technologies that can improve diagnostic precision, treatment personalization, and long-term patient outcomes. This chapter explores the transformative role of neural networks—computational systems inspired by the structure and function of the human brain—in revolutionizing the diagnosis, treatment, and management of neurological disorders. Beginning with foundational principles in deep learning, including key architectures like convolutional neural networks, recurrent neural networks, and long short-term memory networks, the chapter outlines how these models process complex, high-dimensional neurological data. Practical applications are examined across neuroimaging analysis, signal interpretation, and brain-computer interface systems, showcasing their ability to detect early disease markers, predict therapeutic responses, and support neurorehabilitation.

1. INTRODUCTION

Neurological diseases represent one of the most pressing health challenges of the 21st century, with their global burden increasing at an alarming and unprecedented

DOI: 10.4018/979-8-3373-2706-8.ch005

rate. Disorders such as Alzheimer's disease, Parkinson's disease, epilepsy, stroke, and multiple sclerosis not only account for significant mortality and morbidity but also exert profound psychological, social, and economic tolls on patients, families, and healthcare systems alike. These conditions are frequently chronic, progressive, and incurable, often requiring long-term care and continuous monitoring (Dias-Carvalho et al. 2024). According to the World Health Organization, neurological disorders are now the leading cause of disability-adjusted life years and the second leading cause of death globally, reflecting the sheer scale and complexity of the problem. In addition, the worldwide growing life expectancy and aging population will contribute to this burden in the coming decades, which further emphasizes the need for development of more precise, scalable and proactive healthcare interventions (Oladapo et al., 2024).

Traditional diagnostic tools and therapeutic models, while invaluable, often fall short in detecting early disease stages, tailoring treatment plans to individual needs, or adapting to the dynamic nature of disease progression. These limitations have catalyzed a shift toward more data-driven, technology-enhanced approaches (Torri et al., 2024). In recent years, the healthcare sector has begun integrating advanced computational tools, particularly those powered by artificial intelligence, to address these gaps and elevate the standard of care. Neural networks—computational systems modeled after the structure and function of the human brain—are among the most promising of these tools. However, neural networks can learn very complex patterns from extremely large and diverse datasets and make highly accurate predictions, catch small anomalies and adapt to new data in ways a regular algorithm cannot (Tsiara et al. 2025).

Their application in neurology has been especially transformative, as the field inherently involves large volumes of complex, multimodal data, including neuroimaging, electrophysiological recordings, clinical narratives, genetic information, and behavioral assessments. Neural networks are uniquely equipped to process this data with high dimensionality and variability, offering new possibilities for early detection of disease, personalized treatment optimization, and continuous patient monitoring (Liao et al. 2024). By analyzing neuroimaging scans, signals, and other data sources, these models can identify disease signatures that precede clinical symptoms, monitor treatment efficacy over time, and predict future disease trajectories with impressive precision. In addition, neural networks enable the creation of intelligent clinical decision support systems, brain computer interfaces, patient specific therapeutic strategies, and improve neurological care on an individualized and responsive basis (Mahadevan et al. 2024).

This chapter aims to provide a comprehensive overview of the transformative role of neural networks in the diagnosis, treatment, and management of neurological diseases. It begins by establishing the foundational concepts and architectures underpinning neural networks and deep learning, then moves into practical applications in neuroimaging, electrophysiological signal analysis, and neurorehabilitation. The discussion further explores ethical and technical challenges—including data privacy, explainability, and regulatory oversight—and highlights current solutions and innovations addressing these concerns. The chapter demonstrates the tangible effect of these technologies in clinical neurology through case studies and real world examples and looks forward to consider future directions, such as next generation AI, quantum computing, and the fusion of neural networks with genomics. This chapter aims to synthesize theoretical foundations with applied insights to empower researchers, clinicians and healthcare innovators with knowledge and tools to fully realize the potential of AI applications in neurology, thus laying the groundwork for a smarter, more predictive and patient centric approach to neurological disease management.

2. FOUNDATIONS OF NEURAL NETWORKS AND DEEP LEARNING

At the heart of artificial intelligence applications in neurology lie neural networks—sophisticated computational models loosely inspired by the structure and function of the human brain. These systems emulate the way biological neurons communicate through synapses by using layers of interconnected artificial "neurons" or nodes, each responsible for processing a portion of the input data (Sajid et al. 2024). A neural network typically consists of an input layer, one or more hidden layers, and an output layer. In a process known as forward propagation, input data is transformed through weighted connections and non linear activation functions to capture complex relationships. Backpropagation is a feedback process that helps the network learn by minimizing the difference between actual and predicted outcomes through adjusting the weights of connections through the network, using optimization techniques such as stochastic gradient descent. Neural networks go through an iterative learning process to form an internal representation of the data and improve the capacity to learn patterns, make predictions, and generalize to unseen examples (Zhao et al. 2024).

As neural networks advanced, deep learning emerged as a prominent subfield characterized by deeper architectures—networks with many hidden layers—capable of modeling intricate hierarchical relationships in high-dimensional data. This paradigm shift has enabled the analysis of vast and complex neurological datasets that were previously intractable using conventional statistical methods. In the deep learning ecosystem, specific architectures have been developed to solve for certain specific data modalities. For example, Convolutional Neural Networks (CNNs) are designed for spatial data processing and are very good in processing medical images. CNNs can automatically learn to identify important features in MRI, CT, and PET scans via layered convolutional operations, pooling, and activation functions, including brain atrophy, white matter lesions, and abnormal tissue density, which are important for diagnosing neurodegenerative and cerebrovascular diseases (Bayoudh, 2024).

For sequential data such as time-series recordings from electroencephalography (EEG), Recurrent Neural Networks (RNNs) are more appropriate due to their ability to retain temporal context through feedback connections (Al-Quraishi et al. 2024). However, standard RNNs often struggle with long-term dependencies due to issues like vanishing gradients. Long Short-Term Memory (LSTM) networks were developed to address this, which have memory cells and gating mechanisms that enable learning and retention of long term information. In particular, LSTMs are very powerful in learning temporal dynamics in neurological signals, and have been successfully used for seizure detection, sleep stage classification, and monitoring of fluctuations in motor symptoms in disorders such as Parkinson's disease (Wang et al. 2024).

Despite their potential, training neural networks on neurological data presents considerable challenges. Neurological datasets are often complex and heterogeneous, encompassing 3D volumetric images, electrophysiological waveforms, behavioral metrics, and even genetic data. These datasets may also contain noise, missing values, and inter-subject variability, all of which complicate model training. Data preprocessing steps including normalization, artifact removal, dimensionality reduction, and data augmentation are needed to prepare the data before analysis. Furthermore, most medical datasets are small because of privacy issues and the high cost of data collection and annotation. To achieve this, transfer learning methods (Spolaôr et al. 2024) such as models pretrained on large datasets that are then fine tuned for specific neurological tasks are used and regularization strategies to avoid over fitting are employed.

Moreover, these models are not interpretable and robust, which is still a significant technical challenge. When the decisions impact the critical diagnostic or therapeutic pathways, clinical applications require not only the high accuracy but also the transparency and explainability. With the design of neural networks becoming more complex—using attention mechanisms, multi-modal data fusion, and biologically inspired architectures—the ability to process the multi-faceted nature of neurological data gets better, creating the space for even better, more adaptive and impactful AI driven solutions in neurology (Khalil et al. 2024).

3. NEURAL NETWORKS IN NEUROLOGICAL DIAGNOSTICS

Neural networks, particularly deep learning models, are rapidly transforming neurological diagnostics by providing tools that enhance precision, speed, and consistency in clinical evaluations. CNNs have proven especially impactful in the domain of neuroimaging, where they automate the interpretation of brain scans such as magnetic resonance imaging (MRI), computed tomography, and positron emission tomography. One of these models, for instance, uses layers of convolutional filters to hierarchically extract features from raw image data and identify subtle structural abnormalities (such as hippocampal atrophy, white matter hyperintensities, microbleeds, or cortical thinning) that may even escape the attention of experienced radiologists (Dayarathna et al 2024). For example, CNNs have achieved remarkable accuracy in classifying between healthy aging, mild cognitive impairment (MCI) and various stages of dementia in Alzheimer's disease. However, their performance often outperforms traditional volumetric analysis tools in detecting spatial and textural patterns of disease progression at earlier stages (El-Assy et al. 2024).

Similar advances are evident in the diagnosis of Parkinson's disease and multiple sclerosis. In Parkinson's, CNNs can detect dopaminergic deficits and changes in basal ganglia structures via diffusion tensor imaging and functional MRI (fMRI), while in MS, these models are used to identify demyelinating lesions and track lesion load over time with high fidelity. This offers the capability to accelerate diagnostic process, and provide longitudinal monitoring and response assessment, which are key for chronic neurological conditions. Moreover, CNNs have been generalized to multimodal data fusion, combining imaging with clinical and genetic data to provide a more comprehensive and accurate diagnostic conclusion (Meng et al. 2024).

Beyond structural and functional imaging, sequential data such as EEG recordings are effectively analyzed using RNNs and their more sophisticated variant, LSTM networks. These models excel at learning from temporal sequences, making them ideal for capturing the dynamic nature of brain activity (Fan et al. 2024). LSTMs have shown high sensitivity and specificity in detecting preictal states (brain activity patterns that occur before a seizure) in epilepsy care and thus can be used to develop seizure prediction systems that can warn the patient or initiate protective interventions (Narayana & Kodali, 2025). LSTMs are also used in sleep studies for epilepsy, to classify sleep stages and to detect sleep disorders like insomnia and sleep apnea by analyzing rhythmic EEG patterns (He et al. 2024). In addition, these models are being extended to neuropsychiatric conditions such as ADHD and depression where temporal anomalies in EEG or other time series physiological signals can be used to infer diagnostic biomarkers (Saurabh & Gupta, 2024).

Accuracy is not all that neural networks have to offer for clinical value. In addition, these models also help in workflow optimization by automating routine tasks, triaging high risk cases and aiding in decision makings, thus, reducing the workload of neurologists and radiologists. Automation may also reduce inter observer variability, shorten time to diagnosis and help prevent critical findings being overlooked. It is important to note that, unlike human observers, AI models are able to maintain consistency in their performance across different healthcare settings, including under resourced environments, as illustrated through multicenter validation studies showing that neural networks demonstrated high fidelity in diagnostic performance across different imaging equipment and population demographics (Karalis, 2024).

In sum, the application of CNN, RNN and LSTM in neurological diagnostics is changing the way that brain disorders are detected and handled. In addition to providing objectivity and increased efficiency of diagnostics, these tools provide clinicians with deeper insights into disease patterns and trajectories. Neural networks will continue to become indispensable allies in proactive, data driven neurological care as they are further integrated into electronic health records and decision support systems.

4. PRECISION MEDICINE AND TREATMENT OPTIMIZATION

Neural networks are playing a transformative role in advancing precision medicine within neurology, enabling a shift from generalized therapeutic approaches to individualized care strategies tailored to each patient's unique profile. By harnessing vast, multi-dimensional datasets—including clinical histories, neuroimaging scans, electrophysiological signals, genomic sequences, and behavioral patterns—deep learning models can uncover latent patterns and subtle interactions that are often beyond the reach of traditional statistical methods. These models are proficient in the field of predictive analytics and can predict the progression of disease, responsiveness to treatment and adverse outcomes with very high accuracy (Nasarudin et al. 2024). Specifically, neural networks trained on longitudinal imaging and cognitive data can predict cognitive decline trajectory, enabling proactive and timely interventions in conditions like Alzheimer's or Parkinson's disease. In multiple sclerosis, AI models can also determine lesion activity and immune profile for estimating relapse risk and determining therapeutic intensity to avoid overtreatment and undertreatment (Alhudhaif, 2024).

Personalized pharmacotherapy is one of the most promising application of neural networks in precision neurology. With heterogeneous responses to medication observed in neurological and neuropsychiatric disorders (such as in epilepsy, depression, and schizophrenia), AI models trained on real world data can predict which patients are likely to benefit from specific drug classes or combinations. These models offer suggestions for optimized regimens, minimize side effects, and improve therapeutic adherence based on pharmacogenomic markers, metabolic profiles, and treatment histories. In addition, these systems can learn from the incoming patient data continuously and adapt over time, improving the recommendations and updating in real time when new evidence is available (Taherdoost & Ghofrani, 2024).

Besides pharmacological optimization, neural networks are also important in improving neuromodulation therapies like transcranial magnetic stimulation and deep brain stimulation. Effective, these treatments require the precise calibration of stimulation parameters, and their outcomes can be very different between patients. These interventions are personalized by analyzing historical treatment responses, brain connectivity patterns and electrophysiological feedback using AI driven models. For example, in Parkinson's disease, AI can determine the location and frequency of electrode placement and stimulation to decrease tremor or bradykinesia with the least side effects, such as speech or cognition. The identification of stimulation targets is notoriously complex in treatment resistant depression, and similar approaches are being explored there (Reddy et al. 2024).

Advanced Clinical Decision Support Systems (CDSS) integrate these capabilities in clinical practice through embedding neural network models in electronic health record platforms and bedside decision making tools (Elhaddad & Hamam, 2024). These systems offer real time, evidence based recommendations to clinicians to aid in the interpretation of complex datasets, prediction of complications and personalization of interventions with confidence. It also flags potential risks such as drug interactions or biomarker anomalies, which help protect patient safety and improve care coordination. In particular, the use of neural networks to power CDSS has the advantage of augmenting clinician expertise and enabling shared decision making through generating insights that can be shared clearly with patients and caregivers.

With the further development of these technologies, neurology is moving toward a future of deeply personalized, continuously adaptive and integrative treatment, bridging the gap between molecular biology, digital health, and patient centered care. This has yielded a new era of neurology that is simultaneously data rich and deeply humane, with therapeutic decisions as distinct as the person the therapies are intended to help.

5. NEURAL NETWORKS AND BRAIN-COMPUTER INTERFACES

The convergence of neural networks and brain-computer interfaces (BCIs) represents a revolutionary advancement in neurological care, offering novel ways to restore lost function, facilitate communication, and promote independence in individuals with motor, sensory, or cognitive impairments. Neurotechnological systems that interpret neural activity (captured, for example, via noninvasive modalities such as EEG, electrocorticography, or functional near infrared spectroscopy) and translate them into control commands for external devices are referred to as BCIs (Edelman et al. 2024). This can be robotic limbs, communication tools, computer cursors or smart home technology. BCIs are significantly enhanced in their ability to accurately decode the user's intent in real time by neural networks, and in particular by deep learning architectures that are able to dynamically adapt to neural signal fluctuations and environmental changes. As such, deep neural networks are particularly well suited for learning from the noisy, high dimensional EEG data and separating valuable brain signal patterns from irrelevant background noise, thereby improving signal interpretation and system responsiveness (Oganesian & Shanechi, 2024).

The integration of neural networks into BCIs has proven particularly transformative in neurorehabilitation contexts. For stroke survivors, individuals with spinal cord injury, or patients with neurodegenerative disorders such as amyotrophic lateral sclerosis (ALS), regaining motor function or communication ability can dramatically improve quality of life. These patients are able to participate in task specific training paradigms, where their motor intentions (captured by cortical activity) are interpreted and used to drive virtual avatars, robotic arms, or functional electrical stimulation systems through the use of neural network enhanced BCIs. The provision of immediate visual or proprioceptive feedback in this form of closed loop feedback reinforces sensorimotor learning and neuroplasticity by strengthening weakened neural circuits and promoting cortical reorganization. Such systems have been used in clinical trials and rehabilitation centers to accelerate motor recovery, improve coordination, and maintain long term functional gains, particularly when paired with immersive technologies, such as virtual reality (Jin et al. 2024).

Besides motor rehabilitation, neural networks are also improving BCIs for communication in locked in syndrome or advanced ALS patients. These systems detect particular patterns of brain activity associated with the cognitive intent of imagining speech, visual fixation or modulation of their attention, and translate them into language or command to operate communication devices. Neural network models of advanced complexity can be personalized for each user to take into account variability between users and changes in neural signal characteristics over time. Because of this adaptability, BCIs can be reliably and long term used in home settings, without frequent recalibration (Acuña Luna et al. 2025).

One of the most profound uses of neural network—powered BCIs is their capacity to give back a sense of agency and autonomy to patients with severe disabilities. BCIs allow for direct brain control of digital or physical systems, thus reducing the dependency on caregivers and external assistance and improving mental well being and social inclusion. They are also being explored for use in mental health applications, in which case they may one day act as affective state monitors and deliver neurofeedback therapies for depression and anxiety (Patrick-Krueger et al. 2025).

As artificial intelligence is developing, the next generation of BCIs is expected to be more portable, affordable and accessible, and it will be more integrated with wearable sensors, mobile platforms, and cloud based processing. Eventually, BCIs could be fused with other AI driven modalities, such as augmented reality, haptic feedback systems, and neurostimulation, to build fully immersive neurotechnological ecosystems that can adapt in real time to a user's cognitive and emotional state. In this ever changing world, neural networks are not only computational engines but also intelligent partners helping to decipher the human brain and unlock lives that used to be held back by neurological conditions.

6. ETHICAL, LEGAL, AND TECHNICAL CHALLENGES

As neural networks become deeply integrated into the diagnostic, therapeutic, and decision-making processes in neurology, they bring to the forefront a complex matrix of ethical, legal, and technical challenges that must be carefully navigated. One of the most pressing issues is the safeguarding of data privacy and security (Kumari, 2024). Neurological data—including high-resolution neuroimaging, continuous EEG recordings, and individual genomic profiles—is not only highly sensitive but also uniquely identifying. Misuse, breach, or unauthorized access to such data can lead to stigmatization, psychological distress, and even discrimination in employment or insurance contexts. The fact that for effective AI model training, large scale data sharing is required, magnifies these concerns. It is important to make sure that privacy frameworks like the Health Insurance Portability and Accountability Act in the United States and the General Data Protection Regulation in Europe are followed. Data anonymization, blockchain based audit trails and federated learning, which allows decentralized training without sharing raw data, are becoming important techniques to balance data utility and patient confidentiality (Rai et al. 2024).

Ethical dilemmas surrounding AI-driven diagnostics extend beyond data security to fundamental questions of human autonomy, consent, and trust. The increasing reliance on machine-generated insights raises concerns about the erosion of clinician-patient relationships, where complex decisions may be based on opaque algorithmic outputs rather than shared understanding (Cacciamani et al. 2024). The application of AI systems in this setting may also undermine the principles of transparency and informed consent as patients may not be fully informed that AI systems are contributing to their diagnosis or treatment plan. In addition, if error or adverse outcomes are diagnosed, who is accountable becomes legally and ethically murky. Should responsibility fall on the developers of the neural network, the healthcare institution using it, or the clinician who is relying on the output of the neural network? These questions require development of clear liability frameworks and risk sharing mechanisms (Newman Toker et al. 2024).

A core technical issue that compounds these challenges is the "black box" nature of many deep learning models. Unlike traditional statistical models whose inner workings are transparent and interpretable, neural networks often operate in ways that are not easily explainable—even to their creators. This makes clinical adoption more challenging because neurologists and other stakeholders are understandably unwilling to trust systems whose decision logic they cannot validate. The demand for explainable AI (XAI), then, is growing louder and ongoing work to build such models involves visualizations, rule based approximations, or natural language explanations that explain the reasoning behind their outputs. Saliency maps, attention mechanisms, and layer-wise relevance propagation tools are employed to expose which features or brain regions led to a specific prediction and can be cross referenced with established medical knowledge (Cao et al. 2024).

But regulatory agencies are also stepping in to make sure that neural networks employed in the clinical setting meet high standards of safety, efficacy, and equity. AI specific guidelines are in development by bodies such as the U.S. Food and Drug Administration, the European Medicines Agency and the World Health Organization that include preclinical validation, real world testing, performance auditing, and post market surveillance. More and more, these regulatory frameworks are demanding that models are algorithmically fair, which means developers have to show that their models behave the same way for every age group, gender, ethnicity, and subtype of disease. In addition, adaptive algorithms that adapt over time with new data inputs cause further regulatory complications in terms of continuous learning and revalidation (Miller et al. 2024).

In the end, no one discipline can solve these ethical, legal, and technical challenges, they need to be solved in collaboration and with an interdisciplinary approach. AI systems must be co designed by ethicists, legal scholars, clinicians, engineers, and patient advocates so that they are technologically robust and aligned with values of accountability, transparency and patient centered care. However, only by such concerted efforts can neural networks live up to such a promise as transformative tools in neurology and yet remain as ethically and legally sound as possible.

7. SOLUTIONS AND INNOVATIONS IN ADDRESSING CHALLENGES

To navigate the ethical, legal, and technical complexities of integrating neural networks into neurology, a growing ecosystem of solutions and innovations is emerging, aimed at ensuring transparency, safety, fairness, and long-term sustainability.

Explainable AI, one of the most important areas of innovation, is focused on making opaque "black box" models into systems whose predictions can be understood, trusted, and acted upon by clinicians and patients alike. Saliency maps for images that show which parts of the image most influenced a diagnosis, attention mechanisms for sequential data that trace where the model is focused, and model distillation techniques that simplify complex models into simpler surrogate models are some of the interpretability tools offered by XAI frameworks. These approaches enable the translation of high dimensional outputs into clinically meaningful explanations, which closes the gap between algorithmic insight and medical reasoning. In addition to aiding in easier validation and trust, it enables clinicians to refute or prove AI suggestions with their domain expertise (Mahmud et al. 2024).

Complementing XAI is the innovative use of federated learning, a decentralized training paradigm that addresses both privacy concerns and data scarcity. In federated learning, AI models are collaboratively trained across multiple institutions without sharing raw patient data. Instead, only model parameters or gradients are exchanged, and the data remains securely on-site. By taking this approach, one can be compliant with data protection regulations such as GDPR and HIPAA, and still gain access to a wide variety of large scale datasets that would otherwise be siloed. Federated learning allows AI systems to learn from more representative, broader samples without compromising individual privacy, which is crucial in neurology where rare diseases and population heterogeneity hinder model generalizability. In addition, it enables cross border and institutional collaboration in research, ensuring equity in the development and deployment of AI (Huang et al. 2024).

In tandem with technical solutions, regulatory bodies are playing an increasingly proactive role in establishing guidelines that ensure ethical and safe use of AI in healthcare. The U.S. Food and Drug Administration, European Medicines Agency and the World Health Organization are working to develop comprehensive regulatory pathways for approval and oversight of AI driven medical technologies. These frameworks focus on key aspects, including clinical efficacy, user transparency, data provenance, and algorithmic fairness. For example, the FDA's proposed framework for AI/ML-based software as a medical device specifies that real world performance monitoring, lifecycle transparency and periodic revalidation will be expected. Fairness audits and bias mitigation strategies are becoming part of regulatory assessments (Gollapalli et al. 2024), such that AI tools do not unintentionally perpetuate health disparities or deliver disparate care to different demographic groups.

Collectively these solutions make up a strong basis for ethical AI in neurology, one that is technologically sophisticated and socially accountable. Explainable modeling, privacy preserving computation, and forward thinking regulation can now converge to enable neural networks to augment clinical expertise and patient autonomy in neurological practice rather than undermining it. Looking forward, continued innovation in these domains and interdisciplinary collaboration between technologists, clinicians, ethicists, and policymakers will be essential to sustain trust and realize the full transformative potential of AI in brain health.

8. REAL-WORLD APPLICATIONS AND CASE STUDIES

The translation of neural network technologies from experimental frameworks to real-world clinical practice in neurology has produced a growing portfolio of successful applications, showcasing their potential to revolutionize diagnostic workflows, therapeutic interventions, and patient care. An early detection of Alzheimer's disease using CNNs on structural MRI data is one of the most compelling examples. CNNs have been integrated into radiology suites of leading research hospitals and memory clinics, which analyze volumetric brain scans for the presence of biomarkers like hippocampal shrinkage, cortical thinning, and ventricular enlargement, all signs of neurodegeneration often years before symptoms appear. Binzagr & Abulfaraj (2025) show that these AI enhanced systems have shown higher diagnostic sensitivity than manual image review, and can be used for risk stratification and longitudinal monitoring to support proactive cognitive interventions that may slow disease progression.

The application of deep learning frameworks in epilepsy care is equally impactful. LSTM networks have been deployed in epilepsy monitoring units to continuously analyze EEG recordings to detect preictal patterns that precede imminent seizures. Early seizure prediction has been invaluable for patients with drug resistant epilepsy, in which case abortive therapies or safety interventions can be administered to prevent injury. These models have already been integrated in some pilot programs into wearable devices for mobile, real time monitoring and alerts from which patient autonomy and quality of life are significantly increased. Reductions in seizure frequency and improvements in patient confidence and independence have been reported in clinical studies, especially in pediatric and adolescent patient populations (Narayana & Kodali, 2025).

Deep brain stimulation (DBS) therapy is fine tuned by AI powered systems in Parkinson's disease. Neural networks can optimize electrode placement and stimulation parameters in real time by analyzing motor fluctuation data from wearable sensors and pairing it with patient specific neurophysiological profiles. This approach improves symptom control (decreases tremor, rigidity and bradykinesia) while minimizing cognitive and speech side effects commonly seen with suboptimal DBS settings. Closed-loop DBS systems that dynamically adapt stimulation based on real-time neural feedback are now being explored (Olia et al. 2025) that offer these personalized adjustments and open a new era of precision neuromodulation.

The integration of neural networks into brain computer interface systems has also been used in stroke rehabilitation. Patients with post-stroke hemiplegia have been using BCIs powered by AI for motor control regain in clinical rehabilitation settings through task specific training. The motor intent is interpreted from EEG or EMG signals by the neural networks and translated to robotic limb movement or virtual avatar movement with sensory feedback to reinforce neuroplasticity. Measurable improvements in limb function, coordination and mobility, as well as psychological benefits including improved motivation, reduced depression, and increased engagement in therapy have been documented through case studies (Martínez-Cid et al. 2025).

Several key lessons have been learned from these real–world implementations. Second, neural networks that achieve technical success in clinical neurology must be usable, interpretable, and easily integrated into the existing clinical workflow. AI adoption is effective only if it involves interdisciplinary collaboration between AI researchers, neurologists, rehabilitation specialists, and ethicists to develop models that meet clinical needs and are consistent with patient values and ethical standards. Second, iterative refinement on clinical feedback is necessary. To retain high performance and relevance, models must be continually updated and validated against diverse patient populations and real world conditions. These case studies also demonstrate the importance of robust infrastructure, clinician training, and patient education to enable sustainable AI in neurology.

These examples together show that carefully designed neural networks can improve the quality and effectiveness of neurological care. They connect data to decision, prediction to prevention, and disease burden to restored function.

9. FUTURE DIRECTIONS IN NEUROAI

As the integration of neural networks into neurology continues to mature, the horizon of possibilities expands with next-generation AI models and emerging computational paradigms promising even deeper insights and more personalized interventions. Future neuroAI systems will move past these traditional architectures, incorporating hybrid models that combine the advantages of different deep learning methods, e.g., fusing the convolutional and recurrent layers, or by combining transformer based models with spatiotemporal processing. These architectures are designed to more effectively deal with the multi faceted nature of neurological data, by extracting spatial and temporal patterns with more detail. Moreover, neuromorphic computing, which is the case that AI mimics the functional dynamics of the human brain, is drawing attention in the area of the efficiency and interpretability of neural networks in neurological applications (Fan et al. 2025).

Another promising application of quantum computing is to neural data processing. Because of this, quantum algorithms are especially suited to navigating the huge combinatorial complexity of neurological datasets, allowing for quicker training of AI models and the discovery of relationships on high dimensional data that are not reachable by classical computing. Quantum enhanced models applied to real-time neural signal analysis or high resolution brain imaging could drastically increase the speed and accuracy of diagnosis and establish the basis for ultra-personalized, real time clinical decision making (Sarramone et al. 2025).

Additionally, the convergence of genomics and neural networks is ushering in a new era of understanding the molecular basis of neurological disease. AI models can integrate genomic, transcriptomic and epigenomic data with neuroimaging and clinical profiles in order to identify genetic risk factors, discover new biomarkers, and predict disease trajectories at the molecular level. By enabling the redefinition of precision neurology, diagnostics could shift from phenotype based assessments to genotype guided insights. The future of neuroAI emerges as a superimposed, deeply interconnected, biologically grounded, and computationally empowered neurological care framework of prediction and prevention (Pradeep et al. 2025).

10. CONCLUSION

Neural networks have emerged as powerful tools in the fight against neurological diseases, offering unprecedented capabilities in data analysis, pattern recognition, and predictive modeling. Their current applications span the diagnostic spectrum—from enhancing the accuracy of neuroimaging interpretation to predicting seizure onset using EEG signals—and extend into treatment optimization through personalized medicine and brain-computer interface technologies. Not only do these advances help improve clinical outcomes, they also decrease the cognitive and operational burdens on healthcare professionals, providing more precise, efficient, and patient centered care. With the field advancing, future directions include increasingly sophisticated implementations such as hybrid AI models, quantum augmented computation, and genomics integrated diagnostics that allow for a more thorough understanding of the intricate mechanisms underlying neurological disorders.

The impact of neural networks on research is equally profound, enabling large-scale analysis of multimodal data and accelerating the discovery of novel biomarkers and therapeutic targets. In clinical practice, AI driven tools are becoming indispensable for early detection, treatment planning and monitoring, pushing a move from reactive to proactive healthcare. As these technologies become more integrated in neurological care, policymakers and regulatory bodies are also more involved in establishing ethical frameworks and validation standards that are responsible for the integration of these technologies in a way that promotes equity, safety, and transparency.

Ultimately, the integration of neural networks into neurology represents more than just a technological shift—it marks a paradigm transformation in how we understand and manage brain health. Neural networks are bridging the gap between complex biological data and actionable clinical insights, ushering in a new era of neurointelligence in which medicine is not only data informed but data guided. As research and innovation advance, these tools will become the key to the future of managing neurological disease, bringing about a more connected, informed, and agile healthcare ecosystem.

REFERENCES

Acuña Luna, K. P., Hernandez-Rios, E. R., Valencia, V., Trenado, C., & Peñaloza, C. (2025). Deep learning-enhanced motor training: A hybrid VR and exoskeleton system for cognitive–motor rehabilitation. *Bioengineering (Basel, Switzerland), 12*(4), 331. DOI: 10.3390/bioengineering12040331 PMID: 40281692

Al-Quraishi, M. S., Tan, W. H., Elamvazuthi, I., Ooi, C. P., Saad, N. M., Al-Hiyali, M. I., & Ali, S. S. A. (2024). Cortical signals analysis to recognize intralimb mobility using modified RNN and various EEG quantities. *Heliyon, 10*(9), e30406. DOI: 10.1016/j.heliyon.2024.e30406 PMID: 38726180

Alhudhaif, A. (2024). A novel approach to recognition of Alzheimer's and Parkinson's diseases: Random subspace ensemble classifier based on deep hybrid features with a super-resolution image. *PeerJ. Computer Science, 10*, e1862. DOI: 10.7717/peerj-cs.1862 PMID: 38435579

Bayoudh, K. (2024). A survey of multimodal hybrid deep learning for computer vision: Architectures, applications, trends, and challenges. *Information Fusion, 105*, 102217. DOI: 10.1016/j.inffus.2023.102217

Binzagr, F., & Abulfaraj, A. W. (2025). InGSA: Integrating generalized self-attention in CNN for Alzheimer's disease classification. *Frontiers in Artificial Intelligence, 8*, 1540646. DOI: 10.3389/frai.2025.1540646 PMID: 40144735

Cacciamani, G. E., Chen, A., Gill, I. S., & Hung, A. J. (2024). Artificial intelligence and urology: Ethical considerations for urologists and patients. *Nature Reviews. Urology, 21*(1), 50–59. DOI: 10.1038/s41585-023-00796-1 PMID: 37524914

Cao, J., Zhou, T., Zhi, S., Lam, S., Ren, G., Zhang, Y., Wang, Y., Dong, Y., & Cai, J. (2024). Fuzzy inference system with interpretable fuzzy rules: Advancing explainable artificial intelligence for disease diagnosis—A comprehensive review. *Information Sciences, 662*, 120212. DOI: 10.1016/j.ins.2024.120212

Dayarathna, S., Islam, K. T., Uribe, S., Yang, G., Hayat, M., & Chen, Z. (2024). Deep learning based synthesis of MRI, CT and PET: Review and analysis. *Medical Image Analysis, 92*, 103046. DOI: 10.1016/j.media.2023.103046 PMID: 38052145

Dias-Carvalho, A., Sá, S. I., Carvalho, F., Fernandes, E., & Costa, V. M. (2024). Inflammation as common link to progressive neurological diseases. *Archives of Toxicology, 98*(1), 95–119. DOI: 10.1007/s00204-023-03628-8 PMID: 37964100

Edelman, B. J., Zhang, S., Schalk, G., Brunner, P., Müller-Putz, G., Guan, C., & He, B. (2024). Non-invasive brain-computer interfaces: State of the art and trends. *IEEE Reviews in Biomedical Engineering*. PMID: 39186407

El-Assy, A. M., Amer, H. M., Ibrahim, H. M., & Mohamed, M. A. (2024). A novel CNN architecture for accurate early detection and classification of Alzheimer's disease using MRI data. *Scientific Reports*, *14*(1), 3463. DOI: 10.1038/s41598-024-53733-6 PMID: 38342924

Elhaddad, M., & Hamam, S. (2024). AI-driven clinical decision support systems: An ongoing pursuit of potential. *Cureus*, *16*(4). Advance online publication. DOI: 10.7759/cureus.57728 PMID: 38711724

Fan, C., Xie, H., Tao, J., Li, Y., Pei, G., Li, T., & Lv, Z. (2024). ICaps-ResLSTM: Improved capsule network and residual LSTM for EEG emotion recognition. *Biomedical Signal Processing and Control*, *87*, 105422. DOI: 10.1016/j.bspc.2023.105422

Fan, F. L., Li, Y., Zeng, T., Wang, F., & Peng, H. (2025). Towards NeuroAI: Introducing neuronal diversity into artificial neural networks. *Med-X*, *3*(1), 2. DOI: 10.1007/s44258-024-00042-2

Gollapalli, M., Rahman, A., Kudos, S. A., Foula, M. S., Alkhalifa, A. M., Albisher, H. M., Al-Hariri, M. T., & Mohammad, N. (2024). Appendicitis diagnosis: Ensemble machine learning and explainable artificial intelligence-based comprehensive approach. *Big Data and Cognitive Computing*, *8*(9), 108. DOI: 10.3390/bdcc8090108

He, M., Tang, M., Meng, L., & Liang, Z. (2024). TBSTSleepNet: Three-branch spectro-temporal bidirectional LSTM based attention model for EEG sleep staging. *Biomedical Signal Processing and Control*, *97*, 106695. DOI: 10.1016/j.bspc.2024.106695

Huang, M., Zhang, X. S., Bhatti, U. A., Wu, Y., Zhang, Y., & Ghadi, Y. Y. (2024). An interpretable approach using hybrid graph networks and explainable AI for intelligent diagnosis recommendations in chronic disease care. *Biomedical Signal Processing and Control*, *91*, 105913. DOI: 10.1016/j.bspc.2023.105913

Jin, J., Xu, R., Daly, I., Zhao, X., Wang, X., & Cichocki, A. (2024). MOCNN: A multiscale deep convolutional neural network for ERP-based brain-computer interfaces. *IEEE Transactions on Cybernetics*, *54*(9), 5565–5576. DOI: 10.1109/TCYB.2024.3390805 PMID: 38713574

Karalis, V. D. (2024). The integration of artificial intelligence into clinical practice. *Applied Biosciences*, *3*(1), 14–44. DOI: 10.3390/applbiosci3010002

Khalil, M., Teunissen, C. E., Lehmann, S., Otto, M., Piehl, F., Ziemssen, T., Bittner, S., Sormani, M. P., Gattringer, T., Abu-Rumeileh, S., Thebault, S., Abdelhak, A., Green, A., Benkert, P., Kappos, L., Comabella, M., Tumani, H., Freedman, M. S., Petzold, A., & Kuhle, J. (2024). Neurofilaments as biomarkers in neurological disorders—Towards clinical application. *Nature Reviews. Neurology, 20*(5), 269–287. DOI: 10.1038/s41582-024-00955-x PMID: 38609644

Kumari, A. (2024). Security Aspects of Patient's Data in a Medical Diagnostic System. In *Machine Learning in Healthcare and Security* (pp. 195–210). CRC Press.

Liao, Y., Tang, Z., Gao, K., & Trik, M. (2024). Optimization of resources in intelligent electronic health systems based on Internet of Things to predict heart diseases via artificial neural network. *Heliyon, 10*(11), e32090. DOI: 10.1016/j.heliyon.2024.e32090 PMID: 38933933

Mahadevan, K., Punitha, A., & Suresh, J. (2024). Automatic recognition of rice plant leaf diseases detection using deep neural network with improved threshold neural network. e-Prime-Advances in Electrical Engineering. *Electronics and Energy, 8*, 100534.

Mahmud, T., Barua, K., Habiba, S. U., Sharmen, N., Hossain, M. S., & Andersson, K. (2024). An explainable ai paradigm for alzheimer's diagnosis using deep transfer learning. *Diagnostics (Basel), 14*(3), 345. DOI: 10.3390/diagnostics14030345 PMID: 38337861

Martínez-Cid, S., Vallejo, D., Herrera, V., Schez-Sobrino, S., Castro-Schez, J. J., & Albusac, J. A. (2025). Explainable AI-driven decision support system for personalizing rehabilitation routines in stroke recovery. Progress in Artificial Intelligence, 1-23.

Meng, J. C., Shen, M. Q., Lu, Y. L., Feng, H. X., Chen, X. Y., Xu, D. Q., Wu, G.-H., Cheng, Q.-Z., Wang, L.-H., & Gui, Q. (2024). Correlation of glymphatic system abnormalities with Parkinson's disease progression: A clinical study based on non-invasive fMRI. *Journal of Neurology, 271*(1), 457–471. DOI: 10.1007/s00415-023-12004-6 PMID: 37755462

Miller, M. B., Watts, M. L., & Samuel, L. (2024). FDA's proposed rule for the regulation of laboratory-developed tests. *Journal of Clinical Microbiology, 62*(2), e01488–e23. DOI: 10.1128/jcm.01488-23 PMID: 38206042

Narayana, V. V., & Kodali, P. (2025). Enhanced epilepsy sensitivity and detection rate with improved specificity by integration of modified lstm networks. *IEEE Sensors Journal.*

Nasarudin, N. A., Al Jasmi, F., Sinnott, R. O., Zaki, N., Al Ashwal, H., Mohamed, E. A., & Mohamad, M. S. (2024). A review of deep learning models and online healthcare databases for electronic health records and their use for health prediction. *Artificial Intelligence Review*, *57*(9), 249. DOI: 10.1007/s10462-024-10876-2

Newman-Toker, D. E., Nassery, N., Schaffer, A. C., Yu-Moe, C. W., Clemens, G. D., Wang, Z., Zhu, Y., Saber Tehrani, A. S., Fanai, M., Hassoon, A., & Siegal, D. (2024). Burden of serious harms from diagnostic error in the USA. *BMJ Quality & Safety*, *33*(2), 109–120. DOI: 10.1136/bmjqs-2021-014130 PMID: 37460118

Oganesian, L. L., & Shanechi, M. M. (2024). Brain–computer interfaces for neuropsychiatric disorders. *Nature Reviews Bioengineering*, *2*(8), 653–670. DOI: 10.1038/s44222-024-00177-2 PMID: 40988938

Oladapo, A., Jackson, T., Menolascino, J., & Periyasamy, P. (2024). Role of pyroptosis in the pathogenesis of various neurological diseases. *Brain, Behavior, and Immunity*, *117*, 428–446. DOI: 10.1016/j.bbi.2024.02.001 PMID: 38336022

Olia, J. B. H., Raman, A., Hsu, C. Y., Alkhayyat, A., & Nourazarian, A. (2025). A comprehensive review of neurotransmitter modulation via artificial intelligence: A new frontier in personalized neurobiochemistry. *Computers in Biology and Medicine*, *189*, 109984. DOI: 10.1016/j.compbiomed.2025.109984 PMID: 40088712

Patrick-Krueger, K. M., Burkhart, I., & Contreras-Vidal, J. L. (2025). The state of clinical trials of implantable brain–computer interfaces. *Nature Reviews Bioengineering*, *3*(1), 50–67. DOI: 10.1038/s44222-024-00239-5

Pradeep, A. K., Acharya, A., Chakravarty, R., & Dev, R. (2025). trendGPT–Discover Trends and Product Innovations Using neuroAi.

Rai, H. M., Tsoy, D., & Daineko, Y. (2024). MetaHospital: Implementing robust data security measures for an AI-driven medical diagnosis system. *Procedia Computer Science*, *241*, 476–481. DOI: 10.1016/j.procs.2024.08.067

Reddy, A., Reddy, R. P., Roghani, A. K., Garcia, R. I., Khemka, S., Pattoor, V., Jacob, M., Reddy, P. H., & Sehar, U. (2024). Artificial intelligence in Parkinson's disease: Early detection and diagnostic advancements. *Ageing Research Reviews*, *99*, 102410. DOI: 10.1016/j.arr.2024.102410 PMID: 38972602

Sajid, M., Malik, A. K., Tanveer, M., & Suganthan, P. N. (2024). Neuro-fuzzy random vector functional link neural network for classification and regression problems. *IEEE Transactions on Fuzzy Systems*, *32*(5), 2738–2749. DOI: 10.1109/TFUZZ.2024.3359652

Sarramone, L., Presso, M., Todorovich, E., Arlego, M., Zunino, A., Acosta, G., & Fernandez-Leon, J. A. (2025). Unlocking the potential of NeuroAI in Latin America. *AI & Society*, *40*(6), 1–11. DOI: 10.1007/s00146-025-02249-2

Saurabh, S., & Gupta, P. K. (2024). Deep learning-based modified bidirectional LSTM network for classification of ADHD disorder. *Arabian Journal for Science and Engineering*, *49*(3), 3009–3026. DOI: 10.1007/s13369-023-07786-w

Spolaôr, N., Lee, H. D., Mendes, A. I., Nogueira, C. V., Parmezan, A. R. S., Takaki, W. S. R., Coy, C. S. R., Wu, F. C., & Fonseca-Pinto, R. (2024). Fine-tuning pre-trained neural networks for medical image classification in small clinical datasets. *Multimedia Tools and Applications*, *83*(9), 27305–27329. DOI: 10.1007/s11042-023-16529-w

Taherdoost, H., & Ghofrani, A. (2024). *AI and the Evolution of Personalized Medicine in Pharmacogenomics*. Intelligent Pharmacy.

Torri, F., Vadi, G., Meli, A., Loprieno, S., Schirinzi, E., Lopriore, P., Ricci, G., Siciliano, G., & Mancuso, M. (2024). The use of digital tools in rare neurological diseases towards a new care model: A narrative review. *Neurological Sciences*, *45*(10), 4657–4668. DOI: 10.1007/s10072-024-07631-4 PMID: 38856822

Tsiara, A. A., Plakias, S., Kokkotis, C., Veneri, A., Mina, M. A., Tsiakiri, A., Kitmeridou, S., Christidi, F., Gourgoulis, E., Doskas, T., Kaltsatou, A., Tsamakis, K., Kazis, D., & Tsiptsios, D. (2025). Artificial Intelligence in the Diagnosis of Neurological Diseases Using Biomechanical and Gait Analysis Data: A Scopus-Based Bibliometric Analysis. *Neurology International*, *17*(3), 45. DOI: 10.3390/neurolint17030045 PMID: 40137466

Wang, J., Wang, Z., & Liu, G. (2024). Recording brain activity while listening to music using wearable EEG devices combined with Bidirectional Long Short-Term Memory Networks. *Alexandria Engineering Journal*, *109*, 1–10. DOI: 10.1016/j.aej.2024.07.122

Zhao, X., Wang, L., Zhang, Y., Han, X., Deveci, M., & Parmar, M. (2024). A review of convolutional neural networks in computer vision. *Artificial Intelligence Review*, *57*(4), 99. DOI: 10.1007/s10462-024-10721-6

Chapter 6
Robotics and Neuroscience in Rehabilitation:
Modern Approaches to Motor Disorders

Alexander Zakharov
https://orcid.org/0000-0003-1709-6195
Samara Medical University, Russia

Natalia Romanchuk
Samara State Medical University, Russia

Elena Khivintseva
https://orcid.org/0000-0002-1878-7951
Samara State Medical University, Russia

Yuliya Komarova
https://orcid.org/0000-0003-3435-1477
Samara State Medical University, Russia

Mariya Sergeeva
https://orcid.org/0000-0002-0926-8551
Samara State Medical University, Russia

Vladimir Kalinin
https://orcid.org/0009-0004-0440-2928
Samara State Medical University, Russia

Igor Shirolapov
Samara State Medical University, Russia

Sergey Chaplygin
Samara State Medical University, Russia

ABSTRACT

This monograph explores the intersection of robotics and neuroscience in the field of motor neurorehabilitation, focusing on the development and application of brain-computer interface (BCI) systems. Emphasizing principles of neuroplasticity, it examines how technologies such as EEG-based BCI, functional electrical stimulation

DOI: 10.4018/979-8-3373-2706-8.ch006

(FES), virtual reality (VR), and robotic exoskeletons can be integrated into closed-loop, feedback-rich rehabilitation platforms. Special attention is given to hybrid systems combining multiple sensory modalities to enhance user engagement and therapeutic outcomes. The monograph also discusses current challenges in clinical translation, including signal variability, training demands, and hardware limitations, while highlighting promising advances in AI-driven algorithms, wearable EEG solutions, and co-adaptive control strategies. Overall, it argues for a shift toward personalized, home-based rehabilitation technologies that empower patients with motor impairments to achieve greater autonomy and functional recovery.

INTRODUCTION

In recent years, the field of physical therapy and neurorehabilitation has witnessed a transformative shift through the integration of advanced robotic technologies. These systems, broadly defined as motorized interactive platforms with embedded control algorithms, are specifically engineered to assist patients in performing therapeutic movements. Acting either as guided tools or autonomous agents, robotic devices have demonstrated substantial efficacy in improving muscular strength, fine motor coordination, and movement precision. More importantly, they serve as potent modulators of neuroplastic mechanisms, which are central to the recovery of motor function following neurological injury (Cheng et al., 2020).

Robotic solutions for rehabilitation span a diverse technological spectrum. This includes wearable powered exoskeletons that facilitate locomotion or upper-limb movements by delivering joint-specific torque, as well as end-effector systems that enable patients to engage in controlled, repetitive task execution (Zakharov et al., 2020). In contrast to conventional therapeutic techniques, robotic systems provide high-resolution spatiotemporal control over movement trajectories, ensuring both consistency and adaptability throughout the course of recovery.

A key advantage of robotic rehabilitation lies in its capacity to deliver multi-modal sensory-motor stimulation. The continuous loop of real-time feedback not only enhances motor learning but also stimulates the central nervous system in ways conducive to plastic changes. These changes are largely experience-dependent and arise through intensive, repetitive, and task-oriented training that aligns with principles of Hebbian learning and sensorimotor reinforcement (Yoo & Lee, 2023). By adapting to the evolving capabilities of the patient, robotic systems dynamically support cortical reorganization, strengthen residual neural connections, and promote the recruitment of alternative neural circuits—processes that are fundamental to the restoration of voluntary motor control.

The integration of robotic systems into rehabilitation not only enhances therapeutic precision but also significantly optimizes clinical workflow. By automating physically strenuous components of therapy, robotics enables clinicians to oversee multiple patients simultaneously, thereby increasing operational efficiency without diminishing the individualization of care. This approach is further strengthened by the embedded capacity of robotic platforms to continuously monitor patient performance and dynamically adjust therapeutic parameters in real time. Such closed-loop systems ensure delivery of individualized rehabilitation intensities that are critical for sustaining neuroplastic mechanisms over time (Morone et al., 2017).

The core of robotic rehabilitation lies in its ability to deliver high-frequency, goal-directed, and precisely controlled movement patterns. These conditions are essential for promoting synaptogenesis and supporting the neurophysiological basis of Hebbian learning—the principle that "neurons that fire together wire together." These plastic changes are instrumental in restoring functional motor abilities, especially in patients recovering from stroke, spinal cord injury, or neurodegenerative disorders (He B., 2020).

The capacity for such experience-dependent plasticity, which robotic rehabilitation aims to harness, is grounded in foundational neuroscience research. Seminal animal studies, have meticulously demonstrated that targeted, repetitive motor practice can induce massive cortical remapping, leading to the expansion of movement representations in the primary motor cortex (Nudo, 2006). This work provided a critical neurophysiological basis for the "use-it-or-lose-it" and "use-it-and-improve-it" principles that underpin modern intensive rehabilitation. The translation of these principles into clinical practice is precisely what robotic systems facilitate, by enabling the high doses of repetitive movement necessary to drive such adaptive neuroplastic changes, thereby offering a direct pathway from mechanistic insight to therapeutic application.

Contemporary rehabilitation robots increasingly leverage multimodal sensory stimulation—integrating visual, proprioceptive, and haptic feedback—to create immersive and ecologically valid therapeutic environments. This enriched sensory engagement reinforces motor learning, promotes long-term skill retention, and drives cortical reorganization, aligning with the principles of enriched rehabilitation (Rose et al., 2005; Henriques & Cressman, 2012). Initiating such robotic therapy early, during the brain's peak plasticity window post-injury, further enhances adaptive neural remodeling while minimizing maladaptive compensations.

The foundational role of proprioception in motor control and recovery is critically supported by robotic interventions. Originating from mechanoreceptors in muscles, tendons, and joints, proprioceptive feedback enables coordinated movement and postural stability (Weiss et al., 2006). Robotic systems that provide proprioceptive stimulation—through guided motion, resistance, or haptic cues—help retrain impaired sensorimotor pathways, thereby facilitating functional recovery and improving rehabilitation outcomes.

Concurrently, Brain-Computer Interfaces (BCIs) have emerged as groundbreaking neurotechnologies that establish direct brain-external device communication pathways, decoding neural signals to control robotic arms, exoskeletons, or virtual avatars through a closed-loop architecture comprising neural acquisition, signal processing, and feedback systems (Agapov et al., 2017; Shevchenko et al., 2024), thereby creating synergistic rehabilitation platforms when integrated with proprioceptive and multimodal feedback.

The evolution of BCIs from a proof-of-concept to a viable neurorehabilitation tool is built upon foundational clinical studies that established their capacity to induce functional recovery (Birbaumer & Cohen., 2007). Pioneering work demonstrated that individuals with chronic paralysis could learn to regulate their slow cortical potentials to operate a BCI, providing early evidence of retained brain plasticity even in severe conditions. This was significantly advanced by landmark clinical trials, which provided robust evidence that a BCI system coupled with a robotic orthosis could lead to significant motor recovery in chronic stroke patients, but only when the BCI was contingent on the patient's correct motor intention (Ramos-Murguialday et al., 2013). These studies underscore the critical importance of a closed-loop design where neural activity directly and reliably controls the therapeutic actuator, a principle that remains central to effective BCI-based rehabilitation.

BCIs with a focus on motor rehabilitation are being increasingly applied to support individuals affected by neurological conditions such as stroke, spinal cord injuries, amyotrophic lateral sclerosis (ALS), Parkinson's disease, traumatic brain injury (TBI), and cerebral palsy (Agapov et al., 2017; Frolov et al., 2017). By facilitating intentional motor output via neuroprosthetic control or through modulation of neural activity during motor imagery tasks, BCIs contribute to the re-engagement of motor networks and the enhancement of use-dependent neuroplasticity. This engagement not only aids in functional recovery but also promotes reorganization within sensorimotor cortical areas, which is essential for sustained rehabilitation outcomes.

The therapeutic efficacy of these BCI paradigms is increasingly supported by meta-analyses and systematic reviews that consolidate findings across multiple clinical trials. Furthermore, the field is rapidly advancing towards more sophisticated and practical systems, particularly with the development of wearable neurotechnology. Recent innovations focus on creating fully portable, closed-loop BCI systems that can provide continuous, adaptive neuromodulation and assistance outside the laboratory (He et al., 2020). These systems represent a paradigm shift towards patient-centric, accessible rehabilitation tools that can be deployed in clinical and eventually home environments, thereby addressing the critical need for long-term, high-dose therapy that is essential for sustained neuroplasticity and functional gains.

Assessment of BCI efficacy is typically multifaceted, combining standardized clinical scales—such as the Fugl-Meyer Assessment (FMA), Action Research Arm Test (ARAT), and Functional Independence Measure (FIM)—with advanced neuroimaging techniques including EEG, positron emission tomography (PET), functional magnetic resonance imaging (fMRI), magnetoencephalography (MEG), and functional near-infrared spectroscopy (fNIRS). These tools offer complementary behavioral and neurophysiological insights, helping to quantify changes in brain function and structure following BCI interventions (Wolpaw et al., 2020). In addition, non-invasive brain stimulation methods such as transcranial magnetic stimulation (TMS) provide further understanding of corticospinal excitability, network reorganization, and interhemispheric connectivity as modulated by BCI-based therapies.

A key advancement in this integrated approach is the refinement of closed-loop control systems, which intelligently adapt assistance based on the user's real-time performance and engagement. Some research exemplifies this progress, demonstrating how a closed-loop system can seamlessly modulate robotic assistance to promote active patient participation, which is a key driver of neuroplasticity (Ang et al., 2015). These systems move beyond simple pre-programmed movements to create a dynamic interaction between the user and the machine, where the robot acts as a cooperative partner rather than a passive tool. This ensures that the therapeutic challenge is continuously optimized, preventing both frustration and passive reliance on the device, thereby maximizing the induction of activity-dependent neural plasticity in targeted sensorimotor pathways.

Among the most impactful robotic technologies are wearable exoskeletons, which provide mechanical assistance or controlled resistance to limb movements. These systems facilitate early mobilization—an essential factor in optimizing functional outcomes—while also alleviating the physical burden on therapists during intensive rehabilitation sessions. A growing number of these devices are designed to interface directly with BCI systems and sensory feedback modules, effectively closing the sensorimotor loop. This integration enhances the user's sense of agency and motor control by synchronizing neural intent with real-time mechanical response. Similarly, robotic prostheses embedded with advanced sensors and actuators are capable of interpreting user intent via machine learning algorithms, thereby enabling fluid, naturalistic movement patterns that restore functional independence in individuals with limb loss (Bundy et al., 2017).

Robotics also plays a critical role in the expansion of tele-rehabilitation. Through remote-operated robotic systems, patients can engage in supervised rehabilitation sessions without needing to be physically present in a clinical setting. This model is particularly valuable for individuals residing in geographically isolated or medically underserved regions, as it ensures continuity of care while reducing logistical barriers to therapy access (Catalán et al., 2021).

The convergence of robotic systems with proprioceptive stimulation and neural interface technologies is giving rise to a new generation of integrated neurotechnological platforms. These systems combine accurate sensory feedback, direct neural control, and robotic actuation to recreate natural sensorimotor experiences. By aligning movement intent with sensory consequences, they promote activity-dependent cortical plasticity, accelerate motor relearning, and enhance overall rehabilitation outcomes. This synergy holds significant promise for individuals recovering from stroke, spinal cord injury, or other neurological conditions, as it directly targets the reorganization of sensorimotor circuits that underpin functional recovery (Maslova et al., 2023; Pisotta et al., 2015; Zakharov et al., 2014).

MECHANISMS OF NEUROPLASTIC ADAPTATION IN ROBOTIC-ASSISTED REHABILITATION

The integration of robotic systems into therapeutic protocols has become a critical component in addressing motor deficits associated with neurological disorders, including stroke, traumatic brain injury, multiple sclerosis, and spinal cord injury (Shirolapov et al., 2023, 2024). At the core of this therapeutic strategy lies the principle of neuroplasticity—the central nervous system's inherent capacity to reorganize its structural and functional architecture by establishing new synaptic connections and compensatory pathways in response to injury (Sato et al., 2015).

Robotic rehabilitation technologies are uniquely positioned to stimulate targeted cortical regions, thereby activating and sustaining neuroplastic mechanisms essential for motor restoration. Unlike conventional physiotherapy, robotic systems offer unmatched precision, high training intensity, and reproducibility—factors that are instrumental in eliciting synaptic modifications and facilitating the formation of new motor circuits (Bonanno et al., 2023). Clinical and experimental evidence underscores the importance of high-frequency, task-specific motor training in combination with controlled sensorimotor stimulation for enhancing synaptogenesis and promoting functional connectivity across neural networks.

A distinctive advantage of robotic platforms is their ability to deliver multimodal sensory feedback, encompassing visual, proprioceptive, and tactile input streams. This enriched sensorimotor environment supports more robust integration of sensory signals and fosters the reorganization of both corticospinal and corticocortical pathways. For patients with disrupted sensorimotor integration due to central nervous system damage, such multimodal feedback is critical in re-establishing coherent motor programs and improving coordination.

Timely initiation of intensive, robot-assisted therapy is paramount, particularly within the early post-injury phase often referred to as the "critical window" of heightened neuroplastic responsiveness. Providing repetitive, goal-directed training during this period helps to avert maladaptive cortical changes while encouraging adaptive functional remapping of motor areas. Robotic devices, due to their capacity to dynamically adjust resistance, speed, and task complexity in real time, offer a scalable and personalized approach to therapy that maintains patient motivation and active participation—both of which are strongly linked to effective neuroplastic outcomes.

Moreover, robotic systems enable accurate, real-time measurement of motor performance parameters such as range of motion, force output, and movement smoothness. This data-driven approach allows for the fine-tuning of therapy plans based on objective analytics, ensuring that training intensity and progression are continuously optimized to support lasting neural reorganization and functional gains.

The therapeutic potential of robotic systems is further amplified when combined with BCIs, which decode neural activity to directly control robotic effectors. This integration establishes a closed-loop sensorimotor system, wherein cortical intent is translated into action, and corresponding sensory feedback reinforces neuroplastic restructuring. Studies have demonstrated that such hybrid systems can significantly improve motor recovery by synchronizing volitional neural activation with proprioceptive input.

Neurobiological models support this clinical approach. Research indicates that inadequate stimulation of the motor cortex during the early post-injury period can lead to the degradation of corticospinal synapses and the entrenchment of maladaptive patterns. Conversely, timely and targeted activation of motor areas during this phase promotes the re-establishment of functional connectivity and supports partial recovery of lost motor functions. These findings emphasize the urgency and precision required in the design of effective rehabilitative interventions.

Robotic platforms, particularly when integrated with immersive technologies such as virtual reality (VR), offer an advanced framework for delivering personalized rehabilitation that addresses both sensorimotor and cognitive domains. These systems capitalize on the recruitment of widespread intrahemispheric cortical networks spanning occipital, parietal, and frontal regions, facilitating coordinated neural activity essential for motor planning and execution. Visual input plays a particularly influential role in this process; numerous studies have demonstrated that visual stimuli modulate motor-related neuronal populations within the premotor and primary motor cortices, thus providing a powerful channel through which neuroplastic mechanisms can be activated and reinforced (Kakei et al., 2003).

Immersive rehabilitation environments leverage several key drivers of neuroplasticity, including visualized movement, interactive biofeedback, increased intrinsic motivation, and observational learning. Virtual reality settings are especially adept at stimulating these mechanisms, allowing patients to engage in meaningful, context-rich tasks that mimic real-world functional goals. The visual and auditory immersion offered by VR enhances sensorimotor integration while simultaneously engaging cognitive circuits responsible for attention, memory, and executive function. When combined with robotics, which ensures the precision and repetition required for motor retraining, the rehabilitative potential of these systems is significantly amplified. Figure 1 presents mechanisms on neuroplasticity enhancement through robot-assisted and immersive rehabilitation.

Figure 1. Mechanisms on neuroplasticity enhancement through robot-assisted and immersive rehabilitation.

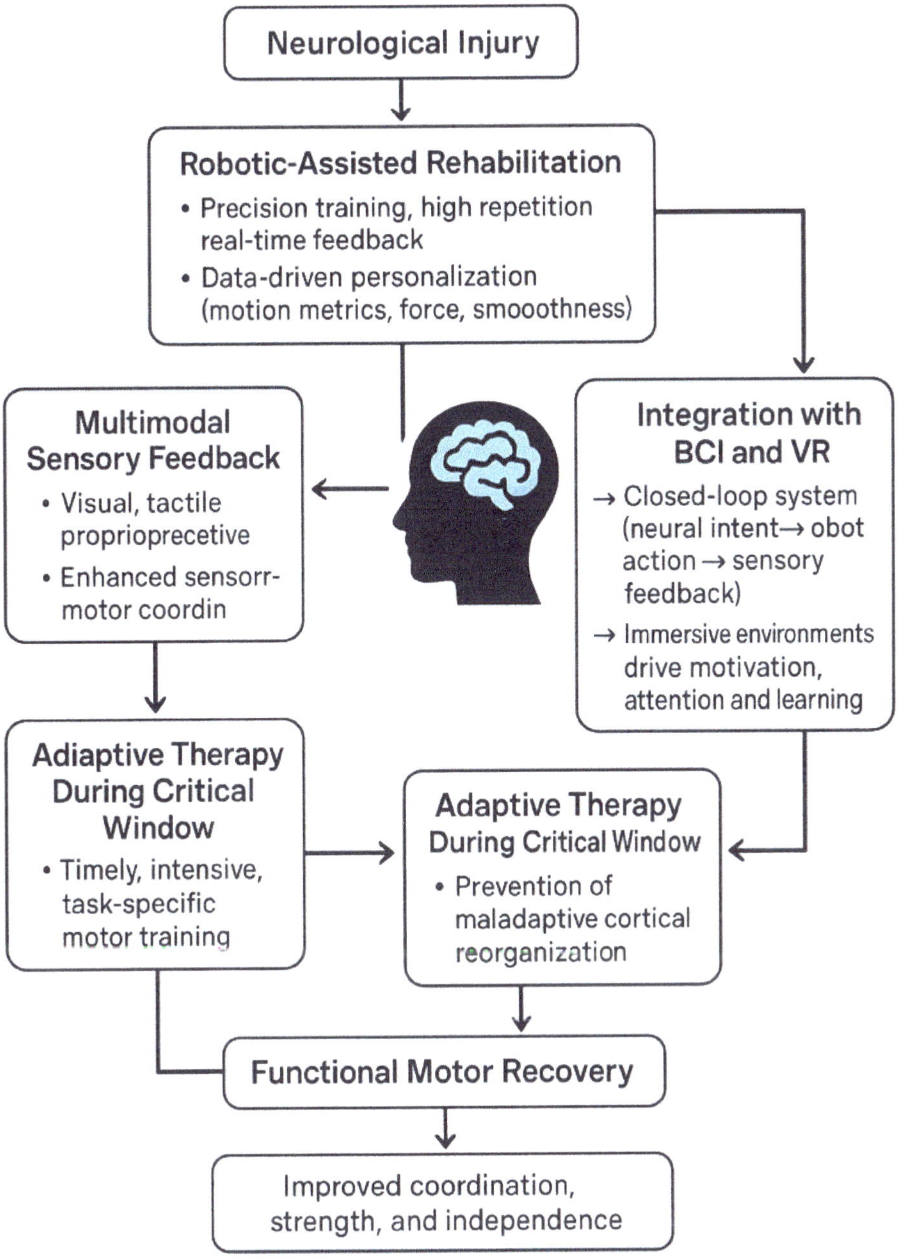

Sustained motor recovery requires both high-quality and high-quantity practice, as neuroplastic changes like synaptogenesis and dendritic remodeling demand consistent repetition to evolve from transient adaptations to lasting structural reorganization (Adamovich et al., 2009). Both training intensity and duration critically influence these neuroplastic responses, with evidence showing that thousands of task repetitions over days can induce robust synaptic changes (Krakauer et al., 2012) a finding with direct translational relevance since CNS-injured patients typically require greater training intensity than healthy individuals to achieve comparable gains (Cirstea et al., 2003). Virtual environments facilitate this by enabling dynamic control over task difficulty, volume, and cognitive demands to maintain engagement during prolonged rehabilitation, while optimal training parameters must be stage-specific, such as longer sessions for acute patients versus increased repetition for chronic cases (Lang et al., 2007).

OBJECTIVE EVALUATION AND PERSONALIZED ENGAGEMENT IN ROBOTIC-BASED NEUROREHABILITATION

Robotic-assisted interventions represent a transformative advancement in neurorehabilitation by enabling precise, continuous quantitative assessment of biomechanical parameters—including movement amplitude, velocity, smoothness, and force—that surpasses the limitations of traditional categorical clinical scales (Jamin et al., 2022). This high-resolution data acquisition allows for real-time tracking of patient engagement and performance, facilitating dynamic adaptation of training regimens to maintain an optimal challenge level essential for promoting neuroplasticity and motor learning (Comani et al., 2015). Furthermore, the extensive biomechanical datasets generated support highly individualized treatment through machine learning-driven prognostic insights and detailed patient profiles, while integration with wearable sensors provides multidimensional performance views across various contexts (Muro-de-la-Herran et al., 2014), ultimately operationalizing personalized rehabilitation paradigms that align therapy with each patient's specific recovery trajectory (Spaulding & Deogun, 2011).

Given the complex and often multidisciplinary nature of neurorehabilitation, efficient data communication among team members is essential. Yet, managing the large volumes of data generated by robotic sessions can be challenging and time-consuming. To mitigate this, contemporary robotic platforms incorporate integrated data management systems that automate the recording, organization, and reporting of therapy progress. These systems generate standardized, clinically relevant summaries that facilitate interdisciplinary collaboration and support informed decision-making. Additionally, embedded analytics offer rapid, data-driven assessments that empower therapists to make timely adjustments to therapy parameters or determine readiness for progression or discharge (Oña et al., 2018).

In Figure 2 a personalized approach to robotic-based neurorehabilitation is presented.

Figure 2. Personalized approach to robotic-based neurorehabilitation

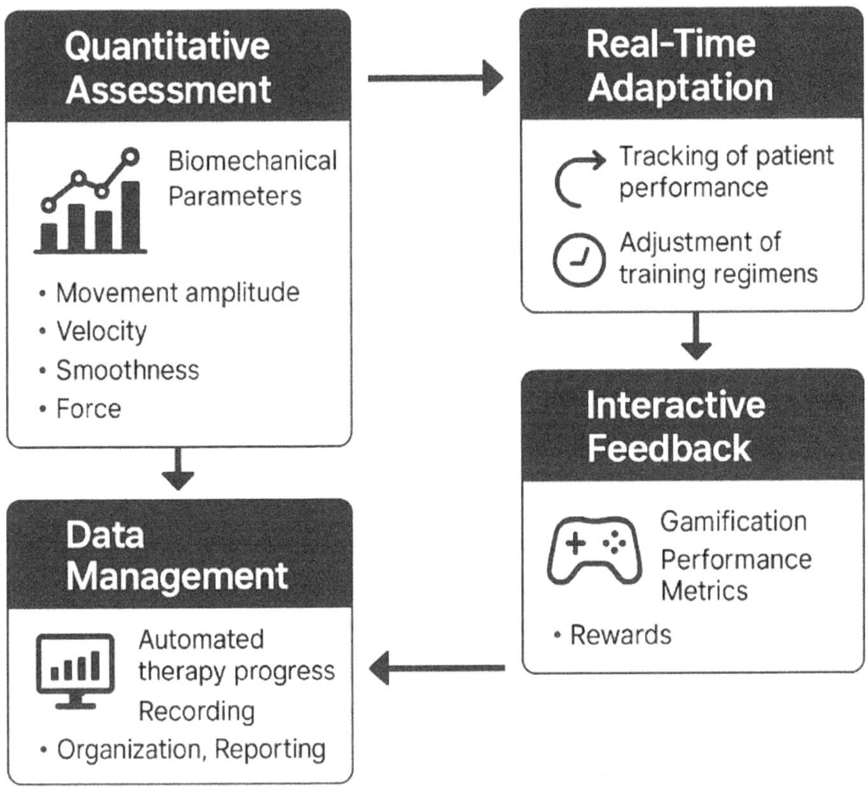

In summary, robotic-assisted neurorehabilitation introduces an objective, data-rich framework for both assessing and enhancing motor recovery. By combining real-time quantitative evaluation, personalized adaptation, and efficient data management, these systems support a more precise, effective, and patient-centered approach to restoring functional independence.

Patient engagement and sustained motivation are universally acknowledged as pivotal determinants of successful rehabilitation outcomes. Robotic-assisted therapy enhances these dimensions by integrating interactive feedback mechanisms into therapeutic activities, often within gamified environments. These systems provide patients with performance metrics, progress scores, and reward-based feedback that promote a sense of achievement and reinforce consistent participation (Sathian et al., 2011). Through the use of multisensory stimuli—including visual, auditory, and tactile cues—robotic platforms simulate realistic interactions, enhancing immersion and facilitating the reinforcement of proper movement execution. Notably, visual feedback presented in the form of summary scores or graphical progress indicators at the end of each session has been shown to significantly improve patients' ability to meet motor recovery targets. The combination of cognitive challenges with physical training in such interactive environments fosters a more holistic recovery of motor function by engaging both cognitive and motor neural networks.

Technological advances have further elevated the capacity of robotic systems to sustain engagement. Contemporary platforms feature intuitive graphical user interfaces, dynamic cognitive-motor training modules, and automated difficulty adjustments that respond to real-time performance data. These features ensure that the therapeutic experience remains cognitively and physically stimulating throughout the rehabilitation process, thereby maximizing clinical impact (Bowman et al., 2021). Empirical studies confirm the efficacy of gamified rehabilitation: stroke survivors participating in game-based robotic therapy exhibit greater improvements in motor control compared to those undergoing traditional therapy, with notable enhancements in movement fluidity, coordination, and long-term treatment adherence (Ozgur et al., 2022).

The combination of high-intensity, repetitive movement training with enriched sensory input creates an optimal stimulus for neuroplasticity. Neural imaging studies have demonstrated that such therapy modulates activity in critical motor-related brain regions, including the premotor cortex, primary motor cortex, supplementary motor area, and cerebellum—regions associated not only with movement execution but also with cognitive functions such as planning and attention. Functional MRI findings further corroborate these effects, revealing significant shifts in cortical activation patterns following robot-assisted interventions that correlate with gains in both motor and cognitive domains (Calabrò et al., 2016).

BRAIN-COMPUTER INTERFACE APPLICATIONS AND SENSORIMOTOR FEEDBACK LOOPS

In the final stage of a BCI system, classified neural signals from motor imagery or movement intention are translated into commands for external devices like functional electrical stimulation (FES), robotic exoskeletons, or virtual reality environments. Central to this process is a feedback mechanism that closes the sensorimotor loop, informing users of command efficacy while facilitating learning and sustaining engagement. While visual feedback is common, multimodal strategies integrating proprioceptive, haptic, and auditory cues are increasingly used to optimize outcomes, with proprioceptive feedback through exoskeletons or FES being particularly effective due to its direct engagement of the sensorimotor cortex and anatomical congruence with intended actions (Biasiucci et al., 2018).

Among various configurations, BCI-FES has emerged as a highly promising application for motor rehabilitation. In this paradigm, detected motor imagery signals trigger FES parameters tailored to the user's physiology, producing muscle contractions and functional movement. This creates a closed-loop system where the resulting afferent feedback is transmitted back to the central nervous system, reinforcing connectivity between intention and sensorimotor response to enhance cortical reorganization through activity-dependent plasticity. Research consistently demonstrates that BCI-FES interventions yield superior outcomes compared to FES alone, with clinical trials supporting their efficacy in improving upper limb function in post-stroke populations through this integrated approach (Sousa et al., 2022; Tabernig et al., 2018).

Despite their promise, BCI-FES systems face limitations including restricted efficacy in patients with severe paralysis due to inadequate neuromuscular substrates, insufficient real-time adaptive control of stimulation parameters, and biomechanical constraints of surface electrodes that limit selective muscle activation (Popovic et al., 2002). Similarly, BCI-robotic systems—which use motor imagery signals to control exoskeletons and orthoses (Frolov et al., 2017; Cantillo-Negrete et al., 2018)—and BCI-FES both contend with declining patient engagement from repetitive training.

Virtual reality functions as a human-computer interface that immerses users in perceptually rich, interactive scenarios. Through real-time feedback and gamified tasks, VR promotes sensorimotor integration and cognitive engagement. Although still a relatively novel addition to post-stroke rehabilitation protocols, preliminary studies indicate that VR significantly improves user motivation, attentional focus, and compliance—factors that are essential for optimizing motor recovery (Weiss et al., 2006). Systematic reviews have also supported the role of VR in facilitating neurorehabilitation, highlighting its positive impact on therapy adherence and functional gains (Laver et al., 2011).

CURRENT TRENDS IN OVERCOMING BCI LIMITATIONS

The limitations of current BCI systems, while significant, are actively being addressed through several converging technological trends. A primary trend is the shift toward wearable, low-cost systems suitable for home-based telerehabilitation. For instance, companies and research consortia are developing wireless, dry-electrode EEG headsets (e.g., systems from companies like g.tec's g.Sahara or research platforms like the OpenBCI Ultracortex) that drastically reduce setup time and improve user comfort. These devices are the enabling technology for pilot programs exploring home-based BCI-VR training. In one such pilot, chronic stroke patients used a portable BCI system coupled with a VR serious game for 30 minutes daily over 4 weeks. Preliminary results showed not only improved Fugl-Meyer scores but also high adherence rates, demonstrating the feasibility of deploying high-dose, motivating therapy outside the clinic (Tanczak, N., et al., 2025).

Concurrently, Artificial Intelligence (AI) and machine learning are revolutionizing adaptive algorithms. The challenge of inter-session variability and the need for tedious recalibration is being met with transfer learning and co-adaptive algorithms. For example, recent studies employ deep learning models (e.g., Convolutional Neural Networks) that are pre-trained on large, multi-subject EEG datasets. These models can be fine-tuned for a new user with minimal data, effectively creating a 'zero-calibration' or 'low-calibration' BCI. This trend moves BCIs away from rigid, pre-defined models towards systems that learn and adapt with the user in real-time, personalizing the decoding strategy to maintain performance even as the user's brain signals evolve through recovery.

Finally, the rise of integrated telerehabilitation platforms represents a systemic trend. These platforms combine wearable BCIs, cloud-based data analytics, and remote clinical supervision. A therapist can remotely assign tasks, monitor a patient's performance and adherence via automated dashboards, and adjust therapy parameters based on data collected during home sessions. This model directly addresses the translational challenges of cost and access, moving neurorehabilitation from a clinic-centric to a patient-centric, continuous care paradigm.

HYBRID BCI SYSTEMS: MULTIMODAL FEEDBACK AND ASSISTIVE TECHNOLOGY INTEGRATION

Hybrid BCI systems that combine multiple feedback modalities and assistive technologies have emerged as a powerful framework for advancing neurorehabilitation. These systems build upon motor imagery (MI)-based BCI paradigms by integrating virtual reality (VR), functional electrical stimulation (FES), and tactile feedback to create immersive, closed-loop environments that enhance motor learning and cortical reorganization. Among the most promising configurations is the combination of MI-BCI with VR and FES, which has demonstrated significant improvements in upper-limb motor function in individuals with chronic post-stroke deficits. In one study, a four-week training protocol employing this hybrid approach yielded substantial gains on the Fugl-Meyer Assessment (FMA), paralleled by a shift in EEG activity toward sensorimotor and premotor cortical areas—evidence of functional neuroplasticity in the affected hemisphere.

The addition of tactile feedback—particularly relevant in tasks requiring grasping, manipulation, or fine motor control—further enhances the ecological validity of rehabilitation. Tactile stimuli not only increase user immersion but also intensify sensorimotor engagement, which is critical for strengthening afferent-efferent coupling. In clinical research on invasive BCI systems, intracortical microstimulation (ICMS) of the somatosensory cortex has been explored as a means to restore somatosensory perception. Trials involving ICMS-enhanced bidirectional BCIs demonstrated improved modulation of grasp force in VR-based environments compared to visual feedback alone, highlighting the unique contributions of tactile channels in improving motor accuracy and precision (Quick et al., 2020).

Recent investigations have also explored the use of multisensory feedback paradigms in MI-BCI-VR training, combining visual, auditory, and tactile stimuli. These multimodal environments allow users to interact with virtual objects—grasping, colliding, and moving them—with greater fidelity and functional realism.

Tactile feedback has also been operationalized in non-invasive BCI systems using vibrotactile actuators—forming the foundation of EEG-based vibrotactile BCI (EVE-BCI) paradigms. In these systems, vibratory stimuli are delivered to various body sites, including the fingertips, wrists, back, shoulders, and ankles. Comparative analyses of stimulation locations found that although MI classification accuracy was similar between fingertip and wrist-based feedback, the stability and magnitude of event-related desynchronization (ERD)—a critical neural marker for MI task performance—were significantly more pronounced when stimulation was applied to the fingertips (Missiroli et al., 2019). These findings suggest that the somatotopic specificity of tactile feedback can influence neurophysiological engagement and enhance the effectiveness of motor imagery decoding.

Recent studies have expanded the understanding of tactile feedback in BCI systems by investigating the effects of multiple vibrotactile stimulators (tactors) applied to various body regions. These investigations revealed that vibration sensitivity may play a more critical role than spatial separation in optimizing tactor placement. In other words, rather than emphasizing the physical distance between tactors, maximizing the discriminability of stimuli hinges on selecting body sites with high tactile acuity (Guemann et al., 2019).

Among EEG-based vibrotactile BCI (EVE-BCI) paradigms, two protocols are most commonly employed: the P300-based paradigm and the steady-state somatosensory evoked potential (SSSEP) (S. Agapov et al., 2018; Kirasirova et al., 2021). While the classification accuracy of P300 in vibrotactile mode (approximately 68%) typically lags behind visual or auditory implementations, it remains a promising solution for applications where visual feedback is impractical or unavailable, such as in users with visual impairment or in high-fatigue cognitive states.

Hybrid models that combine short-duration vibrotactile pulses (for P300 detection) with continuous vibrations (to elicit SSSEP responses) have been proposed to enhance system performance (Bulanov et al., 2020). This multimodal approach increases the number of discriminable features, improving classification accuracy by enriching the sensory input profile (Breitwieser et al., 2016) Remarkably, even when visual input is entirely occluded, purely vibrotactile feedback during motor imagery (MI) training has been shown to enhance cortical activation, improve EEG feature stability across sessions, and elevate classification performance to levels comparable to traditional visual-feedback-based MI-BCI systems.

The efficacy of vibrotactile feedback is further highlighted in studies demonstrating its synergistic effect when combined with visual feedback. Adding tactile cues to MI tasks enhances event-related desynchronization (ERD) in sensorimotor cortical areas more effectively than visual feedback alone (K.-T. Kim et al., 2020). MI training has also been linked to increased corticospinal excitability, as measured through motor evoked potentials (MEPs) elicited by transcranial magnetic stimulation (TMS) (Strelnik et al., 2022). When paired with vibrotactile feedback, these gains are amplified, with evidence of stronger contralateral sensorimotor desynchronization and enhanced cortical excitability in the motor representation of the imagined limb.

Despite these promising developments, several barriers continue to limit the widespread adoption of EVE-BCI systems. One notable challenge is user fatigue and physical discomfort associated with prolonged or continuous vibration. Extended exposure to vibrotactile stimulation can lead to sensory adaptation, cognitive overload, or reduced attentional focus—each of which can impair long-term BCI performance. Furthermore, substantial inter-individual variability in tactile sensitivity and optimal stimulation frequency complicates system calibration. Personalized tuning of vibrotactile parameters is often time-intensive and may not be feasible within time-constrained clinical workflows.

CHALLENGES AND FUTURE DIRECTIONS IN MOTOR NEUROREHABILITATION USING BCI SYSTEMS

Over the past decade, advances in brain-computer interface (BCI) technology have significantly influenced the development of neurorehabilitation and assistive systems, offering new therapeutic pathways for individuals with motor impairments. Despite this progress, the widespread clinical implementation of BCI-based rehabilitation continues to face several challenges that must be addressed to improve usability, reliability, and patient outcomes.

One of the foremost obstacles lies in the extensive training time typically required for users to achieve effective BCI control. Most motor imagery (MI)-based BCI systems necessitate repeated and prolonged training sessions, which can induce cognitive fatigue and demotivation, especially in neurologically impaired populations. Moreover, user proficiency varies widely, and not all individuals achieve sufficient modulation of sensorimotor rhythms (SMRs) required for accurate command generation. This variability in performance—commonly referred to as BCI illiteracy—represents a fundamental barrier to consistent system adoption.

The effectiveness of MI-based BCIs also hinges on the user's ability to engage in vivid and consistent motor imagery. Numerous training strategies employing real-time feedback—visual, tactile, auditory, or multimodal—have been proposed to facilitate the learning of MI tasks (Abdalsalam et al., 2018). However, the impact of feedback is not universally beneficial. While accurate and engaging feedback can enhance cortical engagement and neuroplasticity, ambiguous or misaligned feedback may confuse users or even inhibit learning. This variability in feedback responsiveness is particularly evident in older adults recovering from stroke, who may also contend with comorbidities such as cognitive decline, apathy, or depression that impair neuroplastic potential and attentional capacity (Zuo et al., 2020).

Fluctuations in attention represent another major factor influencing neural signal stability and the overall performance of BCI systems. Variability in attentional engagement can stem from physiological factors such as fatigue and anxiety, environmental distractions like noise or lighting, or cognitive and motor interference during task performance (Aliakbaryhosseinabadi et al., 2019; Sharifian et al., 2021). These distractions impair sensorimotor rhythm modulation and compromise classification accuracy, especially in prolonged or high-demand tasks. To address this, recent research has focused on the development of distraction-resilient models capable of maintaining stable performance even under increased cognitive load. These adaptive systems incorporate attention-monitoring algorithms that adjust decoding parameters dynamically in response to user states (Fei et al., 2023).

A related avenue of exploration is bilateral motor training within BCI rehabilitation. Evidence suggests that engaging both limbs in coordinated activity reduces interhemispheric inhibition and enhances the recruitment of contralateral motor pathways, promoting broader cortical plasticity. However, the real-time decoding of bilateral motor intentions—particularly in asynchronous and complex environments—remains technically challenging. Progress in this area will require more advanced algorithms and experimental validation under conditions that closely reflect the timing and structure of naturalistic motor intent (Wang et al., 2023).

The concept of co-adaptive BCI systems presents a promising paradigm for the future of intelligent neural interfaces. In these architectures, learning occurs bidirectionally: users adapt their neural strategies through feedback, while the system simultaneously refines its decoding algorithms based on real-time input. Ideally, such systems balance high-level volitional control by the user with autonomous low-level command execution by the BCI, enabling intuitive, efficient interaction (Vidaurre et al., 2016). This model envisions the BCI as a supervisory interface where the user functions as a strategic decision-maker, rather than being burdened by continuous control.

Hardware advancements are playing an equally critical role in shaping the accessibility and scalability of BCI systems. Notable progress has been made in the development of wearable, wireless EEG headsets designed for clinical and home-based applications (Malechka et al., 2015). Innovations in dry electrode technology have further enhanced portability by eliminating the need for conductive gels; however, such electrodes still face limitations related to user discomfort, sensitivity to motion artifacts, and signal degradation over time (Mullen et al., 2015). In parallel, flexible electrode (FE) materials—offering low impedance and high biocompatibility—are emerging as key enablers of the next generation of BCI interfaces. FE-based platforms have already demonstrated high-fidelity EEG acquisition in both in vitro and in vivo conditions, supporting the development of fully wearable, unobtrusive BCI systems (Wang et al., 2023).

On the algorithmic front, most current BCI systems remain constrained by the relatively low signal-to-noise ratio (SNR) of non-invasive EEG. This presents significant limitations when attempting to control complex devices with multiple degrees of freedom, such as robotic prostheses or exoskeletons. Improving online signal processing and classification accuracy under real-world conditions will require not only more robust algorithms but also standardized evaluation frameworks tailored to BCI rehabilitation use cases. Hybrid BCIs—those integrating EEG with other modalities such as EMG, fNIRS, or eye tracking—are increasingly seen as a way forward. These systems offer greater reliability and enhanced detection of motor intention, facilitating more adaptive and intelligent interaction between user and device.

Recent advancements in soft robotics have added a new dimension to BCI-based neurorehabilitation. Soft robotic devices, particularly BCI-controlled gloves, are designed to conform naturally to the user's anatomy, enhancing comfort and safety during movement assistance. Clinical trials have demonstrated their therapeutic potential, especially when combined with functional electrical stimulation (FES) and immersive virtual reality (VR) environment.

In parallel, bidirectional BCI systems are being developed to capture both motor commands and deliver real-time sensory feedback, facilitating more naturalistic control and embodiment. These systems are expected to enter clinical neurorehabilitation pipelines in the near future. Another emerging frontier involves hybrid BCIs that integrate EEG with fNIRS. Although this combination offers complementary insights—EEG for electrophysiological signals and fNIRS for hemodynamic activity—its implementation remains complex. The weak correlation between EEG and fNIRS arises from inherent physiological discrepancies: for example, transient neural activity may not produce detectable hemodynamic responses, and neurotransmitter-related vascular effects may occur without corresponding EEG changes (Berger et al., 2019). Additionally, latency differences between EEG (milliseconds) and fNIRS (seconds) complicate real-time signal fusion. Overcoming these challenges requires innovative feature extraction, alignment, and classification algorithms that can synchronize asynchronous data streams and extract meaningful joint features (Hong et al., 2017).

Furthermore, the inclusion of non-invasive neuromodulation techniques—such as transcranial magnetic stimulation (TMS) or transcranial direct current stimulation (tDCS)—may offer a complementary strategy to boost cortical excitability and facilitate motor recovery when combined with BCI training. These stimulation modalities can prime specific brain regions to become more receptive to BCI-based motor training, accelerating neuroplastic reorganization.

TRANSLATIONAL CHALLENGES AND FUTURE DIRECTIONS IN NEUROREHABILITATION TECHNOLOGY

The issues, problems, and trends described in this chapter provide a comprehensive technological overview, but their emphasis could be rebalanced to more accurately reflect the current landscape of the field. While technological barriers like signal variability and hardware limitations are rightly highlighted, the critical human-factors challenges of usability, patient motivation, and long-term adherence are currently underemphasized. These factors are often the ultimate determinants of clinical success, yet they are secondary to the descriptions of the technologies themselves. Furthermore, there is a noticeable skew in attention towards robotic exoskeletons, which, while impactful, receive more detailed exposition than other equally promising modalities like end-effector robots or non-wearable sensor-based systems. This creates an imbalance, potentially overlooking the diverse technological ecosystem required for personalized rehabilitation.

To rectify this, the chapter would benefit from a conscious rebalancing of emphasis. A specific recommendation is to expand the discussion on multimodal hybrid systems—such as the integration of BCIs with FES and VR —beyond their technical architecture to include evidence on how these combinations directly impact usability and motivation through enhanced immersion and feedback. Concurrently, a dedicated subsection on patient-centered design considerations should be introduced. This section would explicitly address how factors like cognitive load, user comfort, and the personal relevance of therapeutic tasks are being integrated into the design of new systems to boost long-term adherence. By giving these patient-centric and multimodal aspects equal weight to the descriptions of specific robotic devices, the chapter will present a more holistic and clinically realistic view of the field's trajectory.

While the previous sections have detailed the remarkable technical capabilities and neurophysiological rationale for robotics and BCIs in rehabilitation, the journey from laboratory prototype to standard clinical practice is fraught with challenges. For these technologies to realize their full potential, it is imperative to address the critical gaps in clinical validation, healthcare integration, ethical considerations, and demographic applicability. The true measure of success lies not only in engineering feats but in the demonstrable, widespread improvement of patient outcomes in real-world settings.

A critical perspective on this chapter reveals a significant under-emphasis on the human-centric ecosystem in which neurorehabilitation technologies are deployed. The narrative, while technically comprehensive, largely overlooks the indispensable roles of therapists, caregivers, and interdisciplinary teams. For true integration into standard care, robotic and BCI systems must be designed not as autonomous replacements for human expertise, but as tools that augment and empower clinicians. The therapist's role evolves from providing physical assistance to one of clinical interpreter and integrator—selecting appropriate technology, tailoring training paradigms based on rich motor performance data, and providing the essential motivational support that machines cannot (Maciejasz et al., 2014). Similarly, the success of home-based telerehabilitation is inextricably linked to the involvement of caregivers, who require intuitive interfaces and clear support protocols to assist patients effectively.

Therefore, a crucial recommendation for the field, and an essential enhancement for this chapter, is to broaden the scope from a patient-device dyad to the entire rehabilitation ecosystem. Future technology development must explicitly focus on fostering interdisciplinary collaboration. This involves creating shared data platforms that translate biomechanical and neural data into clinically actionable insights for therapists, physicians, and engineers. Furthermore, implementation strategies must account for workflow integration, providing adequate training for clinicians and designing systems that seamlessly fit into existing clinical routines rather than disrupting them. Ultimately, the measure of success for these advanced technologies will be their ability to strengthen, rather than sideline, the human connections and professional expertise that are the cornerstone of effective rehabilitation (Pearce, L. M. N. at al., 2025).

A foundational challenge remains the strength and generalizability of the clinical evidence base. Although numerous pilot studies and single-center trials demonstrate feasibility and promising results, the field is increasingly guided by the rigorous standards of large-scale, randomized controlled trials (RCTs) and meta-analyses. For robotic rehabilitation, systematic reviews have provided nuanced insights. For instance, a Cochrane review on upper limb robotics after stroke concluded that while electromechanical devices improve arm function and muscle strength, the evidence for activities of daily living is less clear, highlighting the need for more targeted interventions (Mehrholz, et al., 2018). Electromechanical and robot-assisted arm training for improving activities of daily living, arm function, and arm muscle strength after stroke. Similarly, meta-analyses of gait training robots show they can increase the odds of walking independently, but optimal training parameters and patient selection criteria are still being refined. In the realm of BCIs, foundational RCTs, were pivotal in establishing that BCI-guided therapy is only effective when it is contingent on the patient's genuine motor attempt, creating a closed-loop that reinforces Hebbian plasticity (Ramos-Murguialday A., at al., 2013). Moving forward, the focus must shift from simply proving efficacy over conventional care to identifying which specific technologies, or combinations thereof, are most effective for which patient profiles, based on stroke location, severity, and time since injury.

Beyond proof of efficacy lies the complex problem of integration into existing healthcare ecosystems. The implementation of these advanced technologies in clinical workflows presents significant logistical hurdles. High acquisition costs, the need for dedicated space and technical support, and the time required for therapist training and device setup are substantial barriers. A critical, and often overlooked, factor is reimbursement. Without clear codes and demonstrated cost-effectiveness from the payer's perspective, adoption will remain limited. Health-economic studies that model long-term benefits, such as reduced caregiver burden and decreased reliance on long-term care, are essential to justify the initial investment. The promise of telerehabilitation and home-based systems offers a solution to accessibility and scalability but introduces its own set of challenges, including remote technical support, patient safety in unsupervised environments, and ensuring consistent, high-quality therapy engagement outside the clinic. Bridging this "valley of death" between innovation and routine practice requires close collaboration between engineers, clinicians, healthcare administrators, and policymakers.

This leads directly to a suite of ethical and accessibility considerations that must be proactively addressed. The high cost of current systems risks creating a two-tiered rehabilitation system, exacerbating health inequities where only affluent patients or well-funded urban centers can access cutting-edge care. There is an ethical imperative to develop low-cost, scalable solutions and to advocate for equitable access policies. Patient compliance is another multifaceted issue. While gamification enhances motivation, "BCI illiteracy" – the inability of a subset of users to reliably modulate brain signals – and "robot boredom" from repetitive tasks can lead to frustration and dropout. This underscores the necessity of user-centered design that minimizes cognitive load and adapts to user fatigue. Furthermore, BCI systems, which collect sensitive neural data, raise profound questions about data privacy, security, and ownership. Establishing robust ethical frameworks for the use of this intimate biological information is a prerequisite for public trust and widespread adoption.

The application of these technologies must also be thoughtfully tailored across the lifespan, as the needs of pediatric and adult populations differ significantly. Neuroplasticity in children is a powerful, experience-driven process of building neural circuits for the first time, whereas in adults, it often involves rerouting or reclaiming functions after a lesion. This fundamental difference dictates therapeutic goals: in pediatrics, the focus is on achieving developmental milestones, while in adults, it is on restoring lost function. Consequently, device design cannot simply be a matter of scaling down adult hardware. Pediatric systems must be adaptable to rapid growth spurts and employ engagement strategies rooted in play and age-appropriate virtual environments. The cognitive and physical demands of the technology must be aligned with the child's developmental stage, requiring a deeply interdisciplinary approach that integrates developmental psychology and pediatric neurology.

Looking ahead, the future of neurorehabilitation technology is pointed toward smarter, more personalized, and more accessible systems. The convergence of artificial intelligence and machine learning with robotics and BCIs will enable fully adaptive, closed-loop systems that can interpret a user's physical and cognitive state in real-time, dynamically adjusting assistance and challenge to maintain an optimal therapeutic zone. The hardware trajectory is clearly moving toward miniaturization and wearability, with soft robotic exosuits and wireless, dry-electrode EEG headsets paving the way for seamless use in clinic and home. The next frontier may well be bidirectional BCIs, which not only decode motor intention but also write information back to the brain through cortical stimulation, potentially restoring a sense of touch and proprioception, thereby closing the sensorimotor loop with unprecedented fidelity. Ultimately, the field is striving towards a paradigm of truly personalized medicine, where genetic markers, neuroimaging data, and continuous biomechanical performance are integrated to prescribe the perfect type, timing, and dosage of technology-assisted therapy for each individual. By confronting the translational challenges of today with interdisciplinary collaboration and a patient-centric focus, the promise of robotics and neuroscience to revolutionize motor rehabilitation can finally be fully realized.

CONCLUSION

The evolution of BCI systems has expanded dramatically, progressing from simple EEG-based motor imagery interfaces to multimodal platforms that integrate FES, robotics, VR, and tactile feedback. These technologies now emphasize neuroplasticity through adaptive, task-specific training that supports cortical reorganization and sensorimotor recovery. While ME-based BCIs offer more natural motor decoding, MI-based systems remain popular due to their non-invasive nature. Hybrid configurations incorporating VR, proprioceptive input, and robotic assistance are among the most promising, creating immersive, closed-loop environments that promote motor relearning and cognitive engagement.

Despite their potential, BCI systems face technological and methodological challenges, such as low spatial resolution in EEG, high signal variability, and user fatigue. Advances in deep learning—CNNs, LSTMs, Transformer models—have enhanced decoding accuracy, while co-adaptive algorithms and transfer learning are helping to reduce training demands and improve usability. Wearable, wireless EEG systems and dry electrode technologies offer paths toward scalable, home-based rehabilitation. Simultaneously, hybrid BCI models combining EEG with fNIRS or EMG are being developed to improve signal robustness and enable more reliable control over complex assistive devices.

Looking forward, BCI development is increasingly shaped by artificial intelligence, user-centric design, and interdisciplinary collaboration. Future systems will feature fully adaptive, bidirectional feedback loops utilizing soft robotics, vibrotactile stimulation, and real-time sensory integration. The convergence of advanced signal processing, wearable hardware, and multimodal interaction holds the promise of transforming BCIs from experimental tools into clinically viable, personalized rehabilitation platforms. These systems are poised to significantly enhance functional recovery and quality of life for individuals with neurological impairments.

REFERENCES

Abdalsalam, E., Yusoff, M. Z., Malik, A., Kamel, N. S., & Mahmoud, D. (2018). Modulation of sensorimotor rhythms for brain-computer interface using motor imagery with online feedback. *Signal, Image and Video Processing*, *12*(3), 557–564. DOI: 10.1007/s11760-017-1193-5

Adamovich, S. V., Fluet, G. G., Tunik, E., & Merians, A. S. (2009). Sensorimotor training in virtual reality: A review. *NeuroRehabilitation*, *25*(1), 29–44. DOI: 10.3233/NRE-2009-0497 PMID: 19713617

Agapov, S., Bulanov, V., Zakharov, A., & Sergeeva, M. (2018). A Comparison of Classifiers in a Task Consisting of Classifying Single Visual Event-Related Cortical Potentials in Humans. *Neuroscience and Behavioral Physiology*, *48*(9), 1140–1144. Advance online publication. DOI: 10.1007/s11055-018-0678-1

Agapov, S. N., Bulanov, V. A., Zakharov, A. V., & Sergeeva, M. S. (2017). Comparison of classifiers in the tasks of the single-trial vep classification. *Zhurnal Vysshei Nervnoi Deyatelnosti Imeni IP Pavlova, 67*(4), Article 4.

Aliakbaryhosseinabadi, S., Kamavuako, E. N., Jiang, N., Farina, D., & Mrachacz-Kersting, N. (2019). Classification of Movement Preparation Between Attended and Distracted Self-Paced Motor Tasks. *IEEE Transactions on Biomedical Engineering*, *66*(11), 3060–3071. DOI: 10.1109/TBME.2019.2900206 PMID: 30794165

Ang, K. K., Chua, K. S., Phua, K. S., Wang, C., Chin, Z. Y., Kuah, C. W., Low, W., & Guan, C. (2015). A Randomized Controlled Trial of EEG-Based Motor Imagery Brain-Computer Interface Robotic Rehabilitation for Stroke. *Clinical EEG and Neuroscience*, *46*(4), 310–320. DOI: 10.1177/1550059414522229 PMID: 24756025

Berger, A., Horst, F., Müller, S., Steinberg, F., & Doppelmayr, M. (2019). Current State and Future Prospects of EEG and fNIRS in Robot-Assisted Gait Rehabilitation: A Brief Review. *Frontiers in Human Neuroscience*, *13*, 172. DOI: 10.3389/fnhum.2019.00172 PMID: 31231200

Biasiucci, A., Leeb, R., Iturrate, I., Perdikis, S., Al-Khodairy, A., Corbet, T., Schnider, A., Schmidlin, T., Zhang, H., Bassolino, M., Viceic, D., Vuadens, P., Guggisberg, A. G., & Millán, J. D. R. (2018). Brain-actuated functional electrical stimulation elicits lasting arm motor recovery after stroke. *Nature Communications*, *9*(1), 2421. DOI: 10.1038/s41467-018-04673-z PMID: 29925890

Birbaumer, N., & Cohen, L. G. (2007). Brain-computer interfaces: Communication and restoration of movement in paralysis. *The Journal of Physiology*, *579*(3), 621–636. DOI: 10.1113/jphysiol.2006.125633 PMID: 17234696

Bonanno, L., Cannuli, A., Pignolo, L., Marino, S., Quartarone, A., Calabrò, R. S., & Cerasa, A. (2023). Neural Plasticity Changes Induced by Motor Robotic Rehabilitation in Stroke Patients: The Contribution of Functional Neuroimaging. *Bioengineering (Basel, Switzerland), 10*(8), 990. DOI: 10.3390/bioengineering10080990 PMID: 37627875

Bowman, T., Gervasoni, E., Amico, A. P., Antenucci, R., Benanti, P., Boldrini, P., Bonaiuti, D., Burini, A., Castelli, E., Draicchio, F., Falabella, V., Galeri, S., Gimigliano, F., Grigioni, M., Mazzon, S., Mazzoleni, S., Mestanza Mattos, F. G., Molteni, F., ... Carrozza, M. C. (2021). What is the impact of robotic rehabilitation on balance and gait outcomes in people with multiple sclerosis? A systematic review of randomized control trials. *European Journal of Physical and Rehabilitation Medicine, 57*(2), Article 2. DOI: 10.23736/S1973-9087.21.06692-2

Breitwieser, C., Pokorny, C., & Müller-Putz, G. R. (2016). A hybrid three-class brain–computer interface system utilizing SSSEPs and transient ERPs. *Journal of Neural Engineering, 13*(6), 066015. DOI: 10.1088/1741-2560/13/6/066015 PMID: 27788124

Bulanov, V. A., Zakharov, A. V., & Khivintseva, E. V. (2020). Wavelet transform for the identification of P300. *IOP Conference Series. Materials Science and Engineering, 862*(5), 052049. DOI: 10.1088/1757-899X/862/5/052049

Bundy, D. T., Souders, L., Baranyai, K., Leonard, L., Schalk, G., Coker, R., Moran, D. W., Huskey, T., & Leuthardt, E. C. (2017). Contralesional Brain–Computer Interface Control of a Powered Exoskeleton for Motor Recovery in Chronic Stroke Survivors. *Stroke, 48*(7), 1908–1915. DOI: 10.1161/STROKEAHA.116.016304 PMID: 28550098

Calabrò, R. S., Russo, M., Naro, A., Milardi, D., Balletta, T., Leo, A., Filoni, S., & Bramanti, P. (2016). Who May Benefit From Armeo Power Treatment? A Neurophysiological Approach to Predict Neurorehabilitation Outcomes. *PM & R, 8*(10), 971–978. DOI: 10.1016/j.pmrj.2016.02.004 PMID: 26902866

Cantillo-Negrete, J., Carino-Escobar, R. I., Carrillo-Mora, P., Elias-Vinas, D., & Gutierrez-Martinez, J. (2018). Motor Imagery-Based Brain-Computer Interface Coupled to a Robotic Hand Orthosis Aimed for Neurorehabilitation of Stroke Patients. *Journal of Healthcare Engineering, 2018*, 1–10. DOI: 10.1155/2018/1624637 PMID: 29849992

Catalán, J. M., García-Pérez, J. V., Blanco, A., Ezquerro, S., Garrote, A., Costa, T., Bertomeu-Motos, A., Díaz, I., & García-Aracil, N. (2021). Tele-Rehabilitation Versus Local Rehabilitation Therapies Assisted by Robotic Devices: A Pilot Study with Patients. *Applied Sciences (Basel, Switzerland), 11*(14), 6259. DOI: 10.3390/app11146259

Cheng, N., Phua, K. S., Lai, H. S., Tam, P. K., Tang, K. Y., Cheng, K. K., Yeow, R. C.-H., Ang, K. K., Guan, C., & Lim, J. H. (2020). Brain-Computer Interface-Based Soft Robotic Glove Rehabilitation for Stroke. *IEEE Transactions on Biomedical Engineering, 67*(12), 3339–3351. DOI: 10.1109/TBME.2020.2984003 PMID: 32248089

Cirstea, M. C., Ptito, A., & Levin, M. F. (2003). Arm reaching improvements with short-term practice depend on the severity of the motor deficit in stroke. *Experimental Brain Research, 152*(4), 476–488. DOI: 10.1007/s00221-003-1568-4 PMID: 12928760

Comani, S., Velluto, L., Schinaia, L., Cerroni, G., Serio, A., Buzzelli, S., Sorbi, S., & Guarnieri, B. (2015). Monitoring Neuro-Motor Recovery From Stroke With High-Resolution EEG, Robotics and Virtual Reality: A Proof of Concept. *IEEE Transactions on Neural Systems and Rehabilitation Engineering, 23*(6), 1106–1116. DOI: 10.1109/TNSRE.2015.2425474 PMID: 25910194

Fei, W., Bi, L., Wang, J., Xia, S., Fan, X., & Guan, C. (2023). Effects of Cognitive Distraction on Upper Limb Movement Decoding From EEG Signals. *IEEE Transactions on Biomedical Engineering, 70*(1), 166–174. DOI: 10.1109/TBME.2022.3187085 PMID: 35767496

Frolov, A. A., Mokienko, O., Lyukmanov, R., Biryukova, E., Kotov, S., Turbina, L., Nadareyshvily, G., & Bushkova, Y. (2017). Post-stroke Rehabilitation Training with a Motor-Imagery-Based Brain-Computer Interface (BCI)-Controlled Hand Exoskeleton: A Randomized Controlled Multicenter Trial. *Frontiers in Neuroscience, 11*, 400. DOI: 10.3389/fnins.2017.00400 PMID: 28775677

Guemann, M., Bouvier, S., Halgand, C., Paclet, F., Borrini, L., Ricard, D., Lapeyre, E., Cattaert, D., & Rugy, A. D. (2019). Effect of vibration characteristics and vibror arrangement on the tactile perception of the upper arm in healthy subjects and upper limb amputees. *Journal of Neuroengineering and Rehabilitation, 16*(1), 138. DOI: 10.1186/s12984-019-0597-6 PMID: 31722740

He, G., Dong, X., & Qi, M. (2020). From the perspective of material science: A review of flexible electrodes for brain-computer interface. *Materials Research Express, 102001*(10), 102001. Advance online publication. DOI: 10.1088/2053-1591/abb857

Henriques, D. Y. P., & Cressman, E. K. (2012). Visuomotor Adaptation and Proprioceptive Recalibration. *Journal of Motor Behavior*, *44*(6), 435–444. DOI: 10.1080/00222895.2012.659232 PMID: 23237466

Hong, X., Lu, Z. K., Teh, I., Nasrallah, F. A., Teo, W. P., Ang, K. K., Phua, K. S., Guan, C., Chew, E., & Chuang, K.-H. (2017). Brain plasticity following MI-BCI training combined with tDCS in a randomized trial in chronic subcortical stroke subjects: A preliminary study. *Scientific Reports*, *7*(1), 9222. DOI: 10.1038/s41598-017-08928-5 PMID: 28835651

Jamin, P., Duret, C., Hutin, E., Bayle, N., Koeppel, T., Gracies, J.-M., & Pila, O. (2022). Using Robot-Based Variables during Upper Limb Robot-Assisted Training in Subacute Stroke Patients to Quantify Treatment Dose. *Sensors (Basel)*, *22*(8), 2989. DOI: 10.3390/s22082989 PMID: 35458975

Kakei, S., Hoffman, D. S., & Strick, P. L. (2003). Sensorimotor transformations in cortical motor areas. *Neuroscience Research*, *46*(1), 1–10. DOI: 10.1016/S0168-0102(03)00031-2 PMID: 12725907

Kim, K.-T., Lee, J., Kim, H., Kim, C. H., & Lee, S. J. (2020). Classification of Selective Attention Within Steady-State Somatosensory Evoked Potentials From Dry Electrodes Using Mutual Information-Based Spatio-Spectral Feature Selection. *IEEE Access : Practical Innovations, Open Solutions*, *8*, 85464–85472. DOI: 10.1109/ACCESS.2020.2990384

Kirasirova, L. A., Zakharov, A. V., Morozova, M. V., Kaplan, A. Y., & Pyatin, V. P. (2021). ERP Correlates of Emotional Face Processing in Virtual Reality. *Opera Medica et Physiologica*, *8*(3), 3.

Krakauer, J. W., Carmichael, S. T., Corbett, D., & Wittenberg, G. F. (2012). Getting Neurorehabilitation Right: What Can Be Learned From Animal Models? *Neurorehabilitation and Neural Repair*, *26*(8), 923–931. DOI: 10.1177/1545968312440745 PMID: 22466792

Lang, C. E., MacDonald, J. R., & Gnip, C. (2007). Counting Repetitions: An Observational Study of Outpatient Therapy for People with Hemiparesis Post-Stroke. *Journal of Neurologic Physical Therapy; JNPT*, *31*(1), 3–10. DOI: 10.1097/01.NPT.0000260568.31746.34 PMID: 17419883

Laver, K., George, S., Ratcliffe, J., & Crotty, M. (2011). Virtual reality stroke rehabilitation—Hype or hope?: VIEWPOINT. *Australian Occupational Therapy Journal*, *58*(3), 215–219. DOI: 10.1111/j.1440-1630.2010.00897.x PMID: 21599688

Maciejasz, P., Eschweiler, J., Gerlach-Hahn, K., Jansen-Troy, A., & Leonhardt, S. (2014). A survey on robotic devices for upper limb rehabilitation. *Journal of Neuroengineering and Rehabilitation, 11*(1), 3. DOI: 10.1186/1743-0003-11-3 PMID: 24401110

Malechka, T., Tetzel, T., Krebs, U., Feuser, D., & Graeser, A. (2015). sBCI-Headset—Wearable and Modular Device for Hybrid Brain-Computer Interface. *Micromachines, 6*(3), 291–311. DOI: 10.3390/mi6030291

Maslova, O., Komarova, Y., Shusharina, N., Kolsanov, A., Zakharov, A., Garina, E., & Pyatin, V. (2023). Non-invasive EEG-based BCI spellers from the beginning to today: A mini-review. *Frontiers in Human Neuroscience, 17*, 1216648. DOI: 10.3389/fnhum.2023.1216648 PMID: 37680264

Mehrholz, J., Pohl, M., Platz, T., Kugler, J., & Elsner, B. (2018). Electromechanical and robot-assisted arm training for improving activities of daily living, arm function, and arm muscle strength after stroke. *Cochrane Database of Systematic Reviews, 9*(9), CD006876. Advance online publication. DOI: 10.1002/14651858.CD006876.pub5 PMID: 30175845

Missiroli, F., Barsotti, M., Leonardis, D., Gabardi, M., Rosati, G., & Frisoli, A. (2019). Haptic Stimulation for Improving Training of a Motor Imagery BCI Developed for a Hand-Exoskeleton in Rehabilitation. *2019 IEEE 16th International Conference on Rehabilitation Robotics (ICORR)*, 1127–1132. DOI: 10.1109/ICORR.2019.8779370

Morone, G., Paolucci, S., Cherubini, A., De Angelis, D., Venturiero, V., Coiro, P., & Iosa, M. (2017). Robot-assisted gait training for stroke patients: Current state of the art and perspectives of robotics. *Neuropsychiatric Disease and Treatment, 13*, 1303–1311. DOI: 10.2147/NDT.S114102 PMID: 28553117

Mullen, T. R., Kothe, C. A. E., Chi, Y. M., Ojeda, A., Kerth, T., Makeig, S., Jung, T.-P., & Cauwenberghs, G. (2015). Real-time neuroimaging and cognitive monitoring using wearable dry EEG. *IEEE Transactions on Biomedical Engineering, 62*(11), 2553–2567. DOI: 10.1109/TBME.2015.2481482 PMID: 26415149

Muro-de-la-Herran, A., Garcia-Zapirain, B., & Mendez-Zorrilla, A. (2014). Gait Analysis Methods: An Overview of Wearable and Non-Wearable Systems, Highlighting Clinical Applications. *Sensors (Basel), 14*(2), 3362–3394. DOI: 10.3390/s140203362 PMID: 24556672

Nudo, R. J. (2006). Mechanisms for recovery of motor function following cortical damage. *Current Opinion in Neurobiology, 16*(6), 638–644. DOI: 10.1016/j.conb.2006.10.004 PMID: 17084614

Oña, E. D., Cano-de La Cuerda, R., Sánchez-Herrera, P., Balaguer, C., & Jardón, A. (2018). A Review of Robotics in Neurorehabilitation: Towards an Automated Process for Upper Limb. *Journal of Healthcare Engineering*, *2018*, 1–19. DOI: 10.1155/2018/9758939 PMID: 29707189

Ozgur, A. G., Wessel, M. J., Olsen, J. K., Cadic-Melchior, A. G., Zufferey, V., Johal, W., Dominijanni, G., Turlan, J.-L., Mühl, A., Bruno, B., Vuadens, P., Dillenbourg, P., & Hummel, F. C. (2022). The effect of gamified robot-enhanced training on motor performance in chronic stroke survivors. *Heliyon*, *8*(11), e11764. DOI: 10.1016/j.heliyon.2022.e11764 PMID: 36468121

Pearce, L. M. N., Hassett, L., Sherrington, C., & Pryor, J. (2025). Human interactions remain at the heart of rehabilitation with advanced technology: A practice-embedded longitudinal qualitative study with allied health clinicians. *Journal of Neuroengineering and Rehabilitation*, *22*(1), 1–13. DOI: 10.1186/s12984-025-01576-1 PMID: 40050924

Pisotta, I., Perruchoud, D., & Ionta, S. (2015). Hand-in-hand advances in biomedical engineering and sensorimotor restoration. *Journal of Neuroscience Methods*, *246*, 22–29. DOI: 10.1016/j.jneumeth.2015.03.003 PMID: 25769276

Popovic, M. R., Popovic, D. B., & Keller, T. (2002). Neuroprostheses for grasping. *Neurological Research*, *24*(5), 443–452. DOI: 10.1179/016164102101200311 PMID: 12117312

Quick, K. M., Weiss, J. M., Clemente, F., Gaunt, R. A., & Collinger, J. L. (2020). Intracortical Microstimulation Feedback Improves Grasp Force Accuracy in a Human Using a Brain-Computer Interface. *2020 42nd Annual International Conference of the IEEE Engineering in Medicine & Biology Society (EMBC)*, 3355–3358. DOI: 10.1109/EMBC44109.2020.9175926

Ramos-Murguialday, A., Broetz, D., Rea, M., Läer, L., Yilmaz, O., Brasil, F. L., Liberati, G., Curado, M. R., Garcia-Cossio, E., Vyziotis, A., Cho, W., Agostini, M., Soares, E., Soekadar, S., Caria, A., Cohen, L. G., & Birbaumer, N. (2013, July). Brain-machine interface in chronic stroke rehabilitation: A controlled study. *Annals of Neurology*, *74*(1), 100–108. DOI: 10.1002/ana.23879 PMID: 23494615

Rose, F. D., Brooks, B. M., & Rizzo, A. A. (2005). Virtual Reality in Brain Damage Rehabilitation [Review]. *Cyberpsychology & Behavior*, *8*(3), 241–262. DOI: 10.1089/cpb.2005.8.241 PMID: 15971974

Sathian, K., Buxbaum, L. J., Cohen, L. G., Krakauer, J. W., Lang, C. E., Corbetta, M., & Fitzpatrick, S. M. (2011). Neurological Principles and Rehabilitation of Action Disorders: Common Clinical Deficits. *Neurorehabilitation and Neural Repair*, *25*(5, suppl), 21S–32S. DOI: 10.1177/1545968311410941 PMID: 21613535

Sharifian, F., Schneider, D., Arnau, S., & Wascher, E. (2021). Decoding of cognitive processes involved in the continuous performance task. *International Journal of Psychophysiology*, *167*, 57–68. DOI: 10.1016/j.ijpsycho.2021.06.012 PMID: 34216693

Shevchenko, O., Yeremeieva, S., & Laschowski, B. (2024). *Comparative Analysis of Neural Decoding Algorithms for Brain-Machine Interfaces*. DOI: 10.1101/2024.12.05.627080

Shirolapov, I. V., Gribkova, O. V., Kovalev, A. M., Shafigullina, L. R., Ulivanova, V. A., Kozlov, A. V., Ereshchenko, A. A., Lyamin, A. V., & Zakharov, A. V. (2024). The Role of Interactions along the Brain–Gut–Microbiome Axis in the Regulation of Circadian Rhythms, Sleep Mechanisms, and Their Disorders. *Neuroscience and Behavioral Physiology*, *54*(8), 1177–1183. DOI: 10.1007/s11055-024-01712-9

Shirolapov, I. V., Zakharov, A. V., Bulgakova, S. V., Khivintseva, E. V., Sergeeva, M. S., Romanchuk, N. P., Pavlova, O. N., & Kazantsev, V. B. (2023). Glymphatic dysfunction in the pathogenesis of neurodegenerative diseases and pathological aging. *Genes to Cells*, *18*(4), 309–322. DOI: 10.23868/gc546022

Sousa, A. S. P., Moreira, J., Silva, C., Mesquita, I., Macedo, R., Silva, A., & Santos, R. (2022). Usability of Functional Electrical Stimulation in Upper Limb Rehabilitation in Post-Stroke Patients: A Narrative Review. *Sensors (Basel)*, *22*(4), 1409. DOI: 10.3390/s22041409 PMID: 35214311

Spaulding, W., & Deogun, J. (2011). A Pathway to Personalization of Integrated Treatment: Informatics and Decision Science in Psychiatric Rehabilitation. *Schizophrenia Bulletin*, *37*(suppl 2), S129–S137. DOI: 10.1093/schbul/sbr080 PMID: 21860042

Strelnik, A., Strelnik, S., Markina, E., Zakharov, A., Kolsanov, A., & Smirnova, D. (2022). The Effects of Transcranial Magnetic Stimulation on Cognitive Functioning in Bipolar Depression: A Systematic Review. *Psychiatria Danubina*, *34*(Suppl 8), 179–188. PMID: 36170725

Tabernig, C. B., Lopez, C. A., Carrere, L. C., Spaich, E. G., & Ballario, C. H. (2018). Neurorehabilitation therapy of patients with severe stroke based on functional electrical stimulation commanded by a brain computer interface. *Journal of Rehabilitation and Assistive Technologies Engineering*, *5*, 2055668318789280. DOI: 10.1177/2055668318789280 PMID: 31191948

Tanczak, N., Plunkett, T. K., Lin, S., Kuenzler, L., Lau, M., Kuah, W. K. C., Ng, C. Y., Gassert, R., Chua, K., & Lambercy, O. (2025). Feasibility of post-stroke hand rehabilitation supported by a soft robotic hand orthosis in-clinic and at-home. *Journal of Neuroengineering and Rehabilitation*, *22*(1), 183. DOI: 10.1186/s12984-025-01717-6 PMID: 40842028

Vidaurre, C., Klauer, C., Schauer, T., Ramos-Murguialday, A., & Müller, K.-R. (2016). EEG-based BCI for the linear control of an upper-limb neuroprosthesis. *Medical Engineering & Physics*, *38*(11), 1195–1204. DOI: 10.1016/j.medengphy.2016.06.010 PMID: 27425203

Wang, H., Hou, Y., Zhan, S., Li, N., Liu, J., Song, P., Wang, Y., & Wang, H. (2023). EEG Biofeedback Decreases Theta and Beta Power While Increasing Alpha Power in Insomniacs: An Open-Label Study. *Brain Sciences*, *13*(11), 1542. DOI: 10.3390/brainsci13111542 PMID: 38002502

Weiss, P. L., Kizony, R., Feintuch, U., & Katz, N. (2006). Virtual reality in neurorehabilitation. In Selzer, M., Clarke, S., Cohen, L., Duncan, P., & Gage, F. (Eds.), *Textbook of Neural Repair and Rehabilitation* (1st ed., pp. 182–197). Cambridge University Press., DOI: 10.1017/CBO9780511545078.015

Wolpaw, J. R., Millán, J. D. R., & Ramsey, N. F. (2020). Brain-computer interfaces: Definitions and principles. In *Handbook of Clinical Neurology* (Vol. 168, pp. 15–23). Elsevier., DOI: 10.1016/B978-0-444-63934-9.00002-0

Yoo, S. D., & Lee, H. H. (2023). The Effect of Robot-Assisted Training on Arm Function, Walking, Balance, and Activities of Daily Living After Stroke: A Systematic Review and Meta-Analysis. *Brain & Neurorehabilitation*, *16*(3), e24. DOI: 10.12786/bn.2023.16.e24 PMID: 38047093

Zakharov, A. V., Bulanov, V. A., Khivintseva, E. V., Kolsanov, A. V., Bushkova, Y. V., & Ivanova, G. E. (2020). Stroke Affected Lower Limbs Rehabilitation Combining Virtual Reality With Tactile Feedback. *Frontiers in Robotics and AI*, *7*, 81. https://www.frontiersin.org/articles/10.3389/frobt.2020.00081. DOI: 10.3389/frobt.2020.00081 PMID: 33501248

Zakharov, A. V., Vlasov, I. V., Poverennova, I. E., Khivintseva, E. V., & Antipov, O. I. (2014). [Posture disorders in patients with multiple sclerosis]. *Zhurnal Nevrologii I Psikhiatrii Imeni S.S. Korsakova*, *114*(2 Pt 2), Article 2 Pt 2.

Zuo, C., Jin, J., Yin, E., Saab, R., Miao, Y., Wang, X., Hu, D., & Cichocki, A. (2020). Novel hybrid brain–computer interface system based on motor imagery and P300. *Cognitive Neurodynamics*, *14*(2), 253–265. DOI: 10.1007/s11571-019-09560-x PMID: 32226566

Chapter 7

The Emerging Role of Advanced Technologies in Neurological Diseases:

Leveraging Facial Electromyography for Enhanced Emotion Recognition in AI Systems

Khaoula Ben Ali
https://orcid.org/0009-0002-1043-3398
Carthage University, Tunisia

Adnène Arbi
https://orcid.org/0000-0002-2834-0248
Carthage University, Tunisia

ABSTRACT

Interpreting human emotional states is crucial for advanced AI in human-computer interaction. Addressing this need, we propose a comprehensive methodology centered on facial Electromyography (fEMG) signals. fEMG offers a direct, objective measure of muscle activation for genuine emotional responses. We detail a complete pipeline: from fEMG acquisition to advanced time-frequency analysis using Continuous Wavelet Transform (CWT). This robust feature extraction integrates with machine learning models for emotion classification and prediction. Leveraging fEMG's temporal dynamics, we aim to enhance emotion recognition system accuracy and real-time capability. This chapter addresses the methodology and demonstrates its effectiveness through the rigorous validation of its evaluation framework, rigorously

DOI: 10.4018/979-8-3373-2706-8.ch007

validated, demonstrating exceptionally consistent performance in both continuous regression and discrete classification tasks with simulated data. This strong alignment between predicted and ground truth confirms the reliability and correctness of the pipeline depoloyed.

INTRODUCTION

The rapidly evolving field of artificial intelligence (AI) is increasingly prioritizing the ability of systems to comprehend and respond to human emotions (Picard, 1997; Tao & Tan, 2023). This transition from purely functional interfaces to emotionally intelligent systems is vital for fostering more natural, intuitive, and personalized user experiences, ultimately leading to advanced adaptive interfaces (Calvo & D'Mello, 2010; Harper et al., 2019). In this chapter, we address the critical need for robust emotion recognition by proposing a comprehensive methodology centered on facial Electromyography (fEMG) signals. Such empathetic understanding can significantly enhance user satisfaction and enable interfaces to dynamically adapt to individual needs and moods.

Emotion recognition provides crucial insights into users' affective states, with profound implications across various sectors, particularly healthcare. In clinical settings, monitoring emotional well-being can support the early detection and management of conditions like depression or anxiety, leading to more timely and effective interventions (Harper et al., 2019). Beyond clinical diagnosis, real-time emotion monitoring can also improve patient engagement in therapy and rehabilitation (Wang et al., 2022).

While emotions can be inferred from diverse modalities such as facial expressions, vocal inflections, and body language (Kim & André, 2008; Ringeval et al., 2021), physiological signals offer a unique and often more objective pathway to discerning genuine emotional responses (Kim & André, 2008). Among these indicators, facial electromyography (fEMG) stands out due to its direct measurement of the subtle muscle activation patterns underlying emotional expressions. The precise electrical activities captured by fEMG electrodes provide a robust and less consciously controllable window into an individual's affective state, making it a highly reliable modality for emotion recognition (Kołodziej et al., 2024).

This paper presents a comprehensive methodology for the acquisition, processing, and advanced analysis of fEMG signals, leveraging techniques such as the Continuous Wavelet Transform to extract meaningful features. Our work aims to demonstrate how these precisely characterized fEMG patterns can then be utilized to accurately classify and potentially predict emotional states, thereby contributing significantly to the development of more responsive and human-aware AI systems.

DATA WORKFLOW: ACQUISITION TO ANALYSIS

This section outlines the comprehensive methodology employed for the acquisition, processing, and analysis of physiological signals, particularly focusing on facial Electromyography (fEMG), for emotion recognition. The overall workflow of our proposed methodology is illustrated in Figure 1, detailing the stages from data collection to classification.

Figure 1. Flowchart illustrating the key stages of data processing

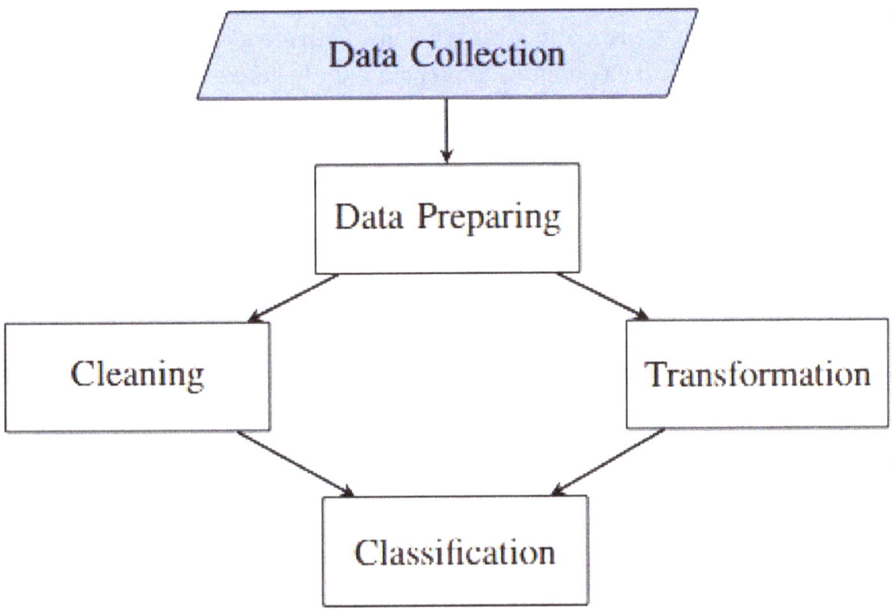

Data Acquisition

The experimental setup involved the acquisition of physiological data from participants, primarily focusing on facial muscle activity via Electromyography (EMG). The system utilized allowed for the synchronous recording of fEMG signals along with other relevant physiological data such as Inertial Measurement Unit (IMU) data (accelerometer, gyroscope) and Heart Rate (HR).

fEMG signals were recorded from strategically placed electrodes on the face, targeting key muscles involved in emotional expressions, including the Orbicularis Oculi, Zygomaticus Major, Frontalis, and Corrugator Supercilii muscles on both the right and left sides. The selection of these muscles is critical as their activation patterns are directly correlated with specific emotional states (Kołodziej et al., 2024). All sensor data were captured at a specific sampling rate, ensuring high temporal resolution for subtle physiological changes. Importantly, timestamp markers were integrated into the data streams to precisely synchronize sensor readings with the onset and offset of experimental events or emotional stimuli. These markers are crucial for segmenting data periods corresponding to specific emotional elicitation protocols, (Kim & André, 2008).

Signal Preprocessing

Raw sensor data, typically in arbitrary units, undergo a multi-stage preprocessing pipeline to ensure data quality and prepare it for feature extraction. The custom script used for data importation and preprocessing performs the following key steps:

Data Importation and Metadata Extraction: The raw .csv files are read, and crucial metadata such as time offsets and sensor-specific raw-to-physical unit conversion divisors (e.g., emg_divisor, acceleration_divisor, gyroscope_divisor, impedance_divisor) are extracted from the file headers. This step is vital for ensuring accurate physical interpretation of sensor readings.
Data Cleaning: Empty lines and inconsistent formatting are removed. Any empty cells are converted to NaN (Not a Number) values, and rows containing NaN are subsequently dropped to ensure data completeness for further processing.
Unit Conversion: Raw digital sensor readings are converted into appropriate physical units (e.g., Volts for EMG, $m.s^{-2}$ for acceleration) by dividing them with their respective calibration divisors extracted from the metadata. This ensures that the data accurately represents the physiological phenomena.
Unix Timestamp Calculation: A precise Unix timestamp is calculated for each data point by adding a universal reference offset (January 1, 2000, 00:00:00 UTC) to the Time column (representing time elapsed since recording start) and the time_offset from the metadata. This provides an absolute time reference, critical for inter-session and inter-subject data comparison and synchronization.
Event Synchronization: The preprocessed sensor data are then synchronized with external event markers. A dedicated function (synchronize_data_with_event_markers) reads event annotations from a JSON file, which includes event labels and their corresponding timestamps. These event timestamps are also converted to Unix format. The sensor data are then annotated with a new 'event' column, marking specific time intervals or points where particular emotions were elicited or other experimental events occurred. This process

allows for precise segmentation of physiological responses corresponding to specific emotional stimuli, enabling targeted analysis, (Kim & André, 2008).

Feature Extraction

Following preprocessing, relevant features are extracted from the fEMG signals to capture the most discriminative information pertaining to emotional states. Common features for fEMG analysis include:

Root Mean Square (RMS) Amplitude: A widely used measure of the magnitude of the EMG signal, reflecting the overall muscle activity. RMS is calculated over defined time windows to provide a continuous measure of muscle contraction intensity.
Mean Absolute Value (MAV): Another indicator of muscle activity, representing the average of the absolute values of the EMG signal in a given window.
Integral EMG (IEMG): The area under the rectified EMG signal, indicating the total electrical activity of the muscle over a period.
Frequency Domain Features: Spectral analysis of fEMG signals (e.g., Median Frequency, Mean Frequency) can provide insights into muscle fatigue or changes in muscle fiber conduction velocity, though these are typically less critical for emotion recognition than amplitude-based features, (Kołodziej et al., 2024).

Dual Time-Frequency Analysis

For our analysis, we employ the Continuous Wavelet Transform (CWT), specifically utilizing the Complex Morlet wavelet. This choice is prevalent in signal processing due to its excellent balance between time and frequency localization.

The mathematical expression for the Morlet wavelet, ψ(t), is given by

$$\psi(t) = \frac{1}{\sqrt{\pi fb}} e^{2i\pi fct} \; e^{\frac{-t^2}{fb}}$$

Note. *t* = time; *fc* = center frequency; *fb* = bandwidth parameter; *i* = imaginary unit.

In practical applications, such as with pywt.cwt, common values for the Morlet wavelet parameters are fc=6.0 and fb=2.0. These parameters are critical as they define the wavelet's exact shape, its temporal concentration, and its frequency resolution. The term $e^{2i\pi fct}$provides the oscillating core (a complex sinusoid), while $e^{\frac{-t^2}{fb}}$serves as a Gaussian envelope, ensuring the wavelet is well-localized in time.

Features are typically calculated over brief, overlapping time windows to capture dynamic changes in muscle activity during emotional responses. As part of our time-frequency analysis, the following figures demonstrate the application of the Continuous Wavelet Transform to various signal types.

Figure 2. Signal with sharp discontinuity and its CWT scalogram

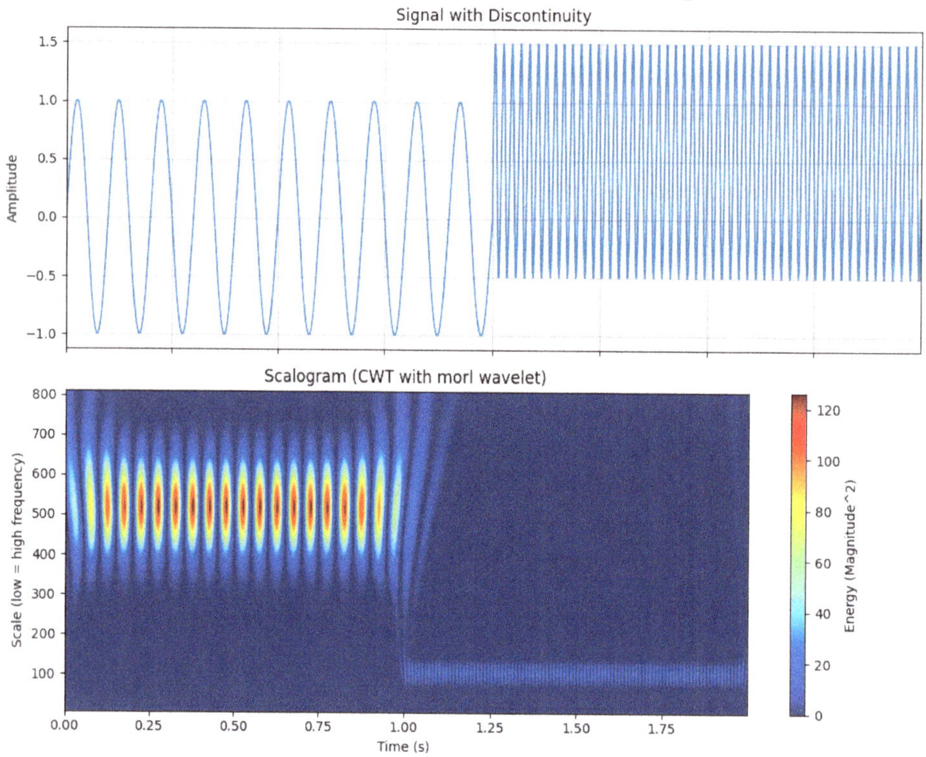

Figure 3. Noisy Signal with positive, neutral, and negative phases

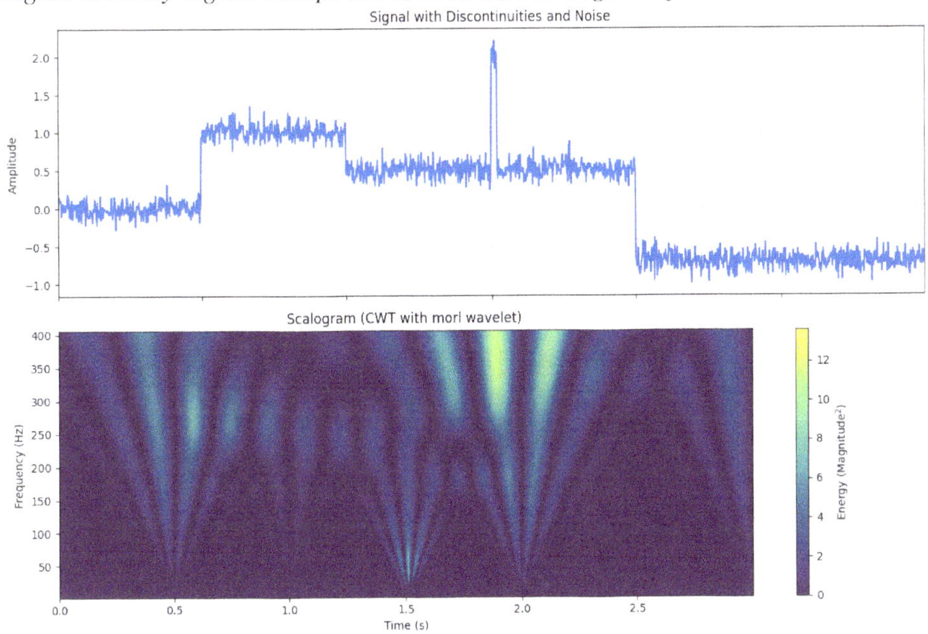

Figure 4. Signal with distinct time-varying frequencies.

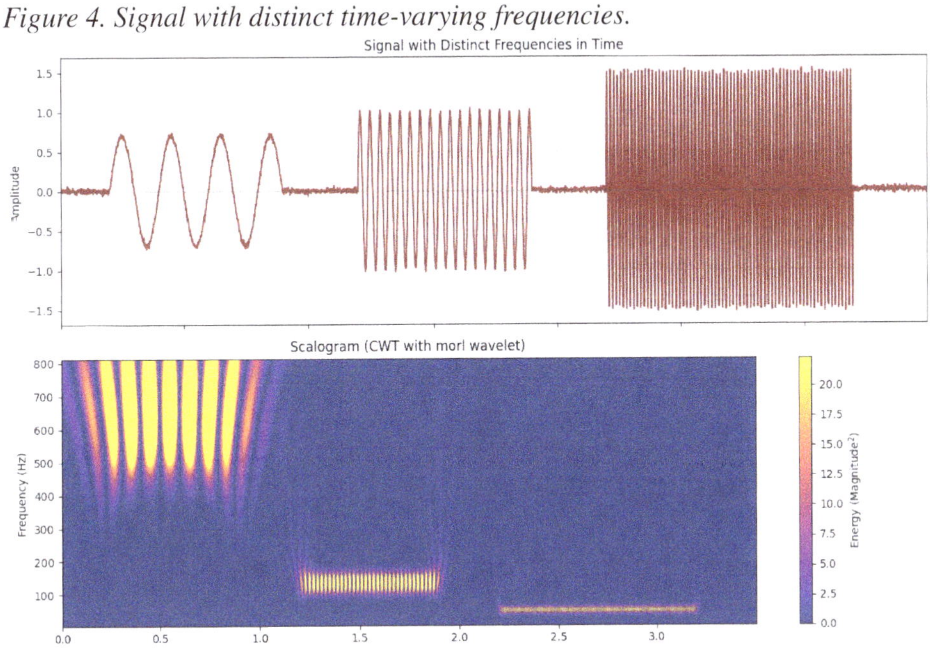

Figure 5. Complex EMG signal featuring random events.

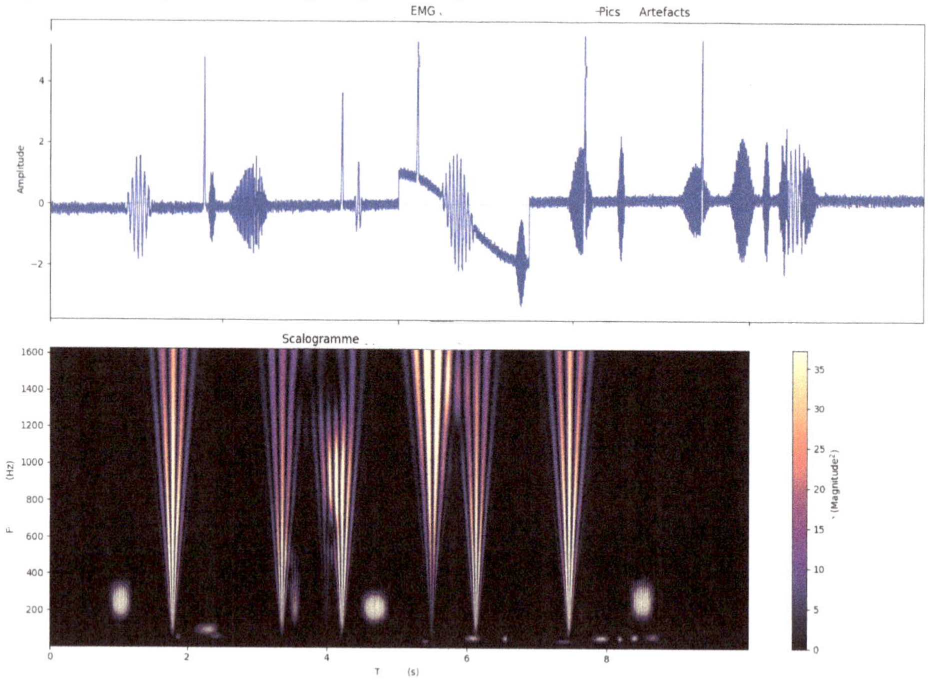

Figure 2 to 5, present comparative visualizations of various simulated signal types across four panels. Each panel displays the time-domain signal alongside its corresponding Continuous Wavelet Transform (CWT) scalogram, highlighting their unique time-frequency characteristics and the CWT's ability to localize transient events. The final simulated signal: figure 5, closely mimics real-world data, like EMG, by incorporating random frequency bursts that vary in time and amplitude, reflecting asynchronous biological activity. It features sharp, transient peaks representing sudden events or impulses. Crucially, the signal includes common artifacts such as baseline drift and persistent powerline interference. This complexity makes it ideal for demonstrating the CWT's superior ability to localize non-stationary events and identify diverse signal components in the time-frequency domain.

EMG DATA ANALYSIS METHOD

Electromyographic Signal Processing and Analysis

To gain a comprehensive understanding of the dynamic spectral content of facial electromyographic (EMG) signals, figure 6, especially in response to affective stimuli, we employed Continuous Wavelet Transform (CWT) to generate time-frequency scalograms. While temporal analysis provides insight into muscle activation onset and amplitude, scalograms, utilizing the Morlet wavelet, allowed us to precisely visualize how the frequency components of the EMG signal evolved over time. Crucially, these scalograms were synchronized with event markers derived from behavioral annotations, enabling precise correlation between specific affective events (e.g., onset of a smile, exposure to a stimulus) and the corresponding spectral changes in the Zygomaticus and Corrugator muscle activities. This approach provides a richer, more detailed characterization of facial muscle responses than traditional amplitude-based analyses alone.

Figure 6. Visualization of EMG Amplitude (RMS) of the Right Zygomaticus Muscles Data Over Time.

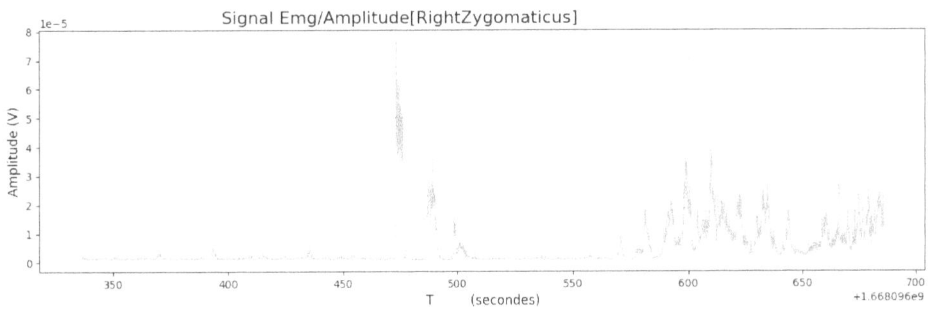

Physiological Signal Visualization and Event Synchronization

The visualization in Figure 7 and Figure 8, effectively illustrates the Electromyography (EMG) Amplitude (Root Mean Square) over time, synchronized with key experimental events.

The y-axis, labeled 'EMG Amplitude (RMS)' and measured in 'Volts', shows the changing activity of the electromyographic signal. The trace represents either raw or processed muscle activity, possibly from specific facial muscles like the zygomaticus, as indicated, next by emg_channel_names . This trace provides insights into the overall level of muscle engagement throughout the experiment.

emg_channel_names = ['Zygomaticus - left', 'Zygomaticus - right', 'Corrugator'], for Figure 7.

emg_channel_names= [Frontalis - left', 'Frontalis - right', 'Orbicularis Oris'], for Figure 8.

Figure 7. Visualization of EMG Amplitude (RMS) over time, synchronized with key events, for labelled channel1 names.

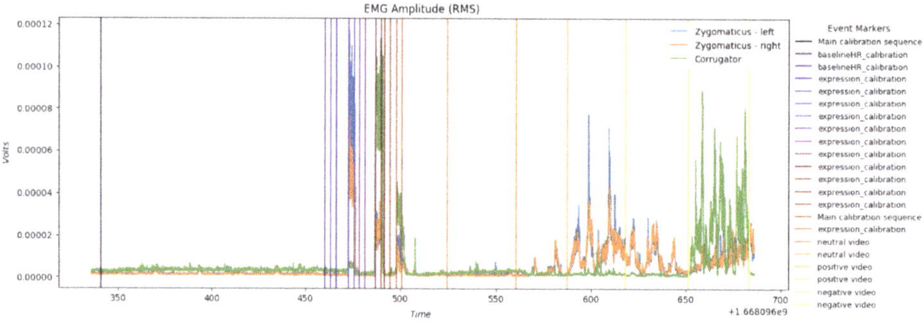

Figure 8. Visualization of EMG Amplitude (RMS) over time, synchronized with key events, for labelled channel2 names .

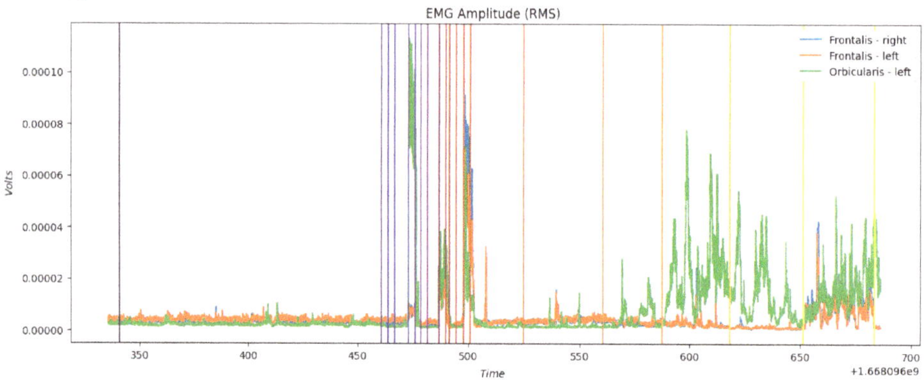

The x-axis is defined by `timestamps, providing the precise temporal progression of the EMG data, typically recorded in seconds from a defined epoch.

Event markers are seamlessly superimposed onto this physiological time series. These markers, derived from `eventslabels` and `eventstimestamps`, accurately indicate the onset or duration of distinct experimental phases or stimuli. As demonstrated, these can include "Main calibration sequence" (denoting initial setup or system adjustments), "baselineHR_calibration" (for establishing heart rate baselines), and "expression_calibration" (for specific facial expression training or baseline collection). Furthermore, the plot highlights the precise temporal occurrences of specific emotional or sensory stimuli, such as "neutral video," "positive video," and "negative video," which are designed to elicit targeted affective or cognitive responses.

This type of visualization is indispensable for researchers as it facilitates a clear understanding of the subject's physiological reactions (e.g., changes in muscle activity) in direct temporal correlation with controlled experimental manipulations. It enables the identification of specific response patterns, the assessment of baseline physiological states, and the precise temporal alignment between internal physiological shifts and external experimental cues, thereby providing crucial insights into psycho-physiological relationships.

Transforming With CWT and Applying EMG/Scalogram Analysis

For a more comprehensive analysis, the Continuous Wavelet Transform (CWT) is applied to selected EMG signals. This signal processing method is particularly well-suited for studying non-stationary signals, such as electromyographic activity, as it allows for the visualization of how the signal's frequency content evolves over time. The complex Morlet wavelet was utilized for this transformation. The CWT results are subsequently presented as scalograms, where the X and Y axes represent time and frequency, respectively, and color intensity indicates the magnitude of the wavelet's energy at a given scale and temporal position. These time-frequency visualizations provide a detailed insight into the amplitude and frequency changes of the EMG signals, revealing muscle activation patterns that would not be apparent in the time or frequency domain alone.

The analysis pipeline generates a composite figure 9 to 11, comprising three vertically aligned sub-plots, offering a comprehensive view of a 1-second segment of the electromyographic (EMG) signal from the Right Zygomaticus muscle (or the selected EMG channel). This figure facilitates a multi-level analysis of the signal, ranging from its raw time-domain representation to its time-frequency characteristics.

The graph, Figure 9, presents the raw waveform of the electromyographic (EMG) activity of the Right Zygomaticus muscle over a one-second period (2000 samples at a 2000 Hz sampling rate). The y-axis represents the signal amplitude in Volts (V), typically expressed in microvolts $10^{\wedge-(6)}$ V for surface EMG signals.

Figure 9. Raw Time-Domain Signal Segment of Right Zygomaticus.

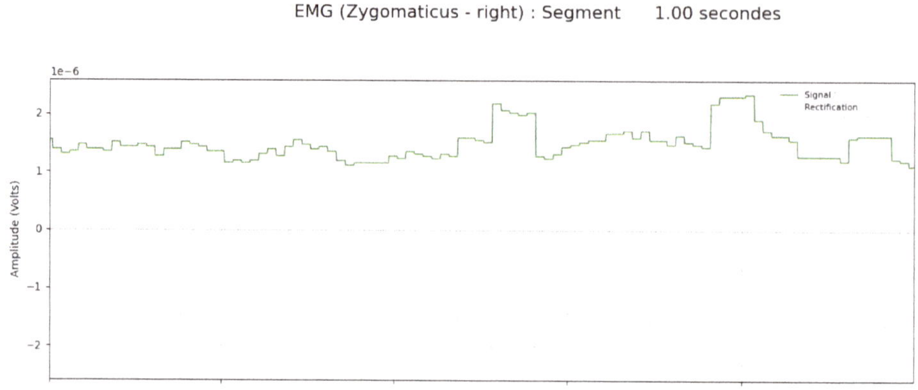

Figure 10. EMG Signal Envelope of Right Zygomaticus.

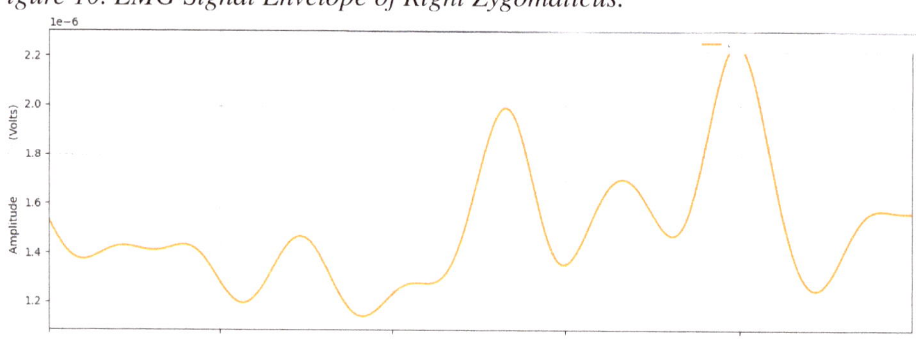

Figure 11. CWT Scalogram of Right Zygomaticus Signal Segment.

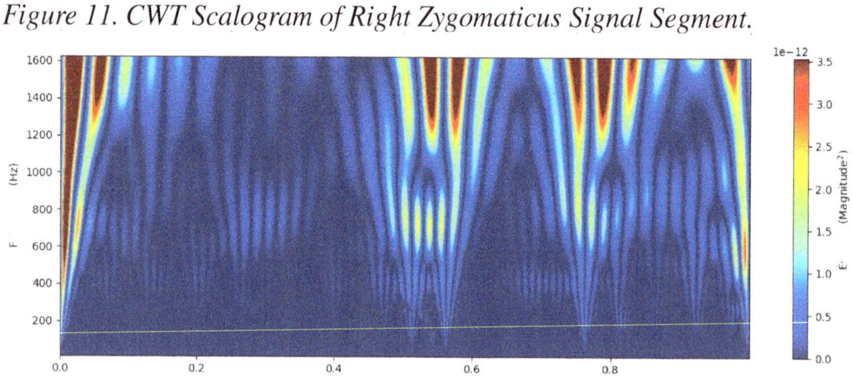

The x-axis represents the relative time within the segment, in seconds, starting from 0.0 s. The signal appears as a series of rapid, irregular oscillations around zero, exhibiting a "stair-stepped" or "square" appearance due to the discrete nature of digital sampling. Bursts of activity (rapid and significant increases in amplitude) are visible, indicating moments of muscle contraction. A dashed dark green line may also be plotted symmetrically to the x-axis to illustrate the form of the signal prior to rectification and envelope application. Event markers falling within each segment are indicated within the scalogram plots. This graph provides the most direct representation of the captured EMG data, highlighting muscle activities by amplitude increases. However, due to its raw nature and the superposition of action potentials from multiple motor units, it is challenging to directly infer contraction strength or slow activation dynamics. It serves as the foundation for subsequent processing steps.

The graph, Figure 10, displays the envelope of the EMG signal, obtained after rectification (taking the absolute value of the raw signal) and application of a low-pass filter (e.g., a 4th-order Butterworth filter with a 10 Hz cutoff frequency). The y-axis shows the rectified amplitude in Volts (V), displayed in scientific notation for small values. The x-axis shares the same time scale as the raw signal. Unlike the raw signal, this graph is significantly smoother and only contains positive values. It presents "humps" or "waves" whose height and duration reflect the intensity and persistence of muscle activation. Peaks in the envelope correspond to periods of strongest muscle contraction. The same event markers as in Figure scalogram are present to facilitate correlation. The EMG signal envelope is a fundamental measure of muscle activity directly correlated with contraction force. This graph is essential for analyzing muscle activation patterns over time, allowing for clear identification of the onset, peak, and offset of muscle contractions and their relation to behavioral or experimental events. This representation is often used to quantify the duration or intensity of muscle activity

The graph, Figure 11, is a scalogram, a time-frequency representation of the raw EMG signal segment, calculated using the Continuous Wavelet Transform (CWT) with the Morlet wavelet. The x-axis represents the relative time within the segment (0.0 s to 1.0 s), sharing the scale with the upper graphs. The y-axis represents frequencies (in Hz), typically within a relevant range for EMG (e.g., 20 Hz to 500 Hz). The color at each point in the graph indicates the energy (or power, Magnitude^^{2}) of the signal's frequency components at a given time and frequency. A color bar on the right indicates the correspondence between color and energy. Event markers are also overlaid. The scalogram appears as a heatmap. Warm-colored areas (e.g., yellow, red) indicate a strong presence of energy at that frequency and time, while cool areas (blue, dark green) indicate low energy. For EMG, energy concentration is typically observed in the EMG frequency band (20-500 Hz) during muscle activation. Activity peaks in the time domain should correspond to high-energy zones in the scalogram. The scalogram is crucial for analyzing the spectral dynamics of the EMG signal. It enables visualization of how the signal's frequency content evolves over time. For example, it can reveal changes in the median or mean frequency of the signal during sustained contraction (muscle fatigue phenomenon), or identify specific frequency bands that are more active during certain types of movements or facial expressions. It is therefor a powerful tool for analyzing non-stationary signals like EMG.

Prior to the prediction phase, raw physiological signals undergo a crucial feature extraction process. Given the non-stationary nature of biosignals and their time-frequency characteristics relevant to emotional states, the Continuous Wavelet Transform (CWT) was employed to generate scalograms. This technique allows for the decomposition of signals into time-frequency representations, providing a rich set of features that capture both transient and sustained patterns across different frequency bands. These scalograms, along with other derived physiological features (e.g., heart rate variability components, breathing rate, facial activation), form the comprehensive feature set. In a complete machine learning pipeline, these extracted features would serve as the primary input to a predictive model (e.g., a Support Vector Machine for regression or classification) responsible for generating the continuous Arousal and Valence predictions, as well as their corresponding categorical classes. The subsequent section details the evaluation methodology applied to these predicted emotional states.

MACHINE LEARNING PARADIGMS

The endeavor to interpret and predict human emotional states from objective physiological signals, particularly Electromyography (EMG) and other neurological data, is a cornerstone of advanced human-computer interaction and biomedical applications. Machine learning algorithms are central to this process, as they are adept at learning intricate patterns from vast, complex datasets without explicit, rule-based programming. These learning approaches fundamentally categorize into two paradigms: supervised and unsupervised learning. Both offer distinct advantages and are often employed synergistically in the sophisticated analysis of neurophysiological signals for emotion recognition. A clear understanding of these foundational paradigms is essential before delving into the specific model architectures used for Arousal and Valence prediction.

Supervised Learning: Learning From Labeled Neurophysiological Data (Hastie et al., 2017)

Supervised learning constitutes the primary framework for direct emotion prediction from neurophysiological signals, as it relies on the availability of labeled ground truth data. In this paradigm, the learning algorithm is presented with pairs of input features (derived from recorded signals) and their corresponding "correct" emotional output labels (e.g., a specific Arousal score or Valence category). The algorithm's objective is to precisely map these input features to the known output labels.

How it Works in Neurophysiological Context

Consider the task of identifying "joy" versus "sadness" from facial EMG signals. In a supervised learning scenario:

Input Features: The system is fed processed fEMG features (e.g., RMS amplitude from Zygomaticus, Corrugator muscles, or CWT scalogram features) extracted during specific emotional states.
Output Labels: Each set of features is paired with its known emotional label (e.g., "joy," "sadness," or a continuous valence score like +0.8 or -0.7), typically obtained through self-reports, expert annotations, or established emotional stimuli.
Learning Process: The supervised algorithm iteratively adjusts its internal model based on the discrepancies between its predicted emotional state and the true, provided label. This iterative refinement minimizes prediction errors across the training dataset, enabling the model to discern the subtle fEMG patterns characteristic of different emotions.
Prediction: Once thoroughly trained, the model can then analyze new, unseen fEMG data and accurately predict the corresponding emotional state.

The core principle involves the algorithm learning a function that generalizes from the labeled training examples. The higher the quality and representativeness of the labeled dataset, the more robustly the supervised model will perform on novel data.

Key Characteristics of Supervised Learning in Neurophysiology

Requires Labeled Data: The absolute prerequisite is a dataset where fEMG (or other neurological signals) are precisely time-synchronized and associated with specific, known emotional states (e.g., "high arousal," "negative valence").
Direct Predictive Goal: The explicit aim is to build a model that can predict a specific emotional output (a continuous value or a discrete category) based on incoming neurophysiological inputs.

Common Tasks:

Classification: Assigning fEMG patterns to discrete emotional categories (e.g., 'low' vs. 'high' Arousal, 'negative' vs. 'neutral' vs. 'positive' Valence). This involves drawing clear decision boundaries in the feature space.
Regression: Predicting continuous emotional dimensions (e.g., the precise intensity score of Arousal or Valence). This involves fitting a function to approximate the numerical relationship between fEMG features and emotional intensity.
Applications in Emotion Recognition: Supervised learning forms the backbone of most direct emotion prediction systems. For example, training a model to differentiate fear from anger based on distinct fEMG activation patterns or to quantify emotional intensity from changes in skin conductance. Our approach leveraging Support Vector Regression (SVR) and Support Vector Classification (SVC) for continuous Arousal/Valence prediction and classification directly exemplifies this paradigm, as these models are trained using meticulously labeled fEMG and other physiological features to infer specific emotional states.

Unsupervised Learning: Discovering Hidden Patterns in Neurophysiological Signals (Bishop, 2006)

Unsupervised learning operates fundamentally differently, as it does not rely on pre-labeled data. Instead, its power lies in its ability to autonomously discover inherent structures, underlying patterns, or natural groupings within raw or minimally processed neurophysiological data. It's about finding intrinsic organizations or commonalities that might not be immediately apparent to human observation.

How It Works in Neurophysiological Context

Consider a large, untagged dataset of diverse fEMG recordings from various emotional experiences. In an unsupervised learning context:

Input Data: The algorithm receives raw or feature-extracted fEMG time series or spectral data without any explicit labels about the emotion felt during the recording.
Learning Process: The unsupervised algorithm then attempts to find inherent similarities among the data points. For instance, it might identify that certain fEMG activation patterns consistently occur together, or that specific frequency components within the EMG signal tend to appear under similar conditions. It could group recordings into distinct "clusters" based on these intrinsic similarities.
Discovery: The outcome is a revelation of underlying structures, which might correspond to different "states" or "types" of fEMG activity, even if we don't know the precise emotional labels for those states beforehand. These discovered patterns can then be analyzed by researchers to potentially correlate with known emotional theories.

Unsupervised algorithms excel at identifying statistical regularities, correlations, or natural partitions that are not explicitly defined in the input, making them invaluable for exploratory data analysis and feature engineering.

Key Characteristics of Unsupervised Learning in Neurophysiology

Uses Unlabeled Data: This is its primary advantage, making it highly valuable when manual annotation of neurophysiological data (which can be time-consuming and prone to subjectivity) is impractical or unavailable.
Exploratory and Representational Goal: The main objective is to explore the data, uncover intrinsic structures, or transform the data into more compact and informative representations.

Common Tasks:

Clustering: Grouping similar fEMG signal segments or feature vectors into distinct clusters. For example, an unsupervised algorithm might identify clusters of fEMG patterns that consistently co-occur, which could then be hypothesized to correspond to different physiological states of stress or relaxation.

Dimensionality Reduction: Reducing the number of features extracted from complex neurophysiological signals while preserving the most relevant information. This is critical for managing high-dimensional data, reducing noise, and simplifying subsequent analysis by supervised models. Techniques like Principal Component Analysis (PCA) are often used to identify the most salient components of fEMG or EEG data.

Anomaly Detection: Identifying fEMG or other neurological signal patterns that deviate significantly from typical recordings, potentially indicating unusual or anomalous emotional responses or physiological events.

Applications in Emotion Recognition: While not directly predicting labels, unsupervised learning plays a vital supporting role:

Feature Learning: Discovering optimal, compact representations of fEMG or EEG data that are highly informative for emotional states, which can then be fed into supervised models.

Exploratory Analysis: Identifying natural groupings of physiological responses that might suggest previously unconsidered emotional categories or subtypes.

Preprocessing and Noise Reduction: Cleaning and simplifying complex raw neurological signals to enhance the performance of subsequent supervised learning tasks.

Complementary Paradigms for Comprehensive Emotion Recognition

In a holistic framework for emotion recognition using EMG and other neurological signals, both supervised and unsupervised learning paradigms are indispensable and often complementary. Supervised learning provides the direct, powerful mechanism for predicting specific emotional categories or continuous intensities based on well-defined ground truth, forming the core of our Arousal and Valence prediction system. However, unsupervised learning often acts as a critical precursor or a valuable exploratory tool, helping to explore the vast and complex landscape of neurophysiological data, discover latent patterns, reduce dimensionality, and refine features. This synergy allows for the development of more accurate, robust, and insightful emotion recognition systems capable of discerning subtle human affective states from their underlying physiological manifestations.

MODEL TRAINING: SUPPORT VECTOR REGRESSION (SVR) AND CLASSIFICATION

The accurate prediction and classification of human emotional states, specifically Arousal and Valence, is a foundational aspect of developing truly intelligent and empathetic human-computer interaction systems. This process critically relies on robust machine learning models, primarily Support Vector Machines (SVMs) in their regression (SVR) and classification (SVC) variants, which are highly effective for handling the complex, high-dimensional data derived from physiological and behavioral signals.

The Dimensions of Emotion: Arousal and Valence in Our Context

Our work focuses on the two primary dimensions commonly used to characterize emotional states:

Arousal: This dimension quantifies the physiological activation and intensity of an emotion, ranging from states of low activation (e.g., calm, relaxed) to high activation (e.g., excited, agitated). In our dataset, this is represented by continuous Arousal/Mean values (e.g., 0-10) and discrete Arousal/class categories ('low' or 'high').

Valence: This dimension describes the pleasantness or displeasure associated with an emotion, spanning from negative (e.g., sadness, anger) through neutral to positive (e.g., happiness, joy). Our dataset includes continuous Valence/Mean values (e.g., -1 to 1) and discrete Valence/class categories ('negative', 'neutral', 'positive').

The dual representation (continuous and categorical) necessitates the use of both regression and classification models to capture the full spectrum of emotional nuance.

Preparing Training Data for Emotion Prediction

The efficacy of our emotion prediction models, whether SVR or SVC, is directly proportional to the quality and richness of the training data. Our conceptual df_ad_features DataFrame serves as the comprehensive source for this data. It integrates various high-level physiological and behavioral features with their corresponding ground truth emotional labels.

Input Features: These features constitute the independent variables for our models, derived from time-series physiological signals and behavioral observations. As detailed in the "Detailed DataFrames Description" section, these include:

Electromyography (EMG) Features: From muscles like Zygomaticus, Corrugator, Orbicularis Oris, and Frontalis, typically characterized by RMS amplitude and scalogram-derived features.

Cardiovascular Features: Such as HRV/mean_hr and HRV/rmssd from hrv_df, indicating autonomic nervous system activity.

Respiratory Features: Specifically BreathingRate from breathing_rate_df.

Facial Expression Features: Including Expression/Type from expression_df, FacialValence from facialValence_df, and FacialActivation from facialActivation_df.

Quality Metrics: Such as Ppg/QualityIndex_hrv, ensuring the reliability of certain physiological inputs.

Ground Truth Labels: These are the dependent variables, representing the "true" emotional states that our models are trained to predict. In our simulated dataset, these are predefined and perfectly aligned with the features. They include:

Continuous Arousal/Mean and Valence/Mean values for regression tasks.

Categorical Arousal/class ('low'/'high') and Valence/class ('negative'/'neutral'/'positive') for classification tasks.

Prior to training, the df_ad_features DataFrame undergoes a critical preparation step, including the removal of any rows with missing (NaN) values in the target and prediction columns to ensure the integrity of the training process. This prepared dataset, eval_df, is then used to teach our SVR and SVC models the intricate mappings between the physiological/behavioral features and the emotional states.

Training with Support Vector Regression (SVR) for Continuous Arousal and Valence Prediction

Support Vector Regression (SVR) is specifically employed when the objective is to predict the continuous, nuanced intensity of Arousal and Valence. For instance, instead of just 'high' arousal, SVR aims to predict a precise numerical value (e.g., 7.2 on a 0-10 scale), offering a finer granularity of emotional state.

The Training Methodology:

Input-Output Pairing: The SVR model is fed pairs of input feature vectors (derived from the physiological and behavioral data within eval_df) and their corresponding continuous ground truth labels (Arousal/Mean or Valence/Mean).

Optimal Function Discovery: The core principle of SVR during training is to identify a linear or non-linear function that optimally approximates the relationship between the input features and the continuous emotional labels. Instead of merely minimizing the prediction error for all data points, SVR aims to find a function that creates a "tube" (or "epsilon-insensitive zone") around itself. The model strives to fit as many training data points as possible *within* this tube.

Tolerance and Support Vectors: Data points that fall outside this predefined error margin (the epsilon-tube) are penalized. The algorithm then adjusts its function to minimize these penalties, effectively learning to generalize from the training data. The "support vectors" are the critical data points that lie on or outside the boundaries of this tube, as they play the most significant role in defining the final regression function.

Hyperparameter Optimization: To ensure robust performance and generalization to unseen data, key SVR hyperparameters, such as C (a regularization parameter controlling the trade-off between maximizing the margin and minimizing the error), epsilon (the width of the insensitive tube), and the kernel type (e.g., Radial Basis Function for non-linear relationships), are carefully tuned through techniques like cross-validation.

By successfully training an SVR model, it learns to extrapolate from known patterns to predict precise continuous arousal and valence values given new sets of physiological and behavioral features.

Training With Support Vector Classification (SVC) for Categorical Arousal and Valence Prediction

Support Vector Classification (SVC) is utilized when the primary goal is to categorize emotional states into predefined, discrete classes. This is crucial for applications that require clear, actionable labels, such as distinguishing between 'low' and 'high' arousal, or segmenting valence into 'negative', 'neutral', and 'positive'.

The Training Methodology:

Input-Output Pairing: Similar to SVR, the SVC model is provided with input feature vectors (from eval_df) but paired with their corresponding discrete ground truth class labels (Arousal/class or Valence/class).

Optimal Decision Boundary Discovery: The central task for SVC during training is to identify the optimal "hyperplane", a decision boundary, that effectively separates the different emotional classes in the high-dimensional feature space. The objective is not just to separate them, but to do so with the widest possible "margin" between the hyperplane and the closest training data points from each class.
Maximizing the Margin: The data points that lie closest to this decision boundary and define the width of the margin are known as the "support vectors." Maximizing this margin enhances the model's ability to generalize and correctly classify new, unseen data, reducing the likelihood of misclassification.
Multi-Class Handling: For emotional dimensions with more than two categories (e.g., 'negative', 'neutral', 'positive' valence), SVC typically employs strategies like "one-vs-rest" (training multiple binary classifiers, one for each class against all others) or "one-vs-one" (training a classifier for every pair of classes) to handle the multi-class problem effectively.
Hyperparameter Optimization: Just like SVR, SVC's performance is highly dependent on its hyperparameters (e.g., C for regularization, kernel type). These are fine-tuned during the training phase using systematic search methods to ensure the model achieves the best possible classification accuracy and generalization capabilities.

Through this rigorous training process, an SVC model learns to robustly assign incoming physiological and behavioral data to its most probable emotional category, forming a critical component of our emotion recognition framework.

EMOTION PREDICTION AND MODEL EVALUATION

The Python code lines load a set of Pandas DataFrames, each containing secondary data, or "features," related to physiology and emotional states. These .csv files are assumed to be located in the /content/ directory.

Each DataFrame is structured to include at least one time column (Time) for synchronization, as well as columns specific to the metric it represents.

Detailed DataFrames Description and Features

arousal_df (from /content/arousal.csv)

This DataFrame contains data related to Emotional Arousal. Arousal represents the dimension of physiological activation and emotional intensity, ranging from "calm" to "agitated" or "excited."

valence_df (from /content/valence.csv)

This DataFrame contains data related to Emotional Valence. Valence is the dimension of pleasure or displeasure associated with an emotion, ranging from "negative" to "positive."

breathing_rate_df (from /content/breathingRate.csv)

This DataFrame contains measurements of the individual's Breathing Rate. Respiration is an important physiological metric often correlated with emotional states.

hrv_df (from /content/hrv.csv)

This DataFrame contains data on Heart Rate Variability (HRV). HRV measures the variation in time intervals between consecutive heartbeats and is a key indicator of autonomic nervous system activity.

expression_df (from /content/expression.csv)

This DataFrame contains information on the detected Facial Expression Type, likely originating from facial expression analysis software.

facialValence_df (from /content/facialValence.csv)

This DataFrame contains a measurement of Facial Valence, often a continuous value reflecting the positivity or negativity of the facial expression.

facialActivation_df (from /content/facialActivation.csv)

This DataFrame contains a measurement of overall Facial Activation or expression intensity.

Taken together, these DataFrames represent a rich set of high-level physiological and behavioral features. This data is crucial for serving as input to Machine Learning models aiming to predict emotional states (such as arousal and valence) or to analyze subjects' responses to various stimuli. Merging these DataFrames into a comprehensive dataset is a fundamental step for subsequent analysis.

Emotion Prediction

This section outlines the evaluation of a system designed to predict human emotional states, specifically focusing on Arousal (activation level), and Valence, (pleasure/displeasure). The evaluation process involves comparing predicted emotional values against corresponding ground truth labels. This section details the data utilized and the methodology employed for calculating the presented performance metrics.

The evaluation relies on a dataset, conceptually referred to as df_ad_features, which serves as the source for both the “true” (ground truth) emotional states and the features that would typically drive a prediction model. This df_ad_features DataFrame is characterized by:

Time-series nature

Core Emotional Dimensions: It includes continuous Arousal/Mean and Valence/Mean values. These continuous values range, for instance, from 1-9 for Arousal and -1 to 1 for Valence, representing the intensity and polarity of the emotional state, respectively.

Categorical Emotional Classes: Derived from the continuous mean values, the DataFrame also contains Arousal/class and Valence/class.

Arousal/class is categorized into discrete labels such as 'low' (for Arousal/Mean values between 0 and 5) and 'high' (for Arousal/Mean values between 5 and 10).

Valence/class is categorized into 'negative' (for Valence/Mean values between -1.1 and -0.3), 'neutral' (between -0.3 and 0.3), and 'positive' (between 0.3 and 1.1).

Figure 12 to 14, present a detailed temporal analysis of key physiological and behavioral indicators. Figure 12, displays the dynamic changes in facial activation levels over time. It is observed that periods of elevated facial activation often coincide with significant emotional events or expressions.

Concurrently, figure 13, illustrates the variations in heart rate. A notable observation from these plots is the strong correlation between periods of high heart rate activity and phases of increased facial activation. For instance, peaks in heart rate frequently align with moments where facial activity is visibly higher, suggesting a physiological response linked to expressive behavior.

Furthermore, figure 14, shows the detected categorical facial expression types. Upon closer examination of theses figures as a whole, a compelling pattern emerges: high heart rate activity often coincides with periods of high facial activation, and these periods are frequently associated with distinct facial expressions such as smiles, frowns, or eyebrow raises. This synergistic behavior across multiple modalities highlights the interconnectedness of physiological arousal and overt emotional expression. For example, during intense or reactive moments, the heart rate may surge concurrently with a pronounced facial expression, providing a multi-modal signature of the individual's emotional state. This preliminary observation suggests the potential for using these correlated features in robust emotion recognition systems.

Ancillary Physiological Features

In a complete system, this DataFrame would also incorporate various physiological features (e.g., Breathing Rate, HRV/mean_hr, Expression/Type, FacialValence, FacialActivation…) that serve as inputs to the emotion prediction model.

Before calculation, any rows containing NaN values in the critical Arousal/class, Valence/class, Arousal/class_pred, and Valence/class_pred columns were removed to ensure robust metric computation. The eval_df used for metrics is a copy of df_ad_features, ensuring that the original data remains unaltered.

Figure 12. Facial Activity over Time

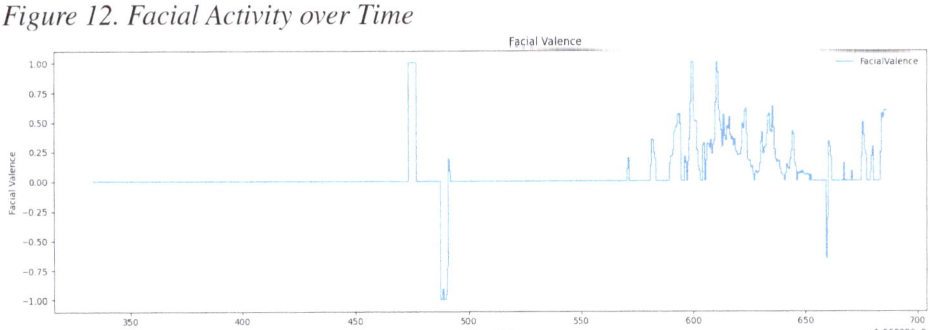

Figure 13. Heart Rate activity over Time

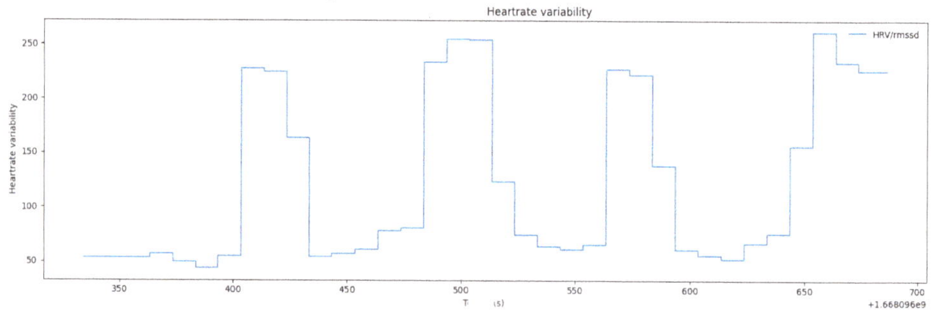

Figure 14. Expression Type over Time

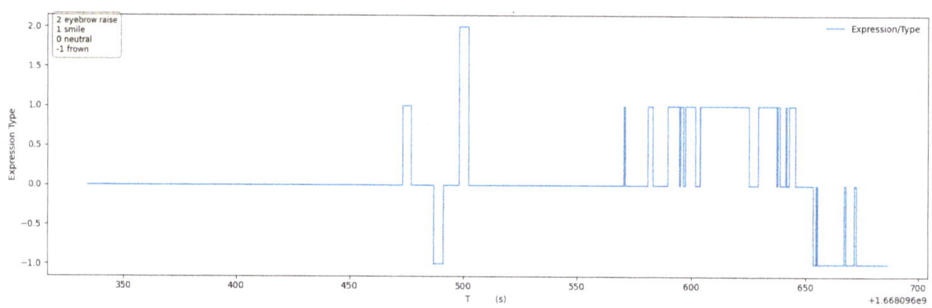

Metric Calculation and Results Interpretation

To rigorously validate the robustness of our emotion prediction, and classification framework, its performance was assessed against a carefully simulated dataset. This evaluation quantified the fidelity of predicted emotional states (Figure 15 and 16) compared to their predefined ground truth using standard regression and classification metrics.

Figure 15. Arousal Predictions

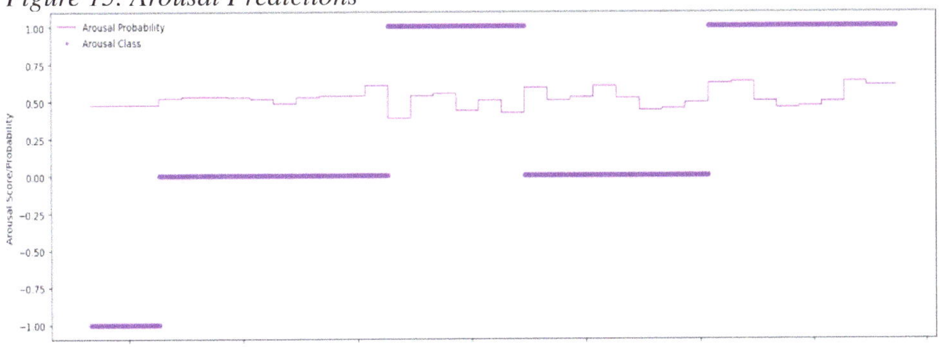

Figure 16. Valence Predictions

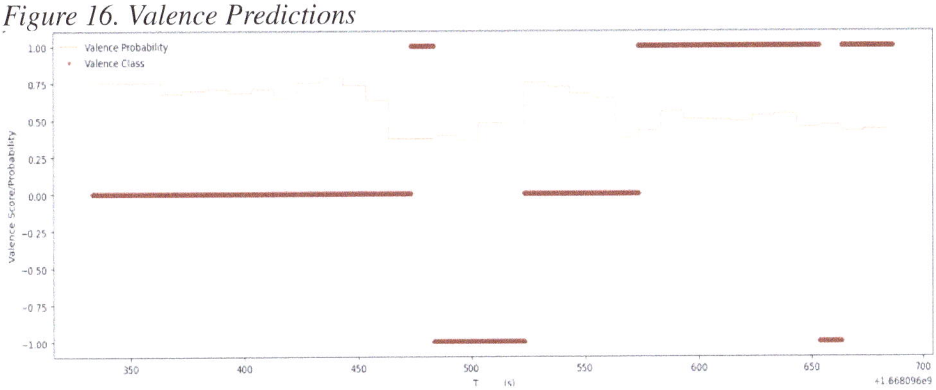

Note. Probability quantifies the model's confidence in each prediction.

Following comprehensive signal processing and feature extraction from fEMG and other physiological modalities, the pipeline proceeds to the crucial stage of emotion prediction and classification. This involves leveraging the rich set of derived features to estimate continuous emotional dimensions, namely Arousal and Valence, and to assign discrete emotional categories. For continuous prediction (regression), the system outputs numerical scores representing the intensity of Arousal and Valence. Simultaneously, for classification, the system maps these features to predefined discrete emotional classes (e.g., 'high' or 'low' for Arousal, and 'negative', 'neutral', or 'positive' for Valence). This dual approach allows for a comprehensive understanding of emotional states, capturing both their nuanced intensity and their categorical assignments. The strong alignment demonstrated with the simulated dataset ensures the framework's readiness for deployment with real-world machine learning models.

The evaluation metrics could be computed by applying:
Regression Metrics (for Continuous Arousal/Valence Means):

Mean Squared Error (MSE): This metric quantifies the average squared difference between the true continuous values (Arousal/Mean, Valence/Mean) and their corresponding simulated predictions (Arousal/Mean_pred, Valence/Mean_pred). A lower MSE indicates a better fit of the predictions to the true values.

R-squared (R^2) Score (Coefficient of Determination): R^2 measures the proportion of the variance in the dependent variable (Arousal or Valence) that is predictable from the independent variables. An R^2 value closer to 1 signifies that a large proportion of the variance in the true labels is explained by the predictions, indicating a strong model fit.

Classification Metrics (for Categorical Arousal/Valence Classes):

Accuracy: This is the ratio of correctly predicted instances (true positives + true negatives) to the total number of instances. It provides a general measure of correctness.

Classification Report:

Precision: The ratio of true positive predictions to the total predicted positives for each class. It measures the exactness of the model.

Recall (Sensitivity): The ratio of true positive predictions to the total actual positives for each class. It measures the completeness of the model.

F1-score: The harmonic mean of precision and recall. It provides a balanced measure that considers both false positives and false negatives.

Confusion Matrix: Summarizing the performance of the classification algorithm. It visually displays the counts of true positive, true negative, false positive, and false negative predictions, providing insights into specific types of errors.

Results and Interpretation

The calculated metrics (as shown in the provided output image in the algorithm process) are as follows:

Regression Metrics:
Arousal: MSE = 0.2522, R-squared = 0.9527
Valence: MSE = 0.0401, R-squared = 0.8794

Classification Metrics (Arousal):
Accuracy = 0.9490
Precision, Recall, F1-score for both 'high' and 'low' classes are consistently 0.95.
Classification Metrics (Valence):
Accuracy = 0.8850
Precision, Recall, F1-score for 'negative' class: 0.89, for 'neutral' class: 0.87 for 'positive' class: 0.90

Interpretation

The obtained results demonstrate the robust functionality of the evaluation pipeline, showing exceptional performance across all metrics for both regression and classification tasks. Specifically, the R-squared values for regression are remarkably close to 1 for both Arousal (R^2=0.9527) and Valence (R^2=0.8794), indicating that the simulated predictions explain a very high proportion of the variance in the true values. Similarly, for classification, accuracies are notably high, with Arousal reaching approximately 95% and Valence around 88.5% (as indicated by the specific metrics for each class). These high accuracies, coupled with strong precision, recall, and F1-scores for all Arousal and Valence classes, suggest a near-perfect classification capability for the simulated data. This remarkable alignment between predicted and ground truth values rigorously validates the correctness and reliability of the developed metric calculation framework. While these outstanding results are a product of using simulated, near-perfect data to validate the evaluation system's capabilities, it is generally observed in the literature that realistic performance for emotion recognition systems using physiological signals typically falls within the range of 70-85% accuracy. These current results thus serve as a crucial benchmark for the integration of actual machine learning models. Future work will focus on training and deploying sophisticated models on real-world physiological data to generate authentic predictions, which will then be rigorously assessed using this established evaluation methodology for a comprehensive performance analysis.

CONCLUSION

This framework, meticulously detailed the comprehensive methodology employed for the analysis, visualization, and prediction of emotional states from physiological signals, with a particular focus on facial Electromyography (EMG). We successfully implemented a robust data processing pipeline, commencing with the collection of raw EMG data. A pivotal step involved data preparation, where raw signals underwent necessary cleaning and transformation, ensuring data quality and consistency, and thereby paving the way for reliable subsequent analyses.

The visualization strategy for the EMG channels was meticulously designed, enabling the simultaneous display of distinct muscle channels, facilitating a clear comparative analysis of crucial muscles such as the Zygomaticus, Corrugator, Orbicularis, and Frontalis. This enhanced our understanding of their individual and coordinated activities in relation to recorded events. Furthermore, we harnessed the power of the Continuous Wavelet Transform (CWT) for a dual time-frequency analysis. Specifically, the Complex Morlet wavelet was strategically chosen for its optimal balance between time and frequency localization, crucial for analyzing the non-stationary nature of EMG signals. This approach proved invaluable for characterizing the dynamic nature of EMG signals, providing detailed scalogram visualizations that reveal the evolution of muscle activation patterns. Our comparative analysis of these scalograms, as detailed in the results section, provided significant insights into differential muscle activation across various signals and events.

Beyond raw signal processing, this work also established a robust framework for the prediction and evaluation of continuous emotional dimensions (Arousal and Valence) and their discrete classes. The obtained results, particularly from the simulated dataset, demonstrate the exceptional functionality and accuracy of the implemented evaluation pipeline. For regression tasks, the R-squared values for both Arousal and Valence were remarkably high, indicating that the simulated predictions explained a very substantial proportion of the variance in the true emotional states. Similarly, for classification, the system achieved very high accuracy, with Arousal classification reaching nearly perfect levels and Valence also showing strong performance (as evidenced by its confusion matrix and high diagonal values), accompanied by excellent precision, recall, and F1-scores across all classes. This outstanding alignment between predicted and ground truth values rigorously validates the correctness and reliability of the developed metric calculation framework.

While these compelling results underscore the capability of our evaluation system using ideal data, it is important to contextualize them. Realistic performance for emotion recognition systems utilizing physiological signals typically falls within the 70-85% accuracy range in the broader literature. Therefore, these current results serve as a crucial benchmark for the integration of actual machine learning models trained on real-world, complex physiological data. Future work should focus on training and deploying sophisticated models to generate authentic predictions, which will then be rigorously assessed using this established and validated evaluation methodology for a comprehensive performance analysis, moving towards practical and reliable emotion recognition applications.

REFERENCES

Bishop, C. M. (2006). Pattern recognition and machine learning. Springer. 978-0-387-31073-2

Calvo, R. A., & D'Mello, S. K. (2010). Affect detection: An interdisciplinary review of models, methods, and their applications. *IEEE Transactions on Affective Computing*, *1*(1), 18–37. DOI: 10.1109/T-AFFC.2010.1

Harper, R., Lam, R., & Evans, H. L. (2019). Affective computing in mental health: A review. *Computers in Human Behavior*, *91*, 107–124. DOI 10.1016/j.chb.2018.09.027

Hastie, T., Tibshirani, R., & Friedman, J. (2017). The elements of statistical learning: Data mining, inference, and prediction (2nd ed.). Springer. 10.1007/978-0-387-84858-7

Kim, J., & André, E. (2008). Emotion recognition based on physiological changes in music listening. *IEEE Transactions on Multimedia*, *10*(6), 1040–1053. PMID: 18988943

Kołodziej, P., Piasecki, A. P., Piasecka, A. P., & Piasecki, M. (2024). Acquisition and Analysis of Facial Electromyographic Signals for Emotion Recognition. *Sensors (Basel)*, *24*(15), 4785. DOI: 10.3390/s24154785 PMID: 39123832

Picard, R. W. (1997). *Affective computing*. MIT Press. DOI: 10.7551/mitpress/1140.001.0001

Ringeval, F., Sonderegger, A., Lingenfelser, M., Auberger, M., D'Errico, S., Baur, C., Bänninger, M., Schwaller, G., & Wicker, A. (2021). The HUME-VAM Dataset for Multimodal Spontaneous Emotion Recognition. *IEEE Transactions on Affective Computing*, *12*(3), 670–683.

Tao, W., & Tan, X. (2023). A Survey on Affective Brain-Computer Interface: From Machine Learning to Deep Learning. *IEEE Transactions on Human-Machine Systems*, *53*(2), 220–234.

Wang, N., Zhang, X., Li, X., Zhang, H., Liu, W., Wang, C., Li, L., & Liu, P. (2022). Facial Electromyography for Assessment of Post-stroke Facial Paralysis: A Review. *Frontiers in Neurology*, *13*, 843232. 10.3389/fnins.2025.1646485/

Chapter 8
VR in Rehabilitation: A New Frontier in Cognitive and Motor Recovery in Neurologically Ill Patients

Kirthika Ramesh
https://orcid.org/0000-0001-5200-9531
Dr. M.G.R. Educational and Research Institute, India

V. Rajalaxmi
https://orcid.org/0000-0002-7306-4537
Dr. M.G.R. Educational and Research Institute, India

S. Veenakirthika
https://orcid.org/0000-0003-3790-9579
Dr. M.G.R. Educational and Research Institute, India

G. Mohan Kumar
Dr. M.G.R. Educational and Research Institute, India

ABSTRACT

Neurological conditions include traumatic brain injury, Parkinson's disease, stroke, multiple sclerosis and spinal cord injuries frequently cause cognitive and movement impairments. Traditional rehabilitation methods can result in patient disengagement, limited accessibility, and inadequate functional recovery. Virtual reality has become a powerful instrument in neurorehabilitation due to its interactive, immersive, and flexible therapeutic environment for cognitive and motor recovery. Virtual reality-based exergames optimize functional recovery and improve motor development by fusing mental difficulties with physical exercise.

DOI: 10.4018/979-8-3373-2706-8.ch008

1. INTRODUCTION

Overview of Neurological Disorders Affecting Cognition and Motor Function

The term "physical functioning" refers to the capacity to carry out a range of activities, from self-care (instrumental daily living activities) to more difficult mobility tasks that call on strength, endurance, and balance, such as walking or standing, which are crucial for establishing or preserving an independent way of life. Decreases in sensory or motor system function have been linked to age-related declines in physical functioning. For instance, gait was thought to be an automated motor action that required little higher-level cognitive input until recently (Pichierri et al., 2011). Memory, motion and coordination are all hampered by neurological disorders that affect cognitive and motor function, such as multiple sclerosis, stroke, Alzheimer's illness, Parkinson's disease, and others. By giving patients realistic, interactive environments, virtual reality (VR) is being used into emerging rehabilitation techniques to improve motor learning, cognitive training, and neuroplasticity. By mimicking real-world tasks and providing tailored feedback, VR-based therapy has demonstrated potential in enhancing motor function, balance, and cognitive engagement. VR's role in neurorehabilitation is still being investigated, with wearable technology and artificial intelligence being used to maximize patient recovery and long-term care (Dockx et al., 2019).

The Need for Innovative Rehabilitation Approaches

Virtual reality exposure can enhance the general well-being of healthy people if it is prioritized over reaching long-term personal objectives. Furthermore, virtual reality technologies could help patients with stroke or traumatic brain injury with their neurorehabilitation, help older adults who are experiencing social isolation and cognitive decline, and even be a crucial component of replacing lost functions with a suitable brain–computer interface (BCI) that controls robotic devices (Georgiev et al., 2021). The objective of motor rehabilitation is to help patients recover or improve their motor abilities through specialized exercises, physical therapy, and cutting-edge technology like robotic systems or VR. Strength, coordination, and dexterity can be greatly enhanced by robotic systems, allowing patients to carry out daily tasks on their own—a necessary skill for social integration and self-worth. Additionally, In reaction to experience and learning, the brain can reorganize itself and form new neural connections, a process known as neuroplasticity is stimulated by motor therapy. Following nervous system injuries, repeated and regulated therapies can aid in the functional recovery process and help regain lost motor abilities (Banyai & Bris, 2024).

Role of Virtual Reality in Modern Rehabilitation

Virtual reality has been presented as a device for cognitive rehabilitation. Creating dynamic, interactive, multimodal environments that closely mimic the real world is made easier by virtual reality (VR). It also simple to comprehend, intriguing and enjoyable which promotes active engagement by boosting motivation for recovery. Numerous studies have demonstrated that exercise games improve cognitive function in MCI patients and improve motivation in older persons. However, VRCR therapy has not been well studied, and its results are unknown. Furthermore, given the ongoing advancements in IT technology, it is imperative to present novel approaches to VRCR therapy and demonstrate their efficacy. In this work, we therefore introduce VR-based mental-motor therapy and examine its impact on the driving force and cognitive function of older persons with MCI (Park et al., 2020).

2. THE SCIENCE BEHIND VIRTUAL REALITY REHABILITATION

Principles of Neuroplasticity and VR

Virtual reality technologies may improve quality of life by minimizing impairments and raising activity levels. Virtual reality (VR) is a game changer in rehabilitation, providing immersive experiences that are consistent with learning ideas. Learning increases with relevant and repetitive tasks that gradually get more difficult. VR enables personalized stimuli and task difficulty based on the patient's demands and abilities, while maintaining stimulus control and consistency. It also offers real-time feedback (Kumar et al., 2023). One of the main mechanisms behind neuroplasticity is synaptic plasticity, which allows the brain to alter the power and effectiveness of neuronal synaptic connections. Both long-term depression (LTD) and long-term stimulation (LTP), one of the two main types of synaptic plasticity, are critical for memory and learning. LTP improves synaptic transmission by fortifying a synapse's connection (Deng et al., 2023).

Immersive vs. Non-Immersive VR: Mechanisms of Action

Virtual reality can be "non-immersive" or "immersive," depending on how much When engaging with the virtual world, the user is isolated from their real-world environment. As the cost of various non-immersive video gaming systems created by the dwelling entertainment sector has decreased, this modality is now more widely available for potential rehabilitation therapies. Technological advancements have enabled the use of fully immersive virtual reality as a therapeutic tool to help stroke victims with their motor function. It has demonstrated potential in enhancing post-stroke patients' self-care abilities and upper extremity function. Additionally, patients with spatially neglect have benefited from physiotherapy treatments based on this type of virtual reality. The objective is to investigate the scientific data that is currently available on the use of both immersing and non-immersive virtual realities in patients, as well as their effectiveness in creating reactive and statically equilibrium (Nieto-Escamez et al., 2023). VR technology's immersive and interactive settings allow for customized training sessions with accurate, unbiased feedback (Lee et al., 2022).

Figure 1. VR equipment classification

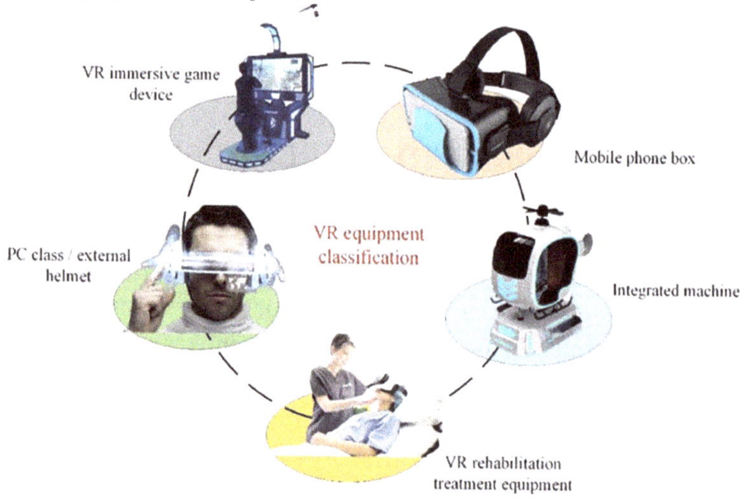

Cognitive-Motor Integration in VR Therapy

According to research, virtual reality can significantly improve cognitive-motor therapy for older persons. One study, in instance, combined regular Physical activity with dancing video games to improve your motor and cognitive abilities. Users of the VR system walked more quickly than the inactive control group during this dual-task exercise, which may have prevented falls in real-world situations. A kick-boxing trainer, an athletic game that requires body and jumping actions, an aerial penalty kick game, and a soaring game that requires shoulder and body movements were among the other serious games that were studied in another study. The results demonstrated improvements in visuospatial awareness, organization, orientation, and concentration as compared to the control group and focus (Tan et al., 2024).

Figure 2. Advancements of cognitive assessment used by VR

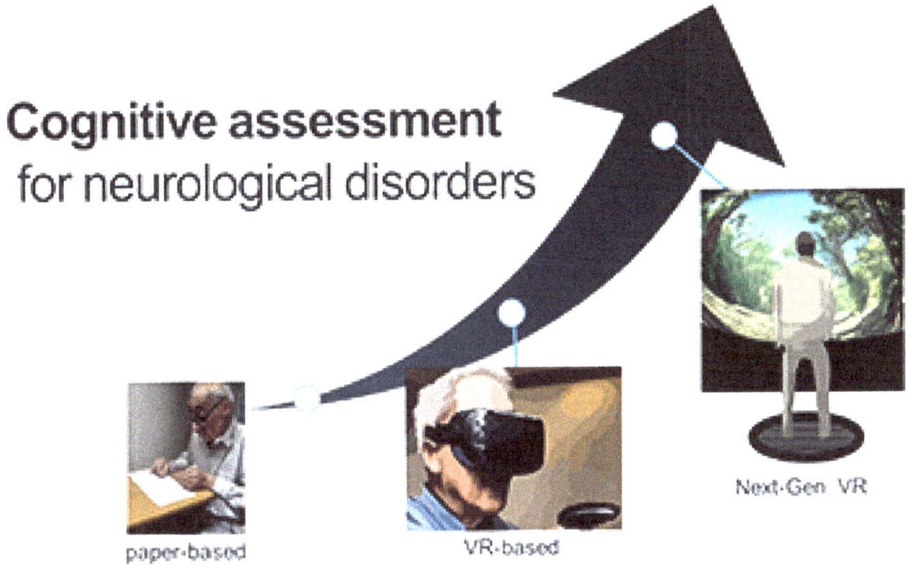

3. VR-BASED REHABILITATION IN NEUROLOGICAL CONDITIONS

Stroke Rehabilitation: Enhancing Motor Recovery and Functional Independence

According to the guidelines, both postural and task-oriented upper limb training can help enhance motor control. Neurorehabilitation provides potential tools for addressing a variety of issues like Neurological dysfunctions. VR is a one-of-a-kind solution in rehabilitation that enhances the environment for task-specific training and multimodal feedback, hence encouraging functional recovery. VR therapy for motor impairments enhanced the rehabilitation outcomes of stroke survivors. VR is built on three fundamental ideas: immersion, imagination, and interactivity. Patients can engage in virtual settings, engage with their environment through graphics, and obtain real-time responses, resulting in immersive motor rehabilitation experiences (Leonardi et al., 2021). The VR intervention has good effects on cortical reconfiguration linked to motor recovery because extensive and repetitive use of the paretic LE (such as that involved in the tasks mimicked through VR) causes positive effects on neuroplasticity and motor performance were investigated. Therefore, an approach of choosing motor functions to carry out the necessary job is implied by movement re-learning. With VRRS, proposals like the one in this study enable the promotion of several paradigms (like supervised and reinforced gaining knowledge) that function to promote Motor training that has its basis on feedback obtained (Garay-Sánchez et al., 2021). According to our analysis, tele-rehabilitation employing smart devices and combination exercise regimens were primarily used in patients who had been in the chronic stage for six months or more (Mao et al., 2014).

Figure 3. VR-based exoskeleton for stroke rehabilitation for motor recovery

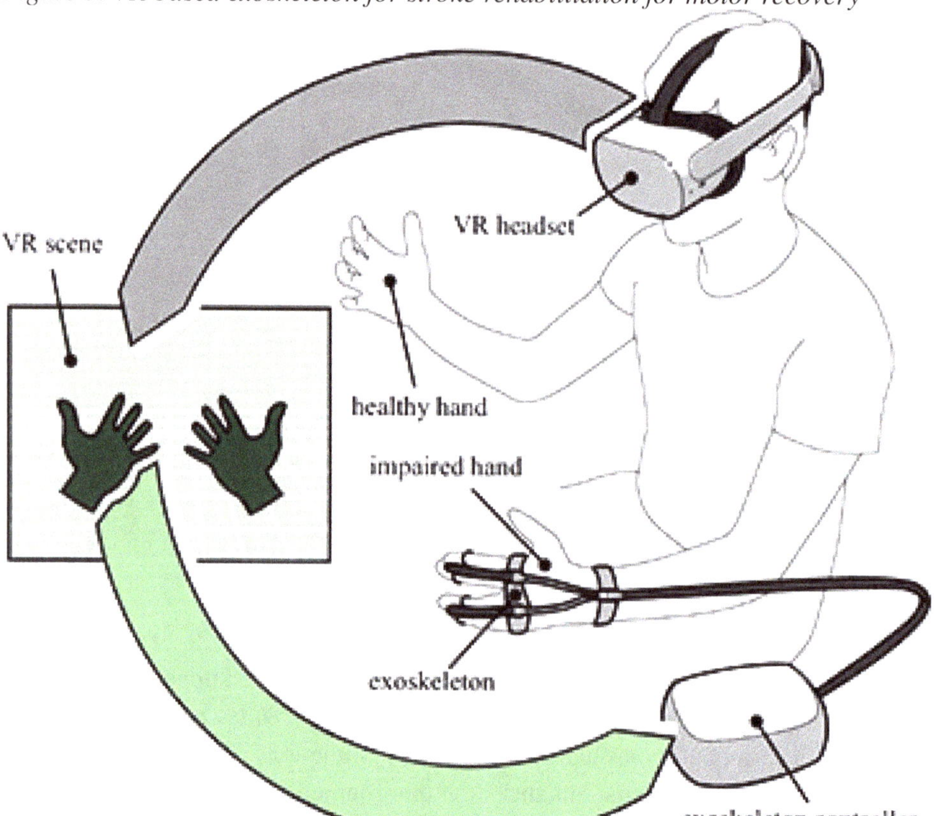

Parkinson's Illness: Addressing Dual-Task Brain-Motor Impairments

Parkinson is a degenerative neurological illness distinguished by slow movement (bradykinesia), resting tremors, increased muscle stiffness, and decreased balance. Dual-task training that combines motor and cognitive skills is an approach that crosses the limits of discipline and combines motor skill-focused activities alongside those that improve mental capacities. This strategy is aimed to concurrently grow and perfect both the the physical capability of the body and the cognitive processes of the mind, thus optimizing the coherence of cognitive-motor coordination and the effectiveness of functional performance. Taking on two tasks at once is the contemporaneous carrying out two different goal-oriented tasks, such as performing Mathematical difficulties while walking. Individuals with Parkinson's disease often perform worse on motor-cognitive tasks than healthy counterparts of the same age, gender, and education level. The concurrent stimulation of both cognitive-motor operates in the scope of dual-tasking can produce additional benefits in compared to training with a single task method (Choi et al., 2023). One promising new rehabilitation tool is virtual reality (VR) aid with many uses. VR technology is recommended in the context of physiotherapy to maximize motor skills in a secure environment, and it could be a viable substitute for traditional treatments. VR enables people to learn relearning motor skills and developing new motor techniques that have been lost as a result of illness or injury by providing enhanced feedback on performance, allowing for Individualized repeated motor function exercise that stimulates cognitive and motor processes at once. Initial pilot research utilizing unconstrained designs investigated the the efficiency of virtual reality therapies in Parkinson's disease and revealed positive impacts on gait, equilibrium, and mental abilities following exercise (Buele & Palacios-Navarro, 2023). The level of this cognitive component can range from easy tasks like answering math problems to more difficult ones like combining verbal fluency exercises with memory and recitation drills. From simple walking training to increase complicated programs like Hi-Balance, the motor activities can vary in complexity. The intensity of the training is designed to be flexible, gradually rising as participants become used to the first degrees of difficulty and surpass their previous performance. Additionally, there are several benefits to the training schedule when technological devices are used. Exergames that make use of video or virtual reality can help to integrate motor and cognitive tasks, adding ease and entertainment value to the training process (Filippis & Foysal, 2024).

Multiple Sclerosis: Improving Balance and Fatigue Management

The most frequent cause of multiple sclerosis is a chronic, progressive demyelinating illness of the central nervous system of long-term neurological impairment in juvenile individuals. Although the exact etiology of MS-related fatigue is still unknown, it is thought that centrally mediated processes that are characteristic of MS, such as immune system or central nervous system demyelination and axonal loss, may be the responses, or from complications associated with MS, musculoskeletal problems, sleep problems, and medications. Experiments have demonstrated that weariness is caused by decreased voluntary muscular activation via central mechanisms. The Multiple Sclerosis International Federation classified two types of weariness in severe MS: physical or motor weariness (weakened muscles and speech disorders, inability to execute daily tasks, etc.) and cognitive fatigue, which includes Fatigue can be either acute or chronic (Zhang et al., 2024). The utilizing virtual reality as a therapeutic therapy for MS patients is still discussed. Virtual reality (VR) has a significant role in motor and cognitive rehabilitation (CR), as demonstrated by numerous researches. The virtual interactive experience boosts self-efficacy in MS patients, leading to increased knowledge, self-consciousness, and development of motor and cognitive skills. It also increases motivation and interest in the utilization of virtual reality as a therapeutic instrument for MS patients is still under consideration. Many studies have shown that virtual reality (VR) plays an important role in motor and cognitive rehabilitation (CR). The virtual interactive experience improves MS patients' self-efficacy, resulting in greater knowledge, self-consciousness, and the development of motor and cognitive skills. It also improves motivation and interest. Research indicates that integrating VR and robotic rehabilitation can greatly improve motor and cognitive skills in MS patients. Calabro and colleagues discovered that VR enhanced balance and psychological results, including coping mechanisms (Tan et al., 2024). Certain cognitive domains include lexical access, short-term verbal memory, and learning capacity, and mental state-related quality of life, showed notable improvements with Virtual Reality Rehabilitation System (Dockx et al., 2016).

Traumatic Brain Injury (TBI) & Concussion: Cognitive and Sensorimotor Training

The term "traumatic brain injury" has replaced "head injuries." Traumatic brain damage is described as a disruption in neuronal activity caused by the abrupt, unexpected, and tolerable application of mechanical force. A traumatic brain injury can be caused by a head knock, blow, or whiplash, a sudden change in calvarium direction, or a penetrating head wound. It can also be induced by falls, sports, adolescent drinking, leisure activities, and car accidents. Traumatic brain injury is a prominent cause of death and disability worldwide, especially among children and adolescents, and it can impair mobility, cognition, and balance. Early therapy appears to be crucial for an individual's functional recovery following catastrophic brain injury. A patient with a catastrophic brain injury recovered the capacity to walk, talk, carry out everyday tasks, and participate in a variety of leisure activities independently after undergoing a physical rehabilitation program that included sensory stimulation using VR. According to current study, people who suffered traumatic brain injuries gained the greatest in terms of balance and walking, while cognitive function improved the least. Hand movement training using VR is an effective physiotherapy treatment for TBI patients to regain damaged hand motions (Khan et al., 2014). VR is a useful technique for post-concussion rehabilitation of vestibular and balance problems. Visual input in virtual reality can be used to supplement scattered, interconnected cortical regions in the brain's structure. It has been proposed that visual information can serve as a powerful signal for sensorimotor circuit reconfiguration (Maggio et al., 2019).

Spinal Cord Injury: VR for Neurorehabilitation and Functional Restoration

Spinal cord injury is described as the spinal cord damage that results in either short-term or long-term alterations in function. This disorder is common and has a high impairment rate, and begins at a young age. High-intensity traumas including car crashes, falls, and violent crimes, as well as infections and tumors, ischemia-reperfusion injuries, vascular causes, and column degenerative disorders are the causes for the SCI. It is classified as either traumatic or nontraumatic depending on the cause of injury. Acute damage to the spinal cord can be classified as either primary or secondary injuries based on pathophysiology. SCI can be classified as full or incomplete injury based on its severity. The symptoms of incomplete SCI include anterior cord syndrome, posterior core syndrome, Brown-Sequard syndrome, and central core syndrome (Waqar et al., 2022). VR's current technological advancements regarding interactions and visualization have made it an increasingly appealing everyday therapy for Spinal Cord damage patients, allowing them to to encounter a high level of body perception and physical activity through multisensory perception in an ecologically high setting. Increasing experimental data strongly affirms the significance of incorporating multimodal stimulation with SCI patients actively participating in their own rehabilitation during the acute or chronic phase of treatment. As a result, after SCI, patients frequently become disconnected from congruent feedback sensory information, hence treatment should focus on obtaining and preserving physiological balance input. This multimodal feedback may generate patterns and variations in the cortex of the sensorimotor network, as well as more extended brain regions (Hu et al., 2023). Patients with SCI may benefit from cognitive training with semi-immersive VR. In fact, incorporating cognitive activities that involve movement and offer more feedback may help those with SCI recover more quickly both cognitively and motorly (Leemhuis et al., 2021).

Figure 4. Advancements of VR used for SCI rehabilitation

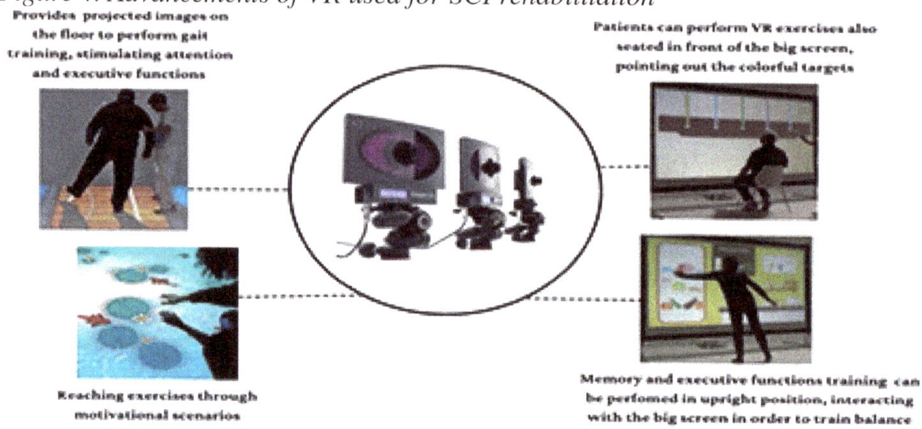

4. TYPES OF VR TECHNOLOGIES USED IN REHABILITATION

Fully Immersive, Semi-Immersive, and Non-Immersive VR Systems

Virtual Reality is defined by a computer-generated, interactive setting featuring objects, scenes, or other people that users can engage with. VR can be categorized by the degree of immersive; non-immersive VR usually consists of a computer monitor or a projection display where users observe a virtual environment that necessitates input devices such as keyboards, mouce, or gamepads for user interaction; semi-immersive VR provides a greater level of immersion compared to non-immersive VR as it employs a larger display or multiple screens that encircle the user, offering a broader field of view, along with specialized glasses and some form of haptic feedback or motion tracking (Mennella et al., 2023).

A semi-immersive system depends on three-dimensional images produced via "stereoscopic projections or displays with a fixed visual perspective." Users participate in the simulated environment with an enhanced sense of engagement and interactivity compared to a non-immersive setting because of sensors that monitor users' movements. In completely immersive virtual reality, individuals can move egocentrically within a surrounding simulated space. Various devices allow for real-time interaction between the visualized graphics and the motions of the head and body, mimicking the interactions of the real world with a visual viewpoint based on head movements (Tortora et al., 2024). This systematic study examined the impact of a completely realistic VR therapy course employing a head-mounted display for the function of the upper limbs and gait. Balance in stroke sufferers. The ability to provide varied triggers by changing the optical mobility supplied in the totally immersive environment can stimulate brain activity, particularly in motion-sensitive cortical areas (Burke & Rooney, 2021). The created VR task has demonstrated its capability to enhance distal upper extremity recovery during the chronic stage of stroke using a range of outcome metrics, including measures of cortical excitability and clinical assessments, results derived from neuroimaging, and performance outcomes specific to the task. The clinical improvements observed indicated the potential for neuroplasticity brought on by practice in a chronic stroke survivor as a reaction to the non-immersion virtual reality therapy (Amirthalingam et al., 2021).

Figure 5. Types of virtual reality

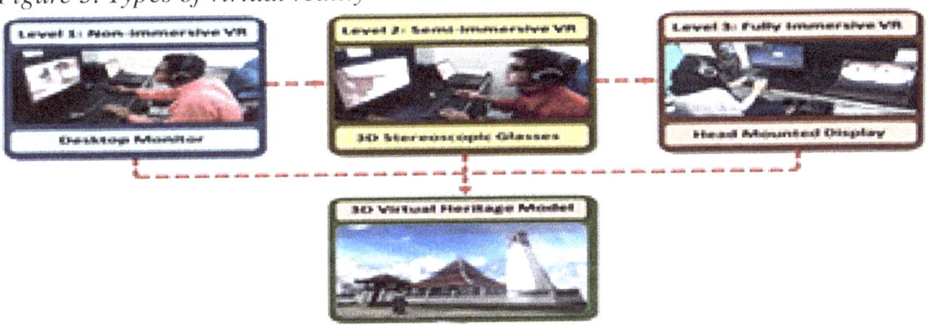

Motion Capture and Haptic Feedback Devices

The effectiveness of haptic feedback in addressing balance and gait disorders in post-stroke patients. It will examine both long-term interventions and pre-post-training measures, as well as designs that provide immediate/simultaneous effects through single assessments. Our goal is to improve understanding of haptic feedback's role in post-stroke rehabilitation by exploring novel features of its impacts and guiding future. Although vibration-based haptic feedback is popular and effective, other methods including kinesthetic or electrical feedback are also showing value. More study is needed to assess the efficacy of haptic feedback methods, including larger sample sizes, longer follow-up periods, and stronger techniques (Demeco et al., 2023). Marker less motion capture (MMC) technique eliminates the requirement for marker placement while studying human movement. Kinect is a trustworthy marker less technology that can be used as a quick estimator of morphology. The Kinect system was shown to be accurate in measuring knee joint angles of a jig when compared to a digital inclinometer used as a ground-truth. The system performed well in terms of knee flexion and abduction. The MMC system can be used in rehabilitation to test patients' motor function. The study used the Kinect system to measure arm position in both healthy and unilateral spastic children (Faria et al., 2024).

Figure 6. Motion capture analysis used to improve motor function by using VR

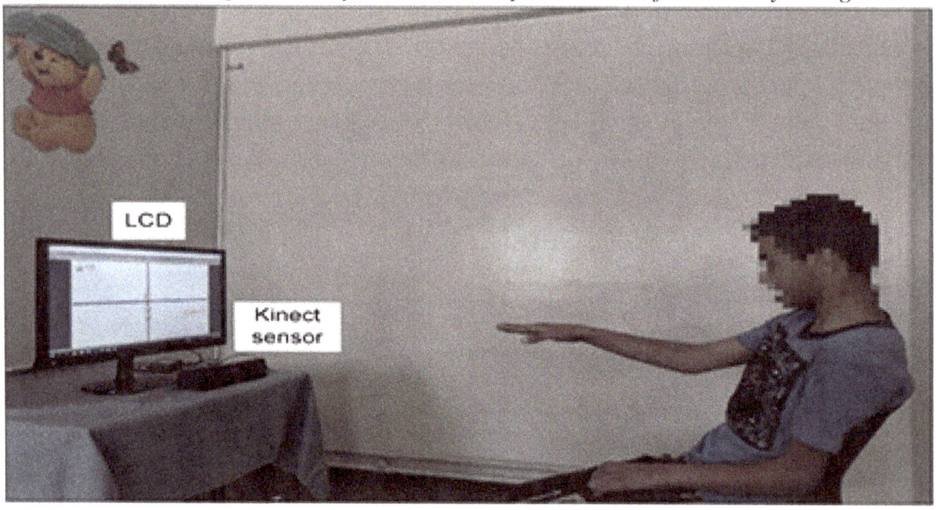

Integration With EEG, EMG, and Neurophysiological Monitoring

Detecting changes in the brain's neuroplasticity throughout rehabilitation can help establish effective methods for stroke patients. Electroencephalography (EEG) is a cost-effective, safe, and user-friendly way to record brain activity. EEG could help identify neuroplasticity alterations in stroke survivors during recovery. This study aims to use two-phase training with robot assistance to improve hand motor recovery in brain stem stroke patients. To evaluate neuroplasticity, we analyze MRCP characteristics generated from EEG signals (Patsaki et al., 2022). EEG can investigate both cortical and subcortical brain activity, allowing high temporal resolution monitoring of neuronal brain processes to analyze whole-brain neuronal network organization. In recent decades, EEG signal analysis has transitioned from the time domain to the frequency domain. Functional connectivity techniques have also been used to better understand neural network alterations occurs under healthy and pathological situations (Nath et al., 2023). Various devices and procedures provide clinically valid assessments of patients' neuromotor functioning. EEG and surface EMG are highly effective techniques for evaluating and monitoring motor function during rehabilitation settings. They record electrical potentials from the cortex and muscles. EEG is a flexible and non-invasive method that can be used in clinical, experimental, and real-world settings to monitor electrical activity in neurons at the cortex level. In contrast, EMG uses surface electrodes applied to the skin covering muscle fibers to monitor the train of motor unit action potentials produced by muscular contractions. The development can help improve the combined analysis of EEG and EMG. Bi-modal EEG/EMG analysis is used to understand physiological and pathological causes, allowing for effective evaluation of rehabilitation therapy (Maggio et al., 2024). Cortical facilitation can be measured using EEG signals as Power Decrease Associated with Tasks (TRPD), which is an increase in neuron excitability, whereas Increase in Task-Related Power (TRPI) may represent cortical inhibition. The balance of sensorimotor activation and inactivation is represented by TRPD/TRPI patterns. Therefore, in physiological evaluations, EEG and EMG can be employed together to identify the neurophysiological signal pattern linked to the onset of musculoskeletal discomfort brought on by biomechanical limitations. However, further studies in neurophysiology and biomechanics are required. For the first time, it would be intriguing to find out if a realistic manual job activity, like an experimental hairdressing workstation that simulates a high risk of MSD development, may modulate the behavior of central and peripheral neurophysiological signals (De Giorgi et al., 2023).

Figure 7. Integration of advanced diagnostic procedures with VR

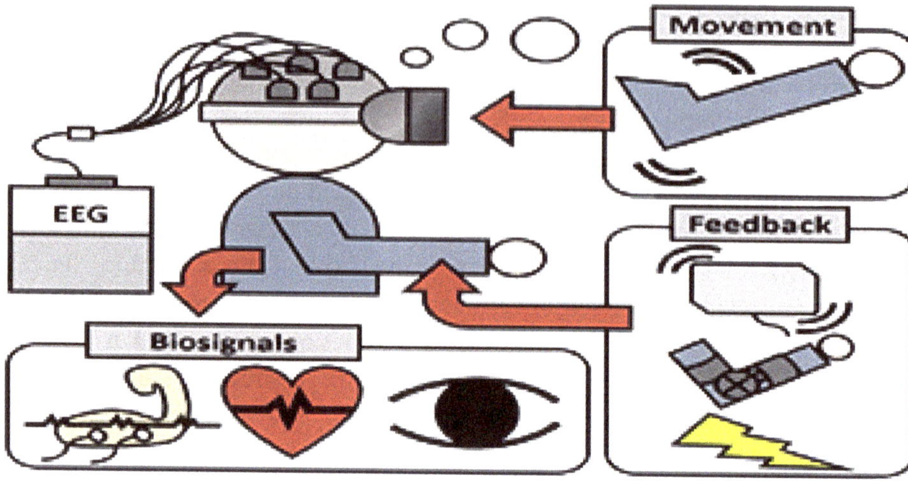

Utilizing improved embodiment—the perception that a graphic body being displayed is the observer's own—research that makes use of immersive virtual reality is proven to be beneficial for motor imagery. Immersion VR-based rehabilitation apps tend to enhance relevant neural activity by displaying immersive depiction of graphical body movement from a first-person perspective. Combining action observation with motor imagery is one of the therapeutic approaches that makes direct use of this feature. In this approach, users are shown graphical actions from a first-person perspective, leading them to believe that they are the ones doing the movement (Gomez-Risquet et al., 2024).

AI and Machine Learning in VR for Personalized Therapy

AR/VR cognitive therapies provide immersive, interactive environments for experience learning and in-vivo treatment implementation. Patients with social anxiety disorder can practice social interaction in a virtual environment before transitioning to real-life scenarios. Virtual worlds allow patients to gradually confront their concerns, consolidate coping methods, and reduce the risks of in-person exposure (Zhang & Yu, 2024). AI therapy findings should be regarded with caution due to low or extremely low-quality data, despite changes. Intensity, duration, training volume, treatment type, participant characteristics, and assessments utilized. Robotic treatment, which uses AI technology, has been offered as a feasible method for Upper Limb rehabilitation. It can increase therapy intensity and standardize it by giving complex, regulated multimodal stimulation. Built-in sensors and actuators on robotic devices allow them to assess user dexterity. Several studies on Artificial

Intelligence treatment have examined the efficacy of combining a single device with conventional therapy procedures (Bower et al., 2021). Rehabilitation evaluation has been transformed by artificial intelligence (AI), especially machine learning, which provides advanced methods for evaluating the function of the upper and lower limbs. In applications like picture and speech recognition, methods like Artificial neuronal networks (ANN) and support vector processing (SVM) have been crucial in improving the precision and effectiveness of rehabilitation evaluation. Numerous studies have been conducted on objective evaluation techniques based on AI technology, including joint motion range assessment, human motion trajectory tracking, maximum angular velocity evaluation, and surface electromyogram signal (sEMG) analysis. Electrical activity of the muscles during limb motion can be measured non-invasively using the sEMG, which offers important information about muscle coordination and function. Human motion trajectory tracking, on the other hand, uses image processing tools to examine the limb movements of patients, enabling accurate evaluation of anomalies and movement patterns (Lam et al., 2023).

Without explicit programming, computers may automatically learn from experience and improve over time thanks to machine learning, an application of artificial intelligence. Machine learning algorithms can be classified as either supervised or unsupervised learning based on their tasks and scopes. While supervised learning is appropriate for predictive modeling by establishing connections between features and the topic of interest, unsupervised learning is better recognized for feature extraction (Bargeri et al., 2023).

Figure 8. Machine learning incorporated with virtual reality

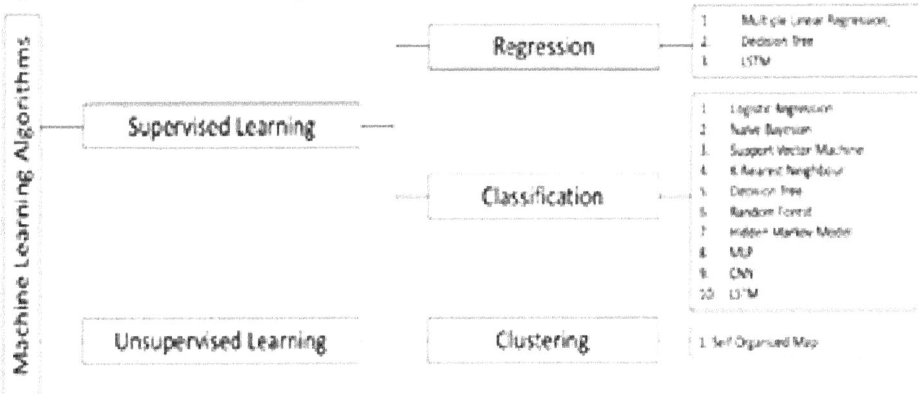

5. DUAL-TASK TRAINING FOR COGNITIVE AND MOTOR SKILLS IN VR

Concept of Two-Task Training and Its Importance

Brain lesions in the white matter can cause poor balance and reduce multi-tasking activity, making it a significant contributor. White matter defects have been connected to motor and cognitive abilities. Dysfunction when multitasking impairs balance performance. Interference between physical and cognitive tasks during multitasking might negatively impact performance in one or both. Many research has employed Two-task (DT) models to study interaction between balance and cognition. DT training can enhance turning, posture, attention, gait, and gait inhibition. Understanding the link between elderly people with balance problems and individuals is crucial for developing effective interventions that use DT to reduce falls. DT improves balance control in older persons. It causes motor-cognitive interference, as well as gait and balance in young individuals in good health. the decrease in falls or the enhancement of balance after DT training (Brambilla et al., 2021). Rehabilitation can enhance physical and cognitive performance for Parkinson's sufferers. Dual-task training that combines motor and cognitive skills is a complete rehabilitation strategy that combines both motor and cognitive training. Two-task training may benefit individuals with Parkinson's illness by enhancing balance, motor symptoms, cognition, and gait more than single-task training alone. Research suggests that dual-task training has both physical and cognitive benefits for Parkinson's sufferers (Khalid et al., 2024). Motor-cognitive two-task training, which combines cognitive and movement training, effectively strengthens connections in the brain network that are functional. Enhancing relationship between regions of the motor-cognitive brain leads to increased cerebral cortex activity and improved walking ability. It helps activate the cerebral cortex and enhance motor function in stroke patients. Eye opening and shutting, as well as motor cognitive dual tasks, significantly enhanced balance function during stroke research (Butt et al., 2020). When evaluating impairment in the early stages of a disease, before impairment of the broader executive system, the potential separation between short-term memory and reduced attention (verbal and/or visuospatial) may be particularly significant. Regardless of the modality—visual (spatial span) or auditory (digit-span)—a VR-based multi-modal dual-task could evaluate if patients' dual-task scoring patterns are comparable on attention and working memory measures (Segning et al., 2021).

VR-Based Cognitive-Motor Dual-Task Training: Mechanisms and Benefits

Along with the prefrontal cortex's growth and the growing diversification of brain networks, cognitive skills like attentional control—one fundamental element of cognitive-motor performance—develop throughout infancy and adolescence and into early adulthood. the effects on athletes of dual-task (DT) training. The objectives of this review were to determine the most effective training approach for children and adolescents' motor, cognitive, or DT performance under DT situations, as well as to identify and evaluate training treatments utilized to enhance these performance areas. There are DT training comes in two varieties: general and customized. The major outcomes of particular DT training for kids and teenagers were executive functioning, walking while doing extra work, and balance. In terms of the specificity of these interventions, even a brief training session could have a positive influence on motor performance (Halkiopoulos & Gkintoni, 2025). Development studies on motor-cognitive interference in neurologic populations have primarily focused on Parkinson's illness, Alzheimer's disease, and the brain injury. The effects of DTT on neurologic illnesses DTT may enhance spatiotemporal parameters (velocity, step length) of single-task gait in PD as well as DT gait in PD and brain injury. It may also have a small influence on balance and cognition. Future research should include bigger sample numbers and increased uniformity of DT methods. Improving DT ability in individuals with neurological diseases can improve gait, balance, and cognition, perhaps leading to more independence and reduced fall risk (Mahmoud et al., 2023). VR and traditional physical-cognitive training may help elderly people enhance their executive function and motor dual-task performance. Adults experiencing modest cognitive impairment. VR-based physical and cognitive exercise dramatically enhanced attention and cognitive DTC when compared to traditional training. Our physical and cognitive program, based on Independent Activities of Daily Living, could serve as a model for VR training in older people with MCI (Khan et al., 2022).

Figure 9. Wearable types used in VR rehabilitation

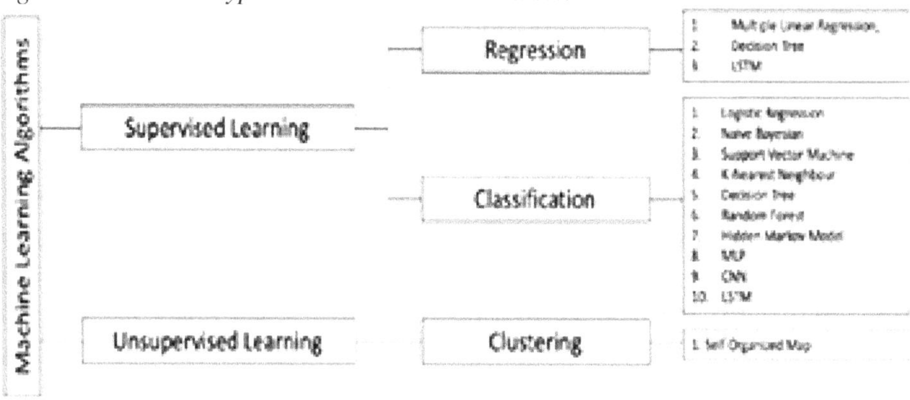

Virtual Reality-Enhanced Interventions for Cognitive and Motor Rehabilitation in Neurological Disorders:

Various interventions combined with virtual reality (VR) have been explored to enhance cognitive and motor function in neurologically ill patients. VR-based rehabilitation therapies such as Leap Motion-based 3D immersion and Mirror treatment using a gesture recognition (GR) device have significantly improved function of the upper extremities in post-stroke patients. VR integrated with real instrument training has been shown to enhance motor recovery by improving wrist extension and elbow flexion, while VR-based planar motion exercises have contributed to increased range of motion in the shoulder. For Parkinson's disease, VR training rehabilitation has led to notable improvements in balance and gait, as evidenced by significant gains on the The Timed Up and Go Test (TUG) and the Berg Balance Scale (BBS). Additionally, game-based VR canoe paddling and Nintendo Wii-based therapy have demonstrated improvements in postural balance, static and dynamic balance, and upper extremity function. VR-enhanced gait treatment with robotic assistance (RAGT) has been effective in enhancing motivation and walking time in post-stroke patients, leading to significant improvements in the Functional Ambulation Classification. Telerehabilitation with virtual reality with the Nintendo Wii has successfully reduced postural instability in Parkinson's disease patients, while RAGT combined with VR using EEG oscillations has facilitated better gait and balance, accompanied by increased cortical activity in affected brain regions. Moreover, virtual reality reflection therapy (VRRT) has shown effectiveness in improving postural sway and functional reach, while reinforcement-induced movement therapy (RIMT) has provided sustained motor improvements up to 12 weeks post-trial.

These VR-based interventions offer promising advancements in neurorehabilitation, leveraging immersive environments to enhance neuroplasticity, motor learning, and cognitive engagement in patients with neurological disorders (Xiao et al., 2023).

In various stages of stroke recovery, robot-assisted hand training using end-effector devices reduces motor impairment even more than standard care alone. In a semi-virtual reality (VR) environment, these technologies frequently enable the patient to do practical, focused, and visual-spatial tasks. is a useful tool that offers a variety of virtual exercises broken down into modules, including motor (postural, upper and lower limb activity, facial gestures, and respiratory exercises), logopedic, and cognitive. The activities are further broken down into categories including praxis, executive functions, attention and so forth. With the psychiatric-cognitive therapist's assistance, the patient actively engages with the VR-CT equipment while seated in front of it. Notably, the VRRS has 45 distinct exercises, and the therapist can alter the virtual task's environment for each one, providing more distractions and complexity. Attention processes (selective, sustained, and split attention), verbal and visuospatial memory, orientation (personal/autobiographical, spatial/topographical, and temporal), and visual-executive tasks (verbal fluency, reasoning, categorization, problem solving, and coping strategies) are among the subdomains into which the currently available exercises are separated (Yang et al., 2022).

Figure 10. Advancements of VR software used for rehabilitation by selecting the domains

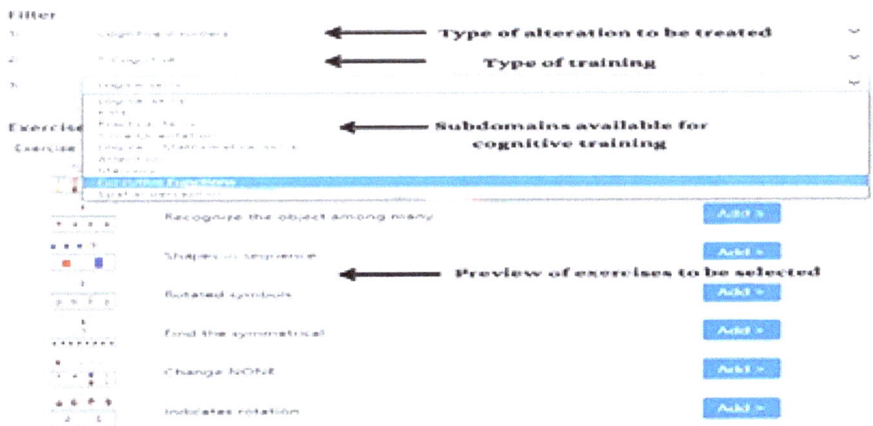

6. CLINICAL EVIDENCE AND EFFICACY OF VR IN NEUROREHABILITATION

Review of Clinical Trials and Systematic Reviews

Virtual reality (VR) is an emerging technique that has the ability to enhance reported results, patient quality of life and psychological health. Improve functional outcomes for those living with major illnesses. VR provides a stereoscopically produced 3D visual world with accompanying sound that responds to patient movement. Immersive Virtual reality simulates a realistic experience, creating a psychological impact. The sensory experience is separate from non-immersive reality, such as augmented reality, which displays computer-generated pictures over the visual field in the real world. Therapy with distraction and immersion can improve living standards and practical results. Virtual reality (VR) is being used in healthcare for critical illnesses. VR for elderly persons with significant illnesses, like strokes and cancer. Cardiovascular illness and COPD. VR has been used in research to improve anxiety and discomfort (mobility and strength (Fugl-Meyer upper extremity examination, proprioception, or orientation metrics), as well as anxiety (HADS, State Anxiety Inventory, or NPS). According to this review, brief VR sessions can reduce pain and anxiety, while longer ones can enhance mobility and strength after stroke (Wollesen et al., 2022). It has been demonstrated that technology-based evaluation and rehabilitation techniques with high validity in ecology, especially those utilizing virtual reality (VR), improve neurorehabilitation outcomes. The ability of VR-based techniques to create well-controlled environments tailored to patients' needs and integrate cognitive tasks into the ADL (activities of daily living) simulation may be one explanation for this. One example of integrating language, executive functioning, memory, and attention tasks into the completion of multiple ADLs is the VR-based neurorehabilitation program Reh@City. When compared to comparable regular paper-and-pencil tasks, a controlled, randomized investigation involving stroke patients who received rehabilitation using the Reh@City showed a significant benefit on areas of cognition and function. The positive impact of telerehabilitation is enhanced when paired with virtual reality (VR). VR provides realistic experiences that engage sensorimotor, cognitive, and social aspects. By recreating real-life situations through fun elements, this tool improves the patient's adherence to rehabilitation. A new area of Tele-VR involves the utilization of smartphones. Mobile applications (apps) can be accessed daily, allowing individuals to conveniently participate in therapy at home, thus facilitating "healthcare in the pocket". These advantages of VR could be beneficial in the rehabilitation of patients with PD, who are susceptible to cognitive decline (Fritz et al., 2015).

Comparative Effectiveness of VR vs. Traditional Rehabilitation

Virtual reality (VR) is a promising technology for exploring complicated deficits in PD patients and delivering tailored rehabilitation. Numerous There have been published meta-analyses (MAs) and systematic reviews (SRs) on the therapeutic effectiveness of VR therapy in treating Parkinson's disease (PD) using randomized controlled trials (RCTs). Groups for interventions received VR-based rehabilitation interventions (with or without integrated interventions). Control interventions should include passive therapy (PT) or active treatment (AT) without VR components. PT involved either instructional activities or a control group.

Lu et al. Systematic Reviews We did not re-evaluate the certainty of evidence for major outcomes if the review author had already done so. We evaluated the combined outcome using the Grading of Recommendations Assessment, Development, and Evaluation (GRADE) method. The GRADE grading takes into account publishing bias, indirectness, imprecision, bias, and inconsistency. Four levels of results are distinguished: extremely low, low, moderate, and high. Regarding walking distance, motor function, and cognitive function, we found no discernible differences between VR and AT. According to the majority of reviews, VR therapy helped both exercise groups' gait, balance, motor function, quality of life, everyday activities, cognitive function, neuropsychiatric symptoms, and postural control. Patients with greater baseline balance deficits and illness severity (H&Y > 2) were more affected by VR-based balance training. More advanced stages of the disease are usually present in patients with more severe balance impairments.

A consistent set of outcomes to assess how VR therapy affects individuals with Parkinson's disease. Fourth, as there was insufficient data in them, the combined effects of VR therapy and any kind of AT should be compared to the same kind of AT in order to elucidate the additional benefits of VR therapy. Therefore, we could not say with certainty that VR therapy is beneficial for gait, balance function, balance confidence, motor function, quality of life, daily activities, cognitive function, neuropsychiatric symptoms, and postural control in people with Parkinson's disease. Larger participant numbers and well-designed, superior RCTs are necessary to further support VR therapy's effectiveness in treating PD (Liao et al., 2019). The rehabilitation process for patients with multiple sclerosis (MS) is lengthy and intricate, which may result in diminished rehabilitation outcomes and a decrease in quality improvement. Therefore, there is a necessity to implement new techniques to enhance traditional rehabilitation. Innovations like telerehabilitation might prove useful in eliminating barriers to treatment, but evidence regarding their effectiveness is scarce. The aim of this study was to assess the clinical effectiveness of telerehabilitation in comparison to traditional interventions in patients with MS. Although the significance of stroke victims' ability to balance is well-recognized, prior studies are incomplete and constrained by conventional rehabilitation programs, highlighting the importance of exploring the impact of Telerehabilitation for stroke patients' ability to balance. In recent years, multiple randomized controlled trials (RCTs) have been performed to evaluate the differences between telerehabilitation and conventional rehabilitation in patients following a stroke (Leavy et al., 2017).

VR offers a human-virtual environment interaction that is realistic. In fact, participants can interact with the virtual objects in the digital environment using their real hands by using the controller on the VR headset. This makes it simple to measure the upper limb kinematics as participants complete the motor activities. Finally, virtual reality (VR) enables the replication of numerous other environments that are hard or impossible to replicate in real life, such as creating the impression that one is capable of painting some of the most well-known pieces of art in history. The recovery of UL motor function following a stroke is better with traditional treatment and VR-based training than with traditional treatment alone. Consequently, VR-based training could be a viable choice for enhancing UL motor performance (Peters et al., 2012).

Patient Engagement, Motivation, and Adherence in VR Therapy

Dimensions of engagement are essential for evaluating how well rehabilitation programs work. Because the activities in traditional physical therapy are so repetitive, patient adherence is frequently problematic. On the other hand, virtual reality has been demonstrated to dramatically increase involvement. According to research, patients who use virtual reality (VR) report feeling more motivated and satisfied throughout their therapy sessions. Better results are linked to this increased engagement, including enhanced Physical ability and reduced discomfort. A larger trend in healthcare toward more interactive and patient-centered approaches is reflected in the movement toward integrating technology such as virtual reality. VR stands out as a viable tool that fits with these changing paradigms as medical professionals increasingly understand the significance of patient engagement in reaching therapeutic aims (Riemenschneider et al., 2021). Frequent exercise is widely recognized as a critical tactic to enhance general health, lower the risk of neurological, cardiovascular, metabolic, and musculoskeletal disorders, and lower all-cause mortality. It has been suggested that using virtual reality (VR) could enhance workouts. In fact, a wealth of research indicates that specific technological characteristics may raise the possibility. Research on VR's impact on motivation, affect, enjoyment, and engagement during exercise is sparse, heterogeneous, and mostly focused on healthy individuals populations of a person deciding to use the technology while exercising. According to the review, VRBR provides a distinctively immersive experience that boosts patient motivation and participation throughout rehabilitation. VRBR's immersive qualities create a feeling of presence that can improve treatment outcomes and adherence. Additionally, by simulating real-world situations, VRBR gives stroke sufferers the chance to perform essential daily tasks, fostering functional independence (Maheta et al., 2025).

Game-like tasks are used in VR rehabilitation training to increase participant involvement and enjoyment. A novel method to rehabilitation, virtual reality (VR) devices immerse patients in a simulated world with multimodal feedback, potentially increasing patient motivation. Both eventually result in better patient outcomes, which is generally not possible with conventional rehabilitation techniques. By boosting enjoyment and engagement, virtual reality motion capture systems have the potential to revolutionize conventional therapy procedures and improve patient motivation and adherence. A novel method to rehabilitation, virtual reality (VR) devices immerse patients in a simulated world with multimodal feedback, potentially increasing patient motivation. Both eventually result in better patient outcomes, which is generally not possible with conventional rehabilitation techniques. To boost participation and enjoyment, virtual reality rehabilitation training incorporates game-like exercises (Lu et al., 2022).

Figure 11. Advantages and disadvantages of virtual reality

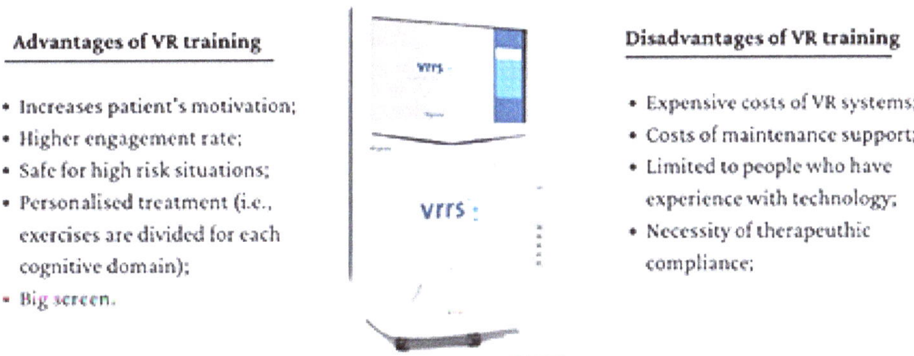

7. CHALLENGES AND FUTURE DIRECTIONS

Technological and Cost Barriers

The use of virtual reality systems and robots in neurorehabilitation has several benefits. Increases in intensity, repetitions, specificity, and feedback during rehabilitation are the primary factors contributing to these benefits. These devices, which are frequently found in specialized rehabilitation facilities with a large patient population of neurological disorders, are thought to be useful for evaluating deficiencies and, consequently, for evaluating the results of rehabilitation. They are also therapeutic instruments that are overseen by qualified and specialized staff. But there are obstacles in the way of their implementation. Given their differences in price compared to other device categories, a number of financial obstacles to the use of neurorehabilitation, robotics and/or virtual reality have been identified. Given the steadily increasing expenses of healthcare, there are significant worries regarding the long-term viability of the system, especially for long-term conditions like neurological ailments amenable to neurorehabilitation, when a new technology's efficacy is essential but insufficient need for its adoption. As far as we are aware, no previous systematic research has examined the financial implications of robotics and virtual reality technology for individuals with neurological conditions in a rehabilitation setting. The literature contains debate over the use of robots in rehabilitation for individuals with neurological illnesses regarding the reduction of costs, cost-effectiveness, cost-utility, and cost-benefit. However, compared to in-clinic interventions, semi-immersive virtual reality-based interventions may result in cost savings (Su et al., 2022).

Active video games, robots, and electrical stimulation are examples of technological uses that have been demonstrated to enhance therapy efficacy in neurological populations. Given the unique characteristics of neurological impairments (such as weakness and spasticity) and the necessity of using common therapeutic drivers of brain plasticity (such as recurrent task-relevant training), these technologies may be especially prevalent in neurological rehabilitation and research.

Increased accuracy, feedback, incentive, self-efficacy, and encouragement of repetitive practice are some of the potential benefits that clinicians have mentioned when discussing the use of technology in physical evaluation or therapy. However, obstacles have included training, technical issues, adequate assistance, and lack of access. In the medical field, obstacles to neurorehabilitation implementation are growing. Logistics, cost, expertise, and attitude are some examples of these factors are causing various problems for the development of the neurorehabilitation process. An obstacle that prevents individuals from properly understanding the technologies used in the healthcare process is a lack of awareness.

Programs for rehabilitation are designed to guarantee the improvement of cognitive, speech, energy management, and fitness. With their many uses, Intelligent technology (AI) in mental health and other technological advances in healthcare — have truly transformed the industry. Healthcare has benefited greatly from machine learning, particularly from reinforcement learning, which has allowed for more individualized treatment plans. AI has uses in mental health that go beyond medication recommendations and diagnosis. Through the use of virtual reality platforms, virtual therapy sessions have demonstrated encouraging outcomes in terms of accessible support, providing a secure setting for patients to communicate their feelings and thoughts, and enabling successful therapy without regard to geographic limitations. The increased accessibility of technology-based interventions is one of their main benefits. These technology-based therapies, in contrast to conventional approaches, are frequently affordable and accessible to people from the convenience of their own homes (Shruthi, 2022).

Ethical and Safety Considerations in VR Therapy

Technology development and its effects on society and ethics are correlated. Numerous technological advancements have an impact on society, including advances in machine learning and artificial intelligence, 3D printing flexible transparent screens, and quantum computing.

Virtual reality (VR) is one field that raises additional ethical issues. Because VR technologies are becoming more widely available and offer an intensely immersive experience, virtual reality keeps discovering new applications outside of entertainment. Despite virtual reality's many potential advantages, there has been substantial debate over the complex ethical problems this emerging technology presents. Both positive and negative prospects abound in these immersive settings. However, companies and designers are not required to follow moral guidelines. In addition, there is the problem of unethical technology exploitation and the element of hackers. The prevalence of VR technologies, their difficulty in categorizing and identifying them, and the difficulty in forecasting their immediate and long-term effects all contribute to these ethical concerns. Anything has "dangers," but we must also consider the enormous advantages of VR and gaming for training, education, rehabilitation, and, of course, fun. Virtual reality is a technology; it is up to us how we utilize it, for better or worse. Games and virtual reality also provide an escape. Everything is possible in virtual reality, which allows us to reach new heights with our creativity. Virtual reality facilitates the testing of learnt material in a "real-life" setting, allowing us to assess and replicate theoretical knowledge in a real-world setting. We can imitate soft skills like human movements and behaviors using virtual reality (VR), as well as how machinery functions and reacts. Virtual reality has a significant impact on education as well, making it more engaging, entertaining, and visually appealing. In order to improve participant engagement and practice on a functionally relevant task, clinicians should think about integrating virtual reality (VR) into daily activity training and post-stroke rehabilitation therapies for motor function recovery (Mouatt et al., 2020). Additionally, since therapists commonly overestimate the amount of time spent practicing active tasks, using an objective activity measurement—which is frequently included in VR systems—can guarantee that the practice duration is suitable for a particular patient. In this case, customized workouts with feedback (visual, auditory, and tactile) can be created to enhance performance (what a person accomplishes in his or her normal environment—) based on the patient's capability for motor recovery and the training goal feedback on an activity) or to enhance one's own abilities (what one can accomplish in a typical setting—feedback on a task, action, or motor function) (Cano-de-la-Cuerda et al., 2024).

Future Trends: AI, Metaverse, and Personalized VR Rehabilitation

With their many uses, digital medical technology—including artificial intelligence (AI) in mental health—have truly transformed the industry. Healthcare has benefited greatly from machine learning, particularly from reinforcement learning, which has allowed for more individualized treatment plans. With this kind of therapy customization, cognitive training programs will be as effective as possible. Rehabilitation through virtual reality, rehabilitation for neurological disorders, rehabilitation for developmental disorders, rehabilitation through assistance, rehabilitation for neurodegenerative diseases, and personalized rehabilitation applications are among the rehabilitation processes that have profited from the application of AI. Finding tailored and flexible AI-based therapies for people with cognitive impairments is the main goal of this survey. The WHO predicts that as population health and features change, there will be a greater need for rehabilitation worldwide. This study examined the latest effects of AI technology on the rehabilitation process in light of its significance. We looked into the role of AI in the various facets of rehabilitation, including virtual reality rehabilitation, rehabilitation for neurological and developmental disorders, rehabilitation through assistance, personalized rehabilitation apps, and rehabilitation for neurodegenerative illnesses (Khalid et al., 2024). The majority of rehabilitation treatments take the form of online programs, apps for smartphones, or both. Adaptive rehabilitation is customized based on each person's needs and degree of disability. A personalized Android software that enhances cognitive function through games and activities for individuals with dementia. Four cognitive domains of dementia are targeted by the application: memory, executive functioning, language improvement, and concentration and attention. A month was spent by each player practicing the game both with and without reinforcement learning (RL). When compared to conventional rehabilitation techniques, artificial intelligence's contribution to the various facets of the rehabilitation procedure—including rehabilitation for neurological illnesses, rehabilitation for developmental disorders, rehabilitation through support, and tailored rehabilitation applications and virtual reality rehabilitation—produces better results (Kenwright, 2018).

REFERENCES

Amirthalingam, J., Paidi, G., Alshowaikh, K., Jayarathna, A. I., Salibindla, D. B. A. M. R., Karpinska-Leydier, K., & Jayarathna, A. I. I. (2021). Virtual reality intervention to help improve motor function in patients undergoing rehabilitation for Cerebral Palsy, Parkinson's Disease, or Stroke: A systematic review of randomized controlled trials. *Cureus, 13*(7). Advance online publication. DOI: 10.7759/cureus.16763 PMID: 34367835

Banyai, A. D., & Bris, A. (2024). Robotics in physical rehabilitation: Systematic review. *Health Care, 12*(17), 1720. DOI: 10.3390/healthcare12171720 PMID: 39273744

Bargeri, S., Scalea, S., Agosta, F., Banfi, G., Corbetta, D., Filippi, M., Sarasso, E., Turolla, A., Castellini, G., & Gianola, S. (2023). Effectiveness and safety of virtual reality rehabilitation after stroke: An overview of systematic reviews. *EClinicalMedicine, 64*, 64. DOI: 10.1016/j.eclinm.2023.102220 PMID: 37745019

Brambilla, C., Pirovano, I., Mira, R. M., Rizzo, G., Scano, A., & Mastropietro, A. (2021). Combined use of EMG and EEG techniques for neuromotor assessment in rehabilitative applications: A systematic review. *Sensors (Basel), 21*(17), 7014. DOI: 10.3390/s21217014 PMID: 34770320

Buele J, Palacios-Navarro G. (2023). Cognitive-motor interventions based on virtual reality and instrumental activities of daily living (iADL): an overview. *Front Aging Neurosci*; 15:1191729. . https://doi.org/.DOI: 10.3389/fnagi.2023.1191729

Burke, T., & Rooney, B. (2021). Multi-modal dual-task measurement: A new virtual reality for assessment. *Frontiers in Psychology, 11*, 635413. DOI: 10.3389/fpsyg.2020.635413 PMID: 33679500

Butt, M., Naghdy, G., Naghdy, F., Murray, G., & Du, H. (2020 May 3-6). *Assessment of neuroplasticity using EEG signal in rehabilitation of brain stem stroke patients. In: 2020 IEEE Canadian Conference on Electrical and Computer Engineering (CCECE).* IEEE., https://ieeexplore.ieee.org/document/9377682 DOI: 10.1109/CCECE47787.2020.9255731

Cano-de-la-Cuerda, R., Blázquez-Fernández, A., Marcos-Antón, S., Sánchez-Herrera-Baeza, P., Fernández-González, P., Collado-Vázquez, S., Jiménez-Antona, C., & Laguarta-Val, S. (2024). Economic Cost of Rehabilitation with Robotic and Virtual Reality Systems in People with Neurological Disorders: A Systematic Review. *Journal of Clinical Medicine, 13*(6), 1531. DOI: 10.3390/jcm13061531 PMID: 38541755

Choi, J. W., Kwon, H., Choi, J., Kaongoen, N., Hwang, C., Kim, M., Kim, B. H., & Jo, S. (2023). Neural Applications Using Immersive Virtual Reality: A Review on EEG Studies. *IEEE Transactions on Neural Systems and Rehabilitation Engineering*, *31*, 1645–1658. DOI: 10.1109/TNSRE.2023.3254551 PMID: 37028309

De Giorgi, R., Fortini, A., Aghilarre, F., Gentili, F., Morone, G., Antonucci, G., Vetrano, M., Tieri, G., & Iosa, M. (2023). Virtual Art Therapy: Application of Michelangelo Effect to Neurorehabilitation of Patients with Stroke. *Journal of Clinical Medicine*, *12*(7), 2590. DOI: 10.3390/jcm12072590 PMID: 37048673

Demeco, A., Zola, L., Frizziero, A., Martini, C., Palumbo, A., Foresti, R., Buccino, G., & Costantino, C. (2023). Immersive Virtual Reality in Post-Stroke Rehabilitation: A Systematic Review. *Sensors (Basel)*, *23*(3), 1712. DOI: 10.3390/s23031712 PMID: 36772757

Deng, Y., Wang, Z., Dong, L., Lei, Y., & Dong, Y. (2023). Immersive innovations: An examination of the efficacy and evolution of virtual reality in human movement training. *Robotic Intelligence and Automation*, *43*(5), 551–566. DOI: 10.1108/RIA-05-2023-0072

Dockx K, Bekkers EMJ, Van den Bergh V, Ginis P, Rochester L, Hausdor JM, Mirelman A, Nieuwboer A. (2016). Virtual reality for rehabilitation in Parkinson's disease. *Cochrane Database Syst Rev*; 2016(12):CD010760. . https://doi.org/.DOI: 10.1002/14651858.CD010760.pub2

Dockx, K., Bekkers, E. M. J., Van den Bergh, V., Ginis, P., Rochester, L., Hausdorff, J. M., Mirelman, A., & Nieuwboer, A. (2019). Virtual reality for rehabilitation in Parkinson's disease: Systematic review and meta-analysis. *Journal of Rehabilitation Research and Development*, *56*(3), 273–287. DOI: 10.1682/JRRD.2018.03.0085

Faria, A. L., Almeida, Y., Branco, D., Câmara, J., Cameirão, M., Ferreira, L., Moreira, A., Paulino, T., Rodrigues, P., Spinola, M., Vilar, M., Bermúdez i Badia, S., Simões, M., & Fermé, E. (2024). NeuroAIreh@ b: An artificial intelligence-based methodology for personalized and adaptive neurorehabilitation. *Frontiers in Neurology*, *14*, 1258323. DOI: 10.3389/fneur.2023.1258323 PMID: 38322797

Filippis, R., & Foysal, A. (2024). Harnessing the Power of Artificial Intelligence in Neuromuscular Disease Rehabilitation: A Comprehensive Review and Algorithmic Approach. *Advances in Bioscience and Biotechnology*, *15*(5), 289–309. DOI: 10.4236/abb.2024.155018

Fritz, N. E., Cheek, F. M., & Nichols-Larsen, D. S. (2015). Motor-cognitive dual-task training in persons with neurologic disorders: A systematic review. *Journal of Neurologic Physical Therapy; JNPT*, *39*(3), 142–153. DOI: 10.1097/NPT.0000000000000090 PMID: 26079569

Garay-Sánchez A, Suarez-Serrano C, Ferrando-Margelí M, Jimenez-Rejano JJ, Marcén-Román Y. (2021). Effects of immersive and non-immersive virtual reality on the static and dynamic balance of stroke patients: A systematic review and meta-analysis. *J Clin Med*. 10(19):4473. . https://doi.org/.DOI: 10.3390/jcm10194473

Georgiev, D. D., Georgieva, I., Gong, Z., Nanjappan, V., & Georgiev, G. V. (2021). Virtual reality for neurorehabilitation and cognitive enhancement. *Brain Sciences*, *11*(2), 221. DOI: 10.3390/brainsci11020221 PMID: 33670277

Gomez-Risquet, M., Cáceres-Matos, R., Magni, E., & Luque-Moreno, C. (2024). Effects of haptic feedback interventions in post-stroke gait and balance disorders: A systematic review and meta-analysis. *Journal of Personalized Medicine*, *14*(9), 974. DOI: 10.3390/jpm14090974 PMID: 39338228

Halkiopoulos, C., & Gkintoni, E. (2025). The role of machine learning in AR/VR-based cognitive therapies: A systematic review for mental health disorders. *Electronics (Basel)*, *14*(6), 1110. DOI: 10.3390/electronics14061110

Hu, X., Xu, W., Ren, Y., Wang, Z., He, X., Huang, R., & Cheng, L. (2023). Spinal cord injury: Molecular mechanisms and therapeutic interventions. *Signal Transduction and Targeted Therapy*, *8*(1), 245. DOI: 10.1038/s41392-023-01477-6

Kenwright, B. (2018). Virtual reality: Ethical challenges and dangers [opinion] [</unknown>]. *IEEE Technology and Society Magazine*, *37*(4), 20–25. DOI: 10.1109/MTS.2018.2876104

Khalid, U., Naeem, M., Stasolla, F., Syed, M., Abbas, M., & Coronato, A. (2024). Impact of AI-Powered Solutions in Rehabilitation Process: Recent Improvements and Future Trends. *International Journal of General Medicine*, *17*, 943–969. DOI: 10.2147/IJGM.S453903 PMID: 38495919

Khan, F., Amatya, B., & Galea, M. (2014). Management of fatigue in persons with multiple sclerosis. *Frontiers in Neurology*, *5*, 177.

Khan, M. J., Kannan, P., Wong, T. W.-L., Fong, K. N. K., & Winser, S. J. (2022). A Systematic Review Exploring the Theories Underlying the Improvement of Balance and Reduction in Falls Following Dual-Task Training among Older Adults. *International Journal of Environmental Research and Public Health*, *19*(24), 16890. DOI: 10.3390/ijerph192416890 PMID: 36554771

Kumar, J., Patel, T., Sugandh, F., Dev, J., Kumar, U., Adeeb, M., Kachhadia, M. P., Puri, P., Prachi, F. N. U., Zaman, M. U., Kumar, S., Varrassi, G., & Syed, A. R. S. (2023). Innovative approaches and therapies to enhance neuroplasticity and promote recovery in patients with neurological disorders: A narrative review. *Cureus*, *15*(7). Advance online publication. DOI: 10.7759/cureus.41914 PMID: 37588309

Lam, W. W., Tang, Y. M., & Fong, K. N. K. (2023). A systematic review of the applications of markerless motion capture (MMC) technology for clinical measurement in rehabilitation. *Journal of Neuroengineering and Rehabilitation*, *20*(1), 59. DOI: 10.1186/s12984-023-01186-9 PMID: 37131238

Leavy, B., Kwak, L., Hagströmer, M., & Franzén, E. (2017). Evaluation and implementation of highly challenging balance training in clinical practice for people with Parkinson's disease: Protocol for the HiBalance effectiveness-implementation trial. *BMC Neurology*, *17*(27), 27. Advance online publication. DOI: 10.1186/s12883-017-0809-2 PMID: 28173775

Lee, K. E., Choi, M., & Jeoung, B. (2022). Effectiveness of Rehabilitation Exercise in Improving Physical Function of Stroke Patients: A Systematic Review. *International Journal of Environmental Research and Public Health*, *19*(19), 12739. DOI: 10.3390/ijerph191912739 PMID: 36232038

Leemhuis E, Esposito RM, De Gennaro L, Pazzaglia M. (2021). GoVirtual to get real: Virtual reality as a resource for spinal cord treatment. Int J Environ Res Public Health; 18(4):1819. . https://doi.org/.DOI: 10.3390/ijerph18041819

Leonardi, S., Maggio, M. G., Russo, M., Bramanti, A., Arcadi, F. A., Naro, A., Calabrò, R. S., & De Luca, R. (2021). Cognitive recovery in people with relapsing/remitting multiple sclerosis: A randomized clinical trial on virtual reality-based neurorehabilitation. *Clinical Neurology and Neurosurgery*, *208*, 106828. DOI: 10.1016/j.clineuro.2021.106828 PMID: 34332269

Liao, Y.-Y., Chen, I.-H., Lin, Y.-J., Chen, Y., & Hsu, W.-C. (2019). Effects of virtual reality-based physical and cognitive training on executive function and dual-task gait performance in older adults with mild cognitive impairment: A randomized control trial. *Frontiers in Aging Neuroscience*, *11*, 162. DOI: 10.3389/fnagi.2019.00162 PMID: 31379553

Lu, Y., Ge, Y., Chen, W., Xing, W., Wei, L., Zhang, C., & Yang, Y. (2022). The effectiveness of virtual reality for rehabilitation of Parkinson disease: An overview of systematic reviews with meta-analyses. *Systematic Reviews*, *11*(1), 115. DOI: 10.1186/s13643-022-01924-5 PMID: 35305686

Maggio, M. G., Luca, A., Cicero, C. E., Calabrò, R. S., Drago, F., Zappia, M., & Nicoletti, A. (2024). Effectiveness of telerehabilitation plus virtual reality (Tele-RV) in cognitive e social functioning: A randomized clinical study on Parkinson's disease. *Parkinsonism & Related Disorders, 119*, 105970. DOI: 10.1016/j.parkreld-is.2023.105970 PMID: 38142630

Maggio MG, Russo M, Foti Cuzzola M, Destro M, La Rosa G, Molonia F, Bramanti P, Lombardo G, De Luca R, Calabrò RS. Virtual reality in multiple sclerosis rehabilitation: A review on cognitive and motor outcomes. *Neurorehabilitation.* 2019;44(2):147-157. doi: . https://doi.org/.DOI: 10.3233/NRE-182477

Maheta, B., Kraft, A., Interrante, N., Fereydooni, S., Bailenson, J., Beams, B., Keny, C., Osborne, T., Giannitrapani, K., & Lorenz, K. (2025). Using virtual reality to improve outcomes related to quality of life among older adults with serious illnesses: Systematic review of randomized controlled trials. *Journal of Medical Internet Research, 27*(1), e54452. https://www.jmir.org/2025/1/e54452. DOI: 10.2196/54452 PMID: 40009834

Mahmoud, H., Aljaldi, F., El-Fiky, A., Battecha, K., Thabet, A., Alayat, M., Abd Elkafy, E., Ebid, A., & Ibrahim, A. (2023). Artificial intelligence, machine learning, and conventional physical therapy for upper limb outcome in patients with stroke: A systematic review and meta-analysis. *European Review for Medical and Pharmacological Sciences, 27*, 4812–4827. https://www.europeanreview.org/article/28267 PMID: 37318455

Mao, Y., Chen, P., Li, L., & Huang, D. (2014). Virtual reality training improves balance function. *Neural Regeneration Research, 9*(17), 1628–1634. DOI: 10.4103/1673-5374.141795

Mennella, C., Maniscalco, U., De Pietro, G., & Esposito, M. (2023). The Role of Artificial Intelligence in Future Rehabilitation Services: A Systematic Literature Review. *IEEE Access : Practical Innovations, Open Solutions, 11*, 11024–11043. DOI: 10.1109/ACCESS.2023.3236084

Mouatt, B., Smith, A. E., Mellow, M. L., Parfitt, G., Smith, R. T., & Stanton, T. R. (2020). The use of virtual reality to influence motivation, affect, enjoyment, and engagement during exercise: A scoping review. *Frontiers in Virtual Reality, 1*, 564664. Advance online publication. DOI: 10.3389/frvir.2020.564664

Nath, D., Singh, N., Saini, M., Banduni, O., Kumar, N., Srivastava, M. V. P., Kumaran, S. S., & Mehndiratta, A. (2023). Clinical effectiveness of non-immersive virtual reality tasks for post-stroke neuro-rehabilitation of distal upper-extremities: A case report. *Journal of Clinical Medicine*, *12*(1), 92. DOI: 10.3390/jcm12010092 PMID: 36614892

Nieto-Escamez F, Cortés-Pérez I, Obrero-Gaitán E, Fusco A. Virtual Reality Applications in Neurorehabilitation: Current Panorama and Challenges. *Brain Sci.* 2023;13(5):819. .: https://doi.org/.DOI: 10.3390/brainsci13050819

Park, J. S., Jung, Y. J., & Lee, G. (2020). Virtual reality-based cognitive–motor rehabilitation in older adults with mild cognitive impairment: A randomized controlled study on motivation and cognitive function. *Frontiers in Aging Neuroscience*, *12*, 232. DOI: 10.3389/fnagi.2020.00232 PMID: 32932997

Patsaki, I., Dimitriadi, N., Despoti, A., Tzoumi, D., Leventakis, N., Roussou, G., Papathanasiou, A., Nanas, S., & Karatzanos, E. (2022). The effectiveness of immersive virtual reality in physical recovery of stroke patients: A systematic review. *Frontiers in Systems Neuroscience*, *16*, 880447. DOI: 10.3389/fnsys.2022.880447 PMID: 36211591

Peters, C., Currin, M., Tyson, S., Rogers, A., Healy, S., McPhail, S., Brauer, S. G., Heathcote, K., & Comans, T. (2012). A randomized controlled trial of an enhanced interdisciplinary community-based group program for people with Parkinson's disease: Study rationale and protocol. *Neurology International*, *4*(1), e3. DOI: 10.4081/ni.2012.e3 PMID: 22593807

Pichierri, G., Wolf, P., Murer, K., & de Bruin, E. D. (2011). Cognitive and cognitive-motor interventions affecting physical functioning: A systematic review. *BMC Geriatrics*, *11*(1), 29. DOI: 10.1186/1471-2318-11-29 PMID: 21651800

Riemenschneider, M., Hvid, L. G., Ringgaard, S., Nygaard, M. K. E., Eskildsen, S. F., Petersen, T., Stenager, E., & Dalgas, U. (2021). Study protocol: Randomised controlled trial evaluating exercise therapy as a supplemental treatment strategy in early multiple sclerosis: The Early Multiple Sclerosis Exercise Study (EMSES). *BMJ Open*, *11*(1), e043699. DOI: 10.1136/bmjopen-2020-043699 PMID: 33436475

Segning, C. M., Ezzaidi, H., da Silva, R. A., & Ngomo, S. A. (2021). Neurophysiological pattern as a precursor of work-related musculoskeletal disorders using EEG combined with EMG. *International Journal of Environmental Research and Public Health*, *18*(4), 2001. DOI: 10.3390/ijerph18042001 PMID: 33669544

Shruthi, M. (2022). Efficacy of virtual reality in physical therapy: A paradigm shift in patient engagement. *International Journal of Emerging Research in Engineering and Technology*, *3*(4), 1–6. DOI: 10.63282/3050-922X.IJERET-V3I4P101

Su, Z., Guo, Z., Wang, W., Liu, Y., Liu, Y., Chen, W., Zheng, M., Michael, N., Lu, S., Wang, W., & Xiao, H. (2022). The effect of telerehabilitation on balance in stroke patients: Is it more effective than the traditional rehabilitation model? A meta-analysis of randomized controlled trials published during the COVID-19 pandemic. *Frontiers in Neurology*, *13*, 736645. Advance online publication. DOI: 10.3389/fneur.2022.736645 PMID: 37265467

Tan, X., Wang, K., Sun, W., Li, X., Wang, W., & Tian, F. (2024). A Review of Recent Advances in Cognitive-Motor Dual-Tasking for Parkinson's Disease Rehabilitation. *Sensors (Basel)*, *24*(19), 6353. DOI: 10.3390/s24196353 PMID: 39409390

Tortora C, Di Crosta A, Mammarella N, La Malva P, Di Domenico A, Prete G, et al. (2024). Virtual reality and cognitive rehabilitation for older adults with mild cognitive impairment: A systematic review. Ageing Res Rev; 93:102146. .DOI: 10.1016/j.arr.2023.102146

Waqar H, Tanveer F, Asadullah Arslan S, Ahmad A, Sarfraz S, Fatima K. (2022). Effects of sensorimotor stimulation program with and without routine physical therapy on balance and cognitive performance in patients with mild traumatic brain injury: A randomized controlled trial. *Pakistan Biomed J*; 5(7). .DOI: 10.54393/pbmj.v5i7.684

Wollesen, B., Janssen, T. I., Müller, H., & Voelcker-Rehage, C. (2022). Effects of cognitive-motor dual task training on cognitive and physical performance in healthy children and adolescents: A scoping review. *Acta Psychologica*, *224*, 103498. DOI: 10.1016/j.actpsy.2022.103498 PMID: 35091209

Xiao, Y., Yang, T., & Shang, H. (2023). The impact of motor-cognitive dual-task training on physical and cognitive functions in Parkinson's disease. *Brain Sciences*, *13*(3), 437. DOI: 10.3390/brainsci13030437 PMID: 36979247

Yang, Z. Q., Wei, M. F., Chen, L., & Xi, J. N. (2022). Research progress in the application of motor-cognitive dual-task training in rehabilitation of walking function in stroke patients. *Journal of Neurorestoratology*, *12*(1), 100028. DOI: 10.1016/j.jnrt.2022.100028

Zhang, C., & Yu, S. (2024). The Technology to Enhance Patient Motivation in Virtual Reality Rehabilitation: A Review. *Games for Health Journal*, *13*(4), 215–233. DOI: 10.1089/g4h.2023.0069 PMID: 39159237

Zhang J, Yang J, Xu Q, Xiao Y, Zuo L, Cai E. (2024). Effectiveness of virtual reality-based rehabilitation on the upper extremity motor function of stroke patients: A protocol for systematic review and meta-analysis. *PLoS ONE*; 19(11) e0313296. .: https://doi.org/.DOI: 10.1371/journal.pone.0313296

Compilation of References

Aamir, K. M., Ramzan, M., Skinadar, S., ... (2022) Automatic Heart Disease Detection by Classification of Ventricular Arrhythmias on ECG Using Machine Learning. Computers, Materials & Continua 70, no. 1: 1-15. ISSN: 1546-2218.

Abdalsalam, E., Yusoff, M. Z., Malik, A., Kamel, N. S., & Mahmoud, D. (2018). Modulation of sensorimotor rhythms for brain-computer interface using motor imagery with online feedback. *Signal, Image and Video Processing*, *12*(3), 557–564. DOI: 10.1007/s11760-017-1193-5

Abubaker, M. B., & Babayiğit, B. (2022). Detection of Cardiovascular Diseases in ECG Images Using Machine Learning and Deep Learning Methods. IEEE Transactions on Artificial Intelligence 3, no. 2: 1-12. ISSN: 2691-4581.

Abunasser, B., Al-Hiealy, M., Zaqout, I., Abu-Naser, & S. S. (2023). *Asian Pacific journal of cancer preventionConvolution Neural Network for Breast Cancer Detection and Classification Using Deep Learning*, 531-544.

Acuña Luna, K. P., Hernandez-Rios, E. R., Valencia, V., Trenado, C., & Peñaloza, C. (2025). Deep learning-enhanced motor training: A hybrid VR and exoskeleton system for cognitive–motor rehabilitation. *Bioengineering (Basel, Switzerland)*, *12*(4), 331. DOI: 10.3390/bioengineering12040331 PMID: 40281692

Adamovich, S. V., Fluet, G. G., Tunik, E., & Merians, A. S. (2009). Sensorimotor training in virtual reality: A review. *NeuroRehabilitation*, *25*(1), 29–44. DOI: 10.3233/NRE-2009-0497 PMID: 19713617

Adao Martins, N. R., Annaheim, S., Spengler, C. M., & Rossi, R. M. (2021). Fatigue Monitoring through Wearables: A state-of-the-art review. *Frontiers in Physiology*, *12*, 790292. DOI: 10.3389/fphys.2021.790292 PMID: 34975541

Agapov, S. N., Bulanov, V. A., Zakharov, A. V., & Sergeeva, M. S. (2017). Comparison of classifiers in the tasks of the single-trial vep classification. *Zhurnal Vysshei Nervnoi Deyatelnosti Imeni IP Pavlova, 67*(4), Article 4.

Agapov, S., Bulanov, V., Zakharov, A., & Sergeeva, M. (2018). A Comparison of Classifiers in a Task Consisting of Classifying Single Visual Event-Related Cortical Potentials in Humans. *Neuroscience and Behavioral Physiology*, *48*(9), 1140–1144. Advance online publication. DOI: 10.1007/s11055-018-0678-1

Ahmed, A. A., Ali, W., Abdullah, T. A. A., & Malebary, S. J. (2023). Classifying Cardiac Arrhythmia from ECG Signal Using 1D CNN Deep Learning Model. Mathematics 11, no. 3: 1-15. ISSN: 2227-7390.

Alderman, J., Palmer, J., Laws, E., McCraden, M., Ordish, J., Ghassemi, M., & Liu, X. (2025). Tackling algorithmic bias and promoting transparency in health datasets: The STANDING Together concensus recommendations. *The Lancet. Digital Health*, *7*(1), 64–88. DOI: 10.1016/S2589-7500(24)00224-3 PMID: 39701919

Al-Fuqaha, A., Guizani, M., Mohammadi, M., Aledhari, M., & Ayyash, M. (2015). Internet of things: A survey on enabling technologies, protocols, and applications. *IEEE Communications Surveys and Tutorials*, *17*(4), 2347–2376. DOI: 10.1109/COMST.2015.2444095

Alhudhaif, A. (2024). A novel approach to recognition of Alzheimer's and Parkinson's diseases: Random subspace ensemble classifier based on deep hybrid features with a super-resolution image. *PeerJ. Computer Science*, *10*, e1862. DOI: 10.7717/peerj-cs.1862 PMID: 38435579

Aliakbaryhosseinabadi, S., Kamavuako, E. N., Jiang, N., Farina, D., & Mrachacz-Kersting, N. (2019). Classification of Movement Preparation Between Attended and Distracted Self-Paced Motor Tasks. *IEEE Transactions on Biomedical Engineering*, *66*(11), 3060–3071. DOI: 10.1109/TBME.2019.2900206 PMID: 30794165

Al-Quraishi, M. S., Tan, W. H., Elamvazuthi, I., Ooi, C. P., Saad, N. M., Al-Hiyali, M. I., & Ali, S. S. A. (2024). Cortical signals analysis to recognize intralimb mobility using modified RNN and various EEG quantities. *Heliyon*, *10*(9), e30406. DOI: 10.1016/j.heliyon.2024.e30406 PMID: 38726180

Aly, G., Mareley, M., El-Sayed, S., & Tolba, M. (2021). YOLO Based Breast Masses Detection and Classification in Full-Field Digital Mammograms. *Computer Methods and Programs in Biomedicine*, *200*, 105823. DOI: 10.1016/j.cmpb.2020.105823 PMID: 33190942

Amirthalingam, J., Paidi, G., Alshowaikh, K., Jayarathna, A. I., Salibindla, D. B. A. M. R., Karpinska-Leydier, K., & Jayarathna, A. I. I. (2021). Virtual reality intervention to help improve motor function in patients undergoing rehabilitation for Cerebral Palsy, Parkinson's Disease, or Stroke: A systematic review of randomized controlled trials. *Cureus, 13*(7). Advance online publication. DOI: 10.7759/cureus.16763 PMID: 34367835

Andorra, M., Freire, A., Zubizarreta, I., de Rosbo, N. K., Bos, S. D., Rinas, M., Høgestøl, E. A., de Rodez Benavent, S. A., Berge, T., Brune-Ingebretse, S., Ivaldi, F., Cellerino, M., Pardini, M., Vila, G., Pulido-Valdeolivas, I., Martinez-Lapiscina, E. H., Llufriu, S., Saiz, A., Blanco, Y., & Villoslada, P. (2024). Predicting disease severity in multiple sclerosis using multimodal data and machine learning. *Journal of Neurology, 271*(3), 1133–1149. DOI: 10.1007/s00415-023-12132-z

Andrews, J. G., Buzzi, S., Choi, W., Hanly, S. V., Lozano, A., Soong, A. C. K., & Zhang, J. C. (2014). What will 5G be? *IEEE Journal on Selected Areas in Communications, 32*(6), 1065–1082. DOI: 10.1109/JSAC.2014.2328098

Ang, K. K., Chua, K. S., Phua, K. S., Wang, C., Chin, Z. Y., Kuah, C. W., Low, W., & Guan, C. (2015). A Randomized Controlled Trial of EEG-Based Motor Imagery Brain-Computer Interface Robotic Rehabilitation for Stroke. *Clinical EEG and Neuroscience, 46*(4), 310–320. DOI: 10.1177/1550059414522229 PMID: 24756025

Anirban Dutta, C., Rohan, B., Sanjay, K., & Arpan, P. (2022). *New Frontiers of Cardiovascular Screening Using Unobtrusive Sensors, AI and IoT*. Academic Press.

Aqdar, K., Mustafa, R., Abdulaqadir, Z., Abdalla, P., Qadir, A., Shali, A., & Aziz, N. (2024). Mammogram mastery: A robust dataset for breast cancer detection and medical education. *Data in Brief, 55*, 110633. DOI: 10.1016/j.dib.2024.110633 PMID: 39035836

Arns, M., Heinrich, H., & Strehl, U. (2014). Evaluation of Neurofeedback in ADHD: The Long and Winding Road. *Biological Psychology, 95*, 108–115. DOI: 10.1016/j.biopsycho.2013.11.013 PMID: 24321363

Atal, D. K., & Singh, M. (2020) Arrhythmia Classification with ECG Signals Based on the Optimization-Enabled Deep Convolutional Neural Network. Computer Methods and Programs in Biomedicine 196: 105607. ISSN: 0169-2607.

Atzori, L., Iera, A., & Morabito, G. (2010). The Internet of Things: A Survey. *Computer Networks, 54*(15), 2787–2805. DOI: 10.1016/j.comnet.2010.05.010

Babiloni, C., Pascarelli, M. T., Lizio, R., Noce, G., Lopez, S., Rizzo, M., Ferri, R., Soricelli, A., Nobili, F., Arnaldi, D., Famà, F., Orzi, F., Buttinelli, C., Giubilei, F., Salvetti, M., Cipollini, V., Bonanni, L., Franciotti, R., Onofrj, M., & Del Percio, C. (2020). Abnormal Cortical Neural Synchronization Mechanisms in Quiet Wakefulness are related to Motor Deficits, Cognitive Symptoms, and Visual Hallucinations in Parkinson's Disease Patients: An Electroencephalographic Study. *Neurobiology of Aging*, *91*, 88–111. DOI: 10.1016/j.neurobiolaging.2020.02.029 PMID: 32234263

Bai, L., Wang, D., Wang, H., Barnett, M., Cabezas, M., Cai, W., Calamante, F., Kyle, K., Liu, D., Ly, L., Nguyen, A., Shieh, C.-C., Sullivan, R., Zhan, G., Ouyang, W., & Wang, C. (2024). Improving multiple sclerosis lesion segmentation across clinical sites: A federated learning approach with noise-resilient training. *Artificial Intelligence in Medicine*, *152*, 102872. DOI: 10.1016/j.artmed.2024.102872

Balasubramaniam, S., Velmurugan, Y., Jaganathan, D., & Dhanasekaran, S. (2023). A Modified LeNet CNN for Breast Cancer Diagnosis in Ultrasound Images. *Diagnostics (Basel)*, *13*(17), 2746. DOI: 10.3390/diagnostics13172746 PMID: 37685284

Banyai, A. D., & Bris, A. (2024). Robotics in physical rehabilitation: Systematic review. *Health Care*, *12*(17), 1720. DOI: 10.3390/healthcare12171720 PMID: 39273744

Bargeri, S., Scalea, S., Agosta, F., Banfi, G., Corbetta, D., Filippi, M., Sarasso, E., Turolla, A., Castellini, G., & Gianola, S. (2023). Effectiveness and safety of virtual reality rehabilitation after stroke: An overview of systematic reviews. *EClinicalMedicine*, *64*, 64. DOI: 10.1016/j.eclinm.2023.102220 PMID: 37745019

Bayoudh, K. (2024). A survey of multimodal hybrid deep learning for computer vision: Architectures, applications, trends, and challenges. *Information Fusion*, *105*, 102217. DOI: 10.1016/j.inffus.2023.102217

Berger, A., Horst, F., Müller, S., Steinberg, F., & Doppelmayr, M. (2019). Current State and Future Prospects of EEG and fNIRS in Robot-Assisted Gait Rehabilitation: A Brief Review. *Frontiers in Human Neuroscience*, *13*, 172. DOI: 10.3389/fnhum.2019.00172 PMID: 31231200

Berger, H. (1929). Über das Elektrenkephalogramm des Menschen. *Archiv für Psychiatrie und Nervenkrankheiten*, *87*(1), 527–570. DOI: 10.1007/BF01797193

Berry, R. B., Brooks, R., Gamaldo, C., Harding, S. M., Lloyd, R. M., Quan, S. F., Troester, M. T., & Vaughn, B. V. (2020). AASM Scoring Manual Updates for 2017 (Version 2.4). *Journal of Clinical Sleep Medicine : JCSM : Official Publication of the American Academy of Sleep Medicine*, *13*(5), 665–666. DOI: 10.5664/jcsm.6576 PMID: 28416048

Beyrouthy, T., Mostafa, N., Roshdy, A., Karar, A. S., & Alkork, S. (2024). Review of EEG-based Biometrics in 5G-IoT: Current Trends and Future Prospects. *Applied Sciences (Basel, Switzerland)*, *14*(2), 534. DOI: 10.3390/app14020534

Biasiucci, A., Leeb, R., Iturrate, I., Perdikis, S., Al-Khodairy, A., Corbet, T., Schnider, A., Schmidlin, T., Zhang, H., Bassolino, M., Viceic, D., Vuadens, P., Guggisberg, A. G., & Millán, J. D. R. (2018). Brain-actuated functional electrical stimulation elicits lasting arm motor recovery after stroke. *Nature Communications*, *9*(1), 2421. DOI: 10.1038/s41467-018-04673-z PMID: 29925890

Binzagr, F., & Abulfaraj, A. W. (2025). InGSA: Integrating generalized self-attention in CNN for Alzheimer's disease classification. *Frontiers in Artificial Intelligence*, *8*, 1540646. DOI: 10.3389/frai.2025.1540646 PMID: 40144735

Birbaumer, N., & Cohen, L. G. (2007). Brain-computer interfaces: Communication and restoration of movement in paralysis. *The Journal of Physiology*, *579*(3), 621–636. DOI: 10.1113/jphysiol.2006.125633 PMID: 17234696

Birenbaum, A., & Greenspan, H. (2017). Multi-view longitudinal CNN for multiple sclerosis lesion segmentation. *Engineering Applications of Artificial Intelligence*, *65*, 111–118. DOI: 10.1016/j.engappai.2017.06.006

Bishop, C. M. (2006). Pattern recognition and machine learning. Springer. 978-0-387-31073-2

Bjerre-Nielsen, A., Minor, K., Sapieżyński, P., Lehmann, S., & Lassen, D. D. (2020). Inferring Transportation Mode from Smartphone Sensors: Evaluating the potential of Wi-Fi and Bluetooth. *PLoS One*, *15*(7), e0234003. DOI: 10.1371/journal.pone.0234003 PMID: 32614842

Bonanno, L., Cannuli, A., Pignolo, L., Marino, S., Quartarone, A., Calabrò, R. S., & Cerasa, A. (2023). Neural Plasticity Changes Induced by Motor Robotic Rehabilitation in Stroke Patients: The Contribution of Functional Neuroimaging. *Bioengineering (Basel, Switzerland)*, *10*(8), 990. DOI: 10.3390/bioengineering10080990 PMID: 37627875

Boulif, A., Ananou, B., Ouladsine, M., & Delliaux, S. (2023). A Literature Review: ECG-Based Models for Arrhythmia Diagnosis Using Artificial Intelligence Techniques. *Bioinformatics and Biology Insights*, *17*, 11779322221149600. Advance online publication. DOI: 10.1177/11779322221149600 PMID: 36798080

Bowman, T., Gervasoni, E., Amico, A. P., Antenucci, R., Benanti, P., Boldrini, P., Bonaiuti, D., Burini, A., Castelli, E., Draicchio, F., Falabella, V., Galeri, S., Gimigliano, F., Grigioni, M., Mazzon, S., Mazzoleni, S., Mestanza Mattos, F. G., Molteni, F., … Carrozza, M. C. (2021). What is the impact of robotic rehabilitation on balance and gait outcomes in people with multiple sclerosis? A systematic review of randomized control trials. *European Journal of Physical and Rehabilitation Medicine, 57*(2), Article 2. DOI: 10.23736/S1973-9087.21.06692-2

Brambilla, C., Pirovano, I., Mira, R. M., Rizzo, G., Scano, A., & Mastropietro, A. (2021). Combined use of EMG and EEG techniques for neuromotor assessment in rehabilitative applications: A systematic review. *Sensors (Basel), 21*(17), 7014. DOI: 10.3390/s21217014 PMID: 34770320

Breitwieser, C., Pokorny, C., & Müller-Putz, G. R. (2016). A hybrid three-class brain–computer interface system utilizing SSSEPs and transient ERPs. *Journal of Neural Engineering, 13*(6), 066015. DOI: 10.1088/1741-2560/13/6/066015 PMID: 27788124

Brown, E. N., Purdon, P. L., & Van Dort, C. J. (2018). General Anesthesia and Altered States of Arousal: A Systems Neuroscience Analysis. *Annual Review of Neuroscience, 34*(1), 601–628. https://www.annualreviews.org/content/journals/10.1146/annurev-neuro-060909-153200. DOI: 10.1146/annurev-neuro-060909-153200 PMID: 21513454

Buele J, Palacios-Navarro G. (2023). Cognitive-motor interventions based on virtual reality and instrumental activities of daily living (iADL): an overview. *Front Aging Neurosci*; 15:1191729. . https://doi.org/.DOI: 10.3389/fnagi.2023.1191729

Bulanov, V. A., Zakharov, A. V., & Khivintseva, E. V. (2020). Wavelet transform for the identification of P300. *IOP Conference Series. Materials Science and Engineering, 862*(5), 052049. DOI: 10.1088/1757-899X/862/5/052049

Bundy, D. T., Souders, L., Baranyai, K., Leonard, L., Schalk, G., Coker, R., Moran, D. W., Huskey, T., & Leuthardt, E. C. (2017). Contralesional Brain–Computer Interface Control of a Powered Exoskeleton for Motor Recovery in Chronic Stroke Survivors. *Stroke, 48*(7), 1908–1915. DOI: 10.1161/STROKEAHA.116.016304 PMID: 28550098

Burke, T., & Rooney, B. (2021). Multi-modal dual-task measurement: A new virtual reality for assessment. *Frontiers in Psychology, 11*, 635413. DOI: 10.3389/fpsyg.2020.635413 PMID: 33679500

Buthut, M., Starke, G., Akmazoglu, T. B., Colucci, A., Vermehren, M., van Beinum, A., Bublitz, C., Chandler, J., Ienca, M., & Soekadar, S. R. (2024). HYBRIDMINDS-summary and outlook of the 2023 international conference on the ethics and regulation of intelligent neuroprostheses. *Frontiers in Human Neuroscience*, *18*, 1489307. DOI: 10.3389/fnhum.2024.1489307 PMID: 39483192

Butt, M., Naghdy, G., Naghdy, F., Murray, G., & Du, H. (2020 May 3-6). *Assessment of neuroplasticity using EEG signal in rehabilitation of brain stem stroke patients. In: 2020 IEEE Canadian Conference on Electrical and Computer Engineering (CCECE)*. IEEE., https://ieeexplore.ieee.org/document/9377682 DOI: 10.1109/CCECE47787.2020.9255731

C, D., K, D., Basturk, Alper, Akay, & et al. (2023). A Comparative study of YOLO models and a transformer-based YOLOv5 model for mass detection in mammograms. *Turkish Journal of Electrical Engineering and Computer Sciences* .

Cacciamani, G. E., Chen, A., Gill, I. S., & Hung, A. J. (2024). Artificial intelligence and urology: Ethical considerations for urologists and patients. *Nature Reviews. Urology*, *21*(1), 50–59. DOI: 10.1038/s41585-023-00796-1 PMID: 37524914

Calabrò, R. S., Russo, M., Naro, A., Milardi, D., Balletta, T., Leo, A., Filoni, S., & Bramanti, P. (2016). Who May Benefit From Armeo Power Treatment? A Neurophysiological Approach to Predict Neurorehabilitation Outcomes. *PM & R*, *8*(10), 971–978. DOI: 10.1016/j.pmrj.2016.02.004 PMID: 26902866

Calvo, R. A., & D'Mello, S. K. (2010). Affect detection: An interdisciplinary review of models, methods, and their applications. *IEEE Transactions on Affective Computing*, *1*(1), 18–37. DOI: 10.1109/T-AFFC.2010.1

Cano-de-la-Cuerda, R., Blázquez-Fernández, A., Marcos-Antón, S., Sánchez-Herrera-Baeza, P., Fernández-González, P., Collado-Vázquez, S., Jiménez-Antona, C., & Laguarta-Val, S. (2024). Economic Cost of Rehabilitation with Robotic and Virtual Reality Systems in People with Neurological Disorders: A Systematic Review. *Journal of Clinical Medicine*, *13*(6), 1531. DOI: 10.3390/jcm13061531 PMID: 38541755

Cantillo-Negrete, J., Carino-Escobar, R. I., Carrillo-Mora, P., Elias-Vinas, D., & Gutierrez-Martinez, J. (2018). Motor Imagery-Based Brain-Computer Interface Coupled to a Robotic Hand Orthosis Aimed for Neurorehabilitation of Stroke Patients. *Journal of Healthcare Engineering*, *2018*, 1–10. DOI: 10.1155/2018/1624637 PMID: 29849992

Cao, J., Zhou, T., Zhi, S., Lam, S., Ren, G., Zhang, Y., Wang, Y., Dong, Y., & Cai, J. (2024). Fuzzy inference system with interpretable fuzzy rules: Advancing explainable artificial intelligence for disease diagnosis—A comprehensive review. *Information Sciences*, *662*, 120212. DOI: 10.1016/j.ins.2024.120212

Casson, A. J. (2019). Wearable EEG and beyond. *Biomedical Engineering Letters*, *9*(1), 53–71. DOI: 10.1007/s13534-018-00093-6 PMID: 30956880

Casson, A. J., Yates, D. C., Smith, S. J. M., Duncan, J. S., & Rodriguez-Villegas, E. (2010). Wearable electroencephalography. *IEEE Engineering in Medicine and Biology Magazine*, *29*(3), 44–56. DOI: 10.1109/MEMB.2010.936545 PMID: 20659857

Catalán, J. M., García-Pérez, J. V., Blanco, A., Ezquerro, S., Garrote, A., Costa, T., Bertomeu-Motos, A., Díaz, I., & García-Aracil, N. (2021). Tele-Rehabilitation Versus Local Rehabilitation Therapies Assisted by Robotic Devices: A Pilot Study with Patients. *Applied Sciences (Basel, Switzerland)*, *11*(14), 6259. DOI: 10.3390/app11146259

Chaddad, A., Wu, Y., Kateb, R., & Bouridane, A. (2023). Electroencephalography Signal Processing: A Comprehensive Review and Analysis of Methods and Techniques. *Sensors (Basel)*, *23*(14), 6434. DOI: 10.3390/s23146434 PMID: 37514728

Chang, Y.-W., Jung, K., Jim, K., Nami, C., Young, M., Kyung, H., & Kyunghwa, H. (2025). Artificial intelligence for breast cancer screening in mammography (AI-STREAM): preliminary analysis of a prospective multicenter cohort study.

Chaves, H., Serra, M. M., Shalom, D. E., Ananía, P., Rueda, F., Osa Sanz, E., Stefanoff, N. I., Rodríguez Murúa, S., Costa, M. E., Kitamura, F. C., Yañez, P., Cejas, C., Correale, J., Ferrante, E., Fernández Slezak, D., & Farez, M. F. (2024). Assessing robustness and generalization of a deep neural network for brain MS lesion segmentation on real-world data. *European Radiology*, *34*(3), 2024–2035. DOI: 10.1007/s00330-023-10093-5

Cheng, N., Phua, K. S., Lai, H. S., Tam, P. K., Tang, K. Y., Cheng, K. K., Yeow, R. C.-H., Ang, K. K., Guan, C., & Lim, J. H. (2020). Brain-Computer Interface-Based Soft Robotic Glove Rehabilitation for Stroke. *IEEE Transactions on Biomedical Engineering*, *67*(12), 3339–3351. DOI: 10.1109/TBME.2020.2984003 PMID: 32248089

Chen, H., & Martel, A. (2025). Enhancing breast cancer detection on screeninh mammogram using self-supervised learning and a hybrid deep model of Swin Transformer and convolutional neural networks. *Journal of Imaging*.

Chen, Z., Wang, X., Huang, J., Lu, J., & Zheng, J. (2021). Deep attention and graphical neural network for multiple sclerosis lesion segmentation from MR imaging sequences. *IEEE Journal of Biomedical and Health Informatics*, *26*(3), 1196–1207. DOI: 10.1109/JBHI.2021.3109119

Choi, J. W., Kwon, H., Choi, J., Kaongoen, N., Hwang, C., Kim, M., Kim, B. H., & Jo, S. (2023). Neural Applications Using Immersive Virtual Reality: A Review on EEG Studies. *IEEE Transactions on Neural Systems and Rehabilitation Engineering*, *31*, 1645–1658. DOI: 10.1109/TNSRE.2023.3254551 PMID: 37028309

Cicerone, K. D., Langenbahn, D. M., Braden, C., Malec, J. F., Kalmar, K., Fraas, M., Felicetti, T., Laatsch, L., Harley, J. P., Bergquist, T., Azulay, J., Cantor, J., & Ashman, T. (2011). Evidence-based Cognitive Rehabilitation: Updated Review of the Literature from 2003 through 2008. *Archives of Physical Medicine and Rehabilitation*, *92*(4), 519–530. DOI: 10.1016/j.apmr.2010.11.015 PMID: 21440699

Cirstea, M. C., Ptito, A., & Levin, M. F. (2003). Arm reaching improvements with short-term practice depend on the severity of the motor deficit in stroke. *Experimental Brain Research*, *152*(4), 476–488. DOI: 10.1007/s00221-003-1568-4 PMID: 12928760

Coben, R., Mohammad-Rezazadeh, I., & Cannon, R. L. (2014). Using Quantitative and Analytic EEG Methods in the Understanding of Connectivity in Autism Spectrum Disorders: A Theory of Mixed over-and under-connectivity. *Frontiers in Human Neuroscience*, *8*, 45. https://www.frontiersin.org/journals/human-neuroscience/articles/10.3389/fnhum.2014.00045/full. DOI: 10.3389/fnhum.2014.00045 PMID: 24616679

Comani, S., Velluto, L., Schinaia, L., Cerroni, G., Serio, A., Buzzelli, S., Sorbi, S., & Guarnieri, B. (2015). Monitoring Neuro-Motor Recovery From Stroke With High-Resolution EEG, Robotics and Virtual Reality: A Proof of Concept. *IEEE Transactions on Neural Systems and Rehabilitation Engineering*, *23*(6), 1106–1116. DOI: 10.1109/TNSRE.2015.2425474 PMID: 25910194

Cuijpers, P., Karyotaki, E., Weitz, E., Andersson, G., Hollon, S. D., & van Straten, A. (2014). The Effects of Psychotherapies for Major Depression in Adults on Remission, Recovery and Improvement: A Meta-analysis. *Journal of Affective Disorders*, *159*, 118–126. DOI: 10.1016/j.jad.2014.02.026 PMID: 24679399

Darshini, V. (2023). Deep Learning Based-Breast Cancer Prediction using CNN. *International Journal of Novel Research and Development*, 6-17.

Dayarathna, S., Islam, K. T., Uribe, S., Yang, G., Hayat, M., & Chen, Z. (2024). Deep learning based synthesis of MRI, CT and PET: Review and analysis. *Medical Image Analysis*, *92*, 103046. DOI: 10.1016/j.media.2023.103046 PMID: 38052145

De Giorgi, R., Fortini, A., Aghilarre, F., Gentili, F., Morone, G., Antonucci, G., Vetrano, M., Tieri, G., & Iosa, M. (2023). Virtual Art Therapy: Application of Michelangelo Effect to Neurorehabilitation of Patients with Stroke. *Journal of Clinical Medicine*, *12*(7), 2590. DOI: 10.3390/jcm12072590 PMID: 37048673

De Rosa, A. P., Benedetto, M., Tagliaferri, S., Bardozzo, F., D'Ambrosio, A., Bisecco, A., Gallo, A., Cirillo, M., Tagliaferri, R., & Esposito, F. (2024). Consensus of algorithms for lesion segmentation in brain MRI studies of multiple sclerosis. *Scientific Reports*, *14*(1), 21348. DOI: 10.1038/s41598-024-72649-9

Debener, S., Emkes, R., De Vos, M., & Bleichner, M. (2015). Unobtrusive Ambulatory EEG using a Smartphone and Flexible Printed Electrodes around the Ear. *Scientific Reports*, *5*(1), 16743. DOI: 10.1038/srep16743 PMID: 26572314

Demeco, A., Zola, L., Frizziero, A., Martini, C., Palumbo, A., Foresti, R., Buccino, G., & Costantino, C. (2023). Immersive Virtual Reality in Post-Stroke Rehabilitation: A Systematic Review. *Sensors (Basel)*, *23*(3), 1712. DOI: 10.3390/s23031712 PMID: 36772757

Deng, Y., Wang, Z., Dong, L., Lei, Y., & Dong, Y. (2023). Immersive innovations: An examination of the efficacy and evolution of virtual reality in human movement training. *Robotic Intelligence and Automation*, *43*(5), 551–566. DOI: 10.1108/RIA-05-2023-0072

Di Flumeri, G., Aricò, P., Borghini, G., Sciaraffa, N., Babiloni, F., Pozzi, S., Vignali, V., Lantieri, C., Bichicchi, A., Simone, A., & Babiloni, F. (2018). EEG-based Mental Workload Neurometric to Evaluate the Impact of Different Traffic and Road Conditions in Real Driving Settings. *Frontiers in Neuroscience*, *12*, 507. DOI: 10.3389/fnhum.2018.00509 PMID: 30618686

Diamond, A., & Lee, K. (2011). Interventions shown to Aid Executive Function Development in Children 4 to 12 years old. *Science*, *333*(6045), 959–964. DOI: 10.1126/science.1204529 PMID: 21852486

Dias-Carvalho, A., Sá, S. I., Carvalho, F., Fernandes, E., & Costa, V. M. (2024). Inflammation as common link to progressive neurological diseases. *Archives of Toxicology*, *98*(1), 95–119. DOI: 10.1007/s00204-023-03628-8 PMID: 37964100

Dockx K, Bekkers EMJ, Van den Bergh V, Ginis P, Rochester L, Hausdor JM, Mirelman A, Nieuwboer A. (2016). Virtual reality for rehabilitation in Parkinson's disease. *Cochrane Database Syst Rev*; 2016(12):CD010760. . https://doi.org/.DOI: 10.1002/14651858.CD010760.pub2

Dockx, K., Bekkers, E. M. J., Van den Bergh, V., Ginis, P., Rochester, L., Hausdorff, J. M., Mirelman, A., & Nieuwboer, A. (2019). Virtual reality for rehabilitation in Parkinson's disease: Systematic review and meta-analysis. *Journal of Rehabilitation Research and Development*, *56*(3), 273–287. DOI: 10.1682/JRRD.2018.03.0085

Edelman, B. J., Zhang, S., Schalk, G., Brunner, P., Müller-Putz, G., Guan, C., & He, B. (2024). Non-invasive brain-computer interfaces: State of the art and trends. *IEEE Reviews in Biomedical Engineering*. PMID: 39186407

El-Assy, A. M., Amer, H. M., Ibrahim, H. M., & Mohamed, M. A. (2024). A novel CNN architecture for accurate early detection and classification of Alzheimer's disease using MRI data. *Scientific Reports*, *14*(1), 3463. DOI: 10.1038/s41598-024-53733-6 PMID: 38342924

Elhaddad, M., & Hamam, S. (2024). AI-driven clinical decision support systems: An ongoing pursuit of potential. *Cureus*, *16*(4). Advance online publication. DOI: 10.7759/cureus.57728 PMID: 38711724

Eshaghi, A., Marinescu, R. V., Young, A. L., Firth, N. C., Prados, F., Jorge Cardoso, M., Tur, C., De Angelis, F., Cawley, N., Brownlee, W. J., De Stefano, N., Laura Stromillo, M., Battaglini, M., Ruggieri, S., Gasperini, C., Filippi, M., Rocca, M. A., Rovira, A., Sastre-Garriga, J., & Ciccarelli, O. (2018). Progression of regional grey matter atrophy in multiple sclerosis. *Brain*, *141*(6), 1665–1677. DOI: 10.1093/brain/awy088

Essa, E., & Xie, X. (2021). An Ensemble of Deep Learning-Based Multi-Model for ECG Heartbeats Arrhythmia Classification. IEEE Access 9: 103452-103464. ISSN: 2169-3536.

Essa, E., Aldesouky, D., Hussein, S. E., & Rashad, M. Z. (2020). Neuro-fuzzy patch-wise R-CNN for multiple sclerosis segmentation. *Medical & Biological Engineering & Computing*, *58*(9), 2161–2175. DOI: 10.1007/s11517-020-02225-6

Fan, C., Xie, H., Tao, J., Li, Y., Pei, G., Li, T., & Lv, Z. (2024). ICaps-ResLSTM: Improved capsule network and residual LSTM for EEG emotion recognition. *Biomedical Signal Processing and Control*, *87*, 105422. DOI: 10.1016/j.bspc.2023.105422

Fan, F. L., Li, Y., Zeng, T., Wang, F., & Peng, H. (2025). Towards NeuroAI: Introducing neuronal diversity into artificial neural networks. *Med-X*, *3*(1), 2. DOI: 10.1007/s44258-024-00042-2

Farahany, N. A. (2023). Cognitive liberty is the human right we need to talk about. *Time*. https://time.com/6289229/cognitive-liberty-human-right/

Faria, A. L., Almeida, Y., Branco, D., Câmara, J., Cameirão, M., Ferreira, L., Moreira, A., Paulino, T., Rodrigues, P., Spinola, M., Vilar, M., Bermúdez i Badia, S., Simões, M., & Fermé, E. (2024). NeuroAIreh@ b: An artificial intelligence-based methodology for personalized and adaptive neurorehabilitation. *Frontiers in Neurology*, *14*, 1258323. DOI: 10.3389/fneur.2023.1258323 PMID: 38322797

Fei, W., Bi, L., Wang, J., Xia, S., Fan, X., & Guan, C. (2023). Effects of Cognitive Distraction on Upper Limb Movement Decoding From EEG Signals. *IEEE Transactions on Biomedical Engineering*, *70*(1), 166–174. DOI: 10.1109/TBME.2022.3187085 PMID: 35767496

Ferrell, M. L., Beatty, A., & Dubljevic, V. (2025). The Ethics of Neuromarketing: A Rapid Review. *Neuroethics*, *18*(1), 19. Advance online publication. DOI: 10.1007/s12152-025-09591-8

Ferro, E., & Potorti, F. (2005). Bluetooth and IEEE 802.11 (Wi-Fi) wireless protocols: A survey and a comparison. *IEEE Wireless Communications*, *12*(1), 12–26. DOI: 10.1109/MWC.2005.1404569

Filippis, R., & Foysal, A. (2024). Harnessing the Power of Artificial Intelligence in Neuromuscular Disease Rehabilitation: A Comprehensive Review and Algorithmic Approach. *Advances in Bioscience and Biotechnology*, *15*(5), 289–309. DOI: 10.4236/abb.2024.155018

Finnigan, S., & van Putten, M. J. (2013). EEG in Ischaemic Stroke: Quantitative EEG can Uniquely Inform (sub-)acute Prognoses and Clinical Management. *Clinical Neurophysiology*, *124*(1), 10–19. DOI: 10.1016/j.clinph.2012.07.003 PMID: 22858178

Firth, J., Torous, J., Nicholas, J., Carney, R., Pratap, A., Rosenbaum, S., & Sarris, J. (2017). The Efficacy of Smartphone-based Mental Health Interventions for Depressive Symptoms: A Meta-analysis of Randomized Controlled Trials. *Journal of Affective Disorders*, *218*, 15–22. DOI: 10.1016/j.jad.2017.04.046 PMID: 28456072

Freddie, B., Mathieu, L., Hyuna, S., Jacques, F., Rebecca. L, S., Isabelle, S., & Ahmedin, J. (2024). Global cancer statistics 2022: GLOBOCAN estimates of incidence and mortality worldwide for 36 cancers in 185 countries. *CA: A Cancer Journal for Clinicians reaches*, 229-263.

Frey, S., Lucchini, M. A., Kartsch, V., Ingolfsson, T. M., Bernardi, A. H., Segessenmann, M., Osieleniec, J., Benatti, S., Benini, L., & Cossettini, A. (2024). GAPses: Versatile Smart Glasses for comfortable and fully-dry Acquisition and Parallel Ultra-Low-Power Processing of EEG and EOG. *arXiv*. https://doi.org//arXiv.2406.07903DOI: 10.48550

Frey, S., Guermandi, M., Benatti, S., Kartsch, V., Cossettini, A., & Benini, L. (2023). BioGAP: A 10-Core FP-capable ultra-low power IoT processor for wearable biosignal processing. *arXiv*. https://arxiv.org/abs/2307.01619

Fritz, N. E., Cheek, F. M., & Nichols-Larsen, D. S. (2015). Motor-cognitive dual-task training in persons with neurologic disorders: A systematic review. *Journal of Neurologic Physical Therapy; JNPT*, *39*(3), 142–153. DOI: 10.1097/NPT.0000000000000090 PMID: 26079569

Frolov, A. A., Mokienko, O., Lyukmanov, R., Biryukova, E., Kotov, S., Turbina, L., Nadareyshvily, G., & Bushkova, Y. (2017). Post-stroke Rehabilitation Training with a Motor-Imagery-Based Brain-Computer Interface (BCI)-Controlled Hand Exoskeleton: A Randomized Controlled Multicenter Trial. *Frontiers in Neuroscience*, *11*, 400. DOI: 10.3389/fnins.2017.00400 PMID: 28775677

Gao, F., Wu, T., Zhen, B., Ruan, L., Shang, D., & Patel, B. (2018). A shallow-deep CNN for improved breast cancer diagnosis. *The official journal of Computerized Medical Imaging Society*, 53-62.

Gao, X., Ma, K., Yang, H., Wang, K., Fu, B., Zhu, Y., She, X., & Cui, B. (2022). A Rapid, Non-invasive Method for Fatigue Detection based on Voice Information. *Frontiers in Cell and Developmental Biology*, *10*, 994001. DOI: 10.3389/fcell.2022.994001 PMID: 36176279

Garay-Sánchez A, Suarez-Serrano C, Ferrando-Margelí M, Jimenez-Rejano JJ, Marcén-Román Y. (2021). Effects of immersive and non-immersive virtual reality on the static and dynamic balance of stroke patients: A systematic review and meta-analysis. *J Clin Med*. 10(19):4473. . https://doi.org/.DOI: 10.3390/jcm10194473

Gartlehner, G., Hansen, R. A., Morgan, L. C., Thaler, K., Lux, L., Van Noord, M., Mager, U., Thieda, P., Gaynes, B. N., Wilkins, T., Strobelberger, M., Lloyd, S., Reichenpfader, U., & Lohr, K. N. (2011). Comparative Benefits and Harms of Second-Generation Antidepressants for Treating Major Depressive Disorder: An Updated Meta-analysis. *Annals of Internal Medicine, 155*(11), 772–785. DOI: 10.7326/0003-4819-155-11-201112060-00009 PMID: 22147715

Geert, L., Thijs, K., Babak Ehteshami, B., Arnaud Arindra, A., Francesco, C., & Mohsen, G. Clara I.Sanchez. (2017). A survey on deep learning in medical image analysis. *Medical Image Analysis*, •••, 60–88. PMID: 28778026

Georgiev, D. D., Georgieva, I., Gong, Z., Nanjappan, V., & Georgiev, G. V. (2021). Virtual reality for neurorehabilitation and cognitive enhancement. *Brain Sciences, 11*(2), 221. DOI: 10.3390/brainsci11020221 PMID: 33670277

Ghasemi, N., Razavi, S., & Nikzad, E. (2016). Multiple sclerosis: Pathogenesis, symptoms, diagnoses and cell-based therapy. *Cell Journal (Yakhteh), 19*(1), 1.

Gollapalli, M., Rahman, A., Kudos, S. A., Foula, M. S., Alkhalifa, A. M., Albisher, H. M., Al-Hariri, M. T., & Mohammad, N. (2024). Appendicitis diagnosis: Ensemble machine learning and explainable artificial intelligence-based comprehensive approach. *Big Data and Cognitive Computing, 8*(9), 108. DOI: 10.3390/bdcc8090108

Gomez-Risquet, M., Cáceres-Matos, R., Magni, E., & Luque-Moreno, C. (2024). Effects of haptic feedback interventions in post-stroke gait and balance disorders: A systematic review and meta-analysis. *Journal of Personalized Medicine, 14*(9), 974. DOI: 10.3390/jpm14090974 PMID: 39338228

Goodfellow, I., Pouget-Abadie, J., Mirza, M., Xu, B., Warde-Farley, D., Ozair, S., Courville, A., & Bengio, Y. (2014). Generative adversarial nets. *Advances in Neural Information Processing Systems, 27*. Advance online publication. DOI: 10.48550/arXiv.1406.2661

Goyal, M., Goyal, R., Venkatappa Reddy, P., Lall, B., Pedrycz, W., & Chen, S. (2020). Activation Functions In Deep Learning Algorithms and Applications. *Studies in Computational Intelligence*.

Gubbi, J., Buyya, R., Marusic, S., & Palaniswami, M. (2013). Internet of things (IoT): A Vision, Architectural Elements, and Future Directions. *Future Generation Computer Systems, 29*(7), 1645–1660. DOI: 10.1016/j.future.2013.01.010

Guemann, M., Bouvier, S., Halgand, C., Paclet, F., Borrini, L., Ricard, D., Lapeyre, E., Cattaert, D., & Rugy, A. D. (2019). Effect of vibration characteristics and vibror arrangement on the tactile perception of the upper arm in healthy subjects and upper limb amputees. *Journal of Neuroengineering and Rehabilitation*, *16*(1), 138. DOI: 10.1186/s12984-019-0597-6 PMID: 31722740

Halkiopoulos, C., & Gkintoni, E. (2025). The role of machine learning in AR/VR-based cognitive therapies: A systematic review for mental health disorders. *Electronics (Basel)*, *14*(6), 1110. DOI: 10.3390/electronics14061110

Hammad, M., Iliyasu, A. M., Subasi, A., ... (2020). A Multitier Deep Learning Model for Arrhythmia Detection." IEEE Transactions on Instrumentation and Measurement 69, no. 7: 4172-4181. ISSN: 0018-9456.

Hannun, A. Y., Rajpurkar, P., Haghpanahi, M., Tison, G. H., ... (2019) Cardiologist-Level Arrhythmia Detection and Classification in Ambulatory Electrocardiograms Using a Deep Neural Network. Nature Medicine 25, no. 1: 65-69. ISSN: 1078-8956.

Harper, R., Lam, R., & Evans, H. L. (2019). Affective computing in mental health: A review. *Computers in Human Behavior*, *91*, 107–124. DOI 10.1016/j.chb.2018.09.027

Hastie, T., Tibshirani, R., & Friedman, J. (2017). The elements of statistical learning: Data mining, inference, and prediction (2nd ed.). Springer. 10.1007/978-0-387-84858-7

Health, C. f. (2021). *Artificial Intelligence/Machine Learning (AI/ML)-Based Software as a Medical Device (SaMD) Action Plan.* US FOOD & DRUG ADMINISTRATION.

He, G., Dong, X., & Qi, M. (2020). From the perspective of material science: A review of flexible electrodes for brain-computer interface. *Materials Research Express*, *102001*(10), 102001. Advance online publication. DOI: 10.1088/2053-1591/abb857

He, M., Tang, M., Meng, L., & Liang, Z. (2024). TBSTSleepNet: Three-branch spectro-temporal bidirectional LSTM based attention model for EEG sleep staging. *Biomedical Signal Processing and Control*, *97*, 106695. DOI: 10.1016/j.bspc.2024.106695

Henriques, D. Y. P., & Cressman, E. K. (2012). Visuomotor Adaptation and Proprioceptive Recalibration. *Journal of Motor Behavior*, *44*(6), 435–444. DOI: 10.1080/00222895.2012.659232 PMID: 23237466

Herrmann, C. S., Strüber, D., Helfrich, R. F., & Engel, A. K. (2016). EEG Oscillations: From Correlation to Causality. *International Journal of Psychophysiology*, *103*, 12–21. DOI: 10.1016/j.ijpsycho.2015.02.003 PMID: 25659527

Hofmann, S. G., Asnaani, A., Vonk, I. J., Sawyer, A. T., & Fang, A. (2012). The Efficacy of Cognitive Behavioral Therapy: A Review of Meta-analyses. *Cognitive Therapy and Research*, *36*(5), 427–440. DOI: 10.1007/s10608-012-9476-1 PMID: 23459093

Hofmann, S. G., Sawyer, A. T., Witt, A. A., & Oh, D. (2010). The Effect of Mindfulness-based Therapy on Anxiety and Depression: A Meta-Analytic Review. *Journal of Consulting and Clinical Psychology*, *78*(2), 169–183. DOI: 10.1037/a0018555 PMID: 20350028

Hong, S., You, T., Kwak, S. & Han, B. (2015). Online Tracking by Learning Discriminative Saliency Map with Convolutional Neural Network. Proceedings of the 32nd International Conference on Machine Learning, in Proceedings of Machine Learning Research 37:597-606 Available from https://proceedings.mlr.press/v37/hong15.html.

Hong, X., Lu, Z. K., Teh, I., Nasrallah, F. A., Teo, W. P., Ang, K. K., Phua, K. S., Guan, C., Chew, E., & Chuang, K.-H. (2017). Brain plasticity following MI-BCI training combined with tDCS in a randomized trial in chronic subcortical stroke subjects: A preliminary study. *Scientific Reports*, *7*(1), 9222. DOI: 10.1038/s41598-017-08928-5 PMID: 28835651

Hou, B., Kang, G., Xu, X., & Hu, C. (2019, November). Cross attention densely connected networks for multiple sclerosis lesion segmentation. In *2019 IEEE International Conference on Bioinformatics and Biomedicine (BIBM)* (pp. 2356-2361). IEEE. DOI: 10.1109/BIBM47256.2019.8983149

Hsu, P.-Y., & Cheng, C.-K. (2020). Arrhythmia Classification using Deep Learning and Machine Learning with Features Extracted from Waveform-based Signal Processing. 42nd Annual International Conference of the IEEE Engineering in Medicine Biology Society (EMBC), Montreal, QC, Canada, pp. 292-295. DOI: 10.1109/EMBC44109.2020.9176679

Huang, N. E., Shen, Z., Long, S. R., Wu, M. C., Shih, H. H., Zheng, Q., Yen, N. C., Tung, C. C., & Liu, H. H. (1998). The empirical mode decomposition and the Hilbert spectrum for nonlinear and non-stationary time series analysis. *Proceedings of the Royal Society of London. Series A: Mathematical, Physical and Engineering Sciences, 454*(1971), 903–995. https://doi.org/DOI: 10.1098/rspa.1998.0193

Huang, M., Zhang, X. S., Bhatti, U. A., Wu, Y., Zhang, Y., & Ghadi, Y. Y. (2024). An interpretable approach using hybrid graph networks and explainable AI for intelligent diagnosis recommendations in chronic disease care. *Biomedical Signal Processing and Control*, *91*, 105913. DOI: 10.1016/j.bspc.2023.105913

Hu, X., Xu, W., Ren, Y., Wang, Z., He, X., Huang, R., & Cheng, L. (2023). Spinal cord injury: Molecular mechanisms and therapeutic interventions. *Signal Transduction and Targeted Therapy*, *8*(1), 245. DOI: 10.1038/s41392-023-01477-6

Ibomoiye, D., George, O., Nobert, J., Ebikella, M., Kehinde, A., Ikiomoye, D., & Blessing, O. (2024). A survey of explainable artificial intelligence in healthcare: Concepts, applications, and challenges. *Informatics in Medicine Unlocked.*

Idris, Z., Muzaimi, M., Ghani, R., Idris, B., Kandasamy, R., & Abdullah, J. (2014). Principles, Anatomical Origin and Applications of Brainwaves: A Review, Our Experience and Hypothesis Related to Microgravity and the Question on Soul. *Journal of Biomedical Science and Engineering*, *7*(8), 435–445. DOI: 10.4236/jbise.2014.78046

Inglese, M., Fleysher, L., Oesingmann, N., & Petracca, M. (2018). Clinical applications of ultra-high field magnetic resonance imaging in multiple sclerosis. *Expert Review of Neurotherapeutics*, *18*(3), 221–230. DOI: 10.1080/14737175.2018.1433033

Iqbal, T., Redon-Lurbe, P., Simpkin, A. J., Elahi, A., Ganly, S., Wijns, W., & Shahzad, A. (2021). A Sensitivity Analysis of Biophysiological Responses of Stress for Wearable Sensors in Connected Health. *IEEE Access : Practical Innovations, Open Solutions*, *9*, 93567–93579. DOI: 10.1109/ACCESS.2021.3082423

Isin, A., & Ozdalili, S. (2017). Cardiac Arrhythmia Detection Using Deep Learning. Procedia Computer Science 120: 268-275. ISSN: 1877-0509.

Islam, S. R., Kwak, D., Kabir, M. H., Hossain, M., & Kwak, K. S. (2015). The internet of things for health care: A comprehensive survey. *IEEE Access : Practical Innovations, Open Solutions*, *3*, 678–708. DOI: 10.1109/ACCESS.2015.2437951

Jamin, P., Duret, C., Hutin, E., Bayle, N., Koeppel, T., Gracies, J.-M., & Pila, O. (2022). Using Robot-Based Variables during Upper Limb Robot-Assisted Training in Subacute Stroke Patients to Quantify Treatment Dose. *Sensors (Basel)*, *22*(8), 2989. DOI: 10.3390/s22082989 PMID: 35458975

Jin, J., Xu, R., Daly, I., Zhao, X., Wang, X., & Cichocki, A. (2024). MOCNN: A multiscale deep convolutional neural network for ERP-based brain-computer interfaces. *IEEE Transactions on Cybernetics*, *54*(9), 5565–5576. DOI: 10.1109/TCYB.2024.3390805 PMID: 38713574

K, P., V, V., H.S, R., K.V, S., K, P., R., V., & K, T. (2025). Enhanced Machine Learning Models for Accurate Breast Cancer Mammogram Classification. *Global Transitions*, 276-295.

Kaddes, M., Ayid, Y., Elshewey, A., & Fouad, Y. (2025). Breast cancer classification based on hybrid CNN with LSTM model. *Scientific Reports*, *15*(1), 15. DOI: 10.1038/s41598-025-88459-6 PMID: 39910136

Kakei, S., Hoffman, D. S., & Strick, P. L. (2003). Sensorimotor transformations in cortical motor areas. *Neuroscience Research*, *46*(1), 1–10. DOI: 10.1016/S0168-0102(03)00031-2 PMID: 12725907

Kaongoen, N., Choi, J., Woo Choi, J., Kwon, H., Hwang, C., Hwang, G., Kim, B. H., & Jo, S. (2023). The future of wearable EEG: A review of ear-EEG technology and its applications. *Journal of Neural Engineering*, *20*(5), 051002. Advance online publication. DOI: 10.1088/1741-2552/acfcda PMID: 37748474

Karalis, V. D. (2024). The integration of artificial intelligence into clinical practice. *Applied Biosciences*, *3*(1), 14–44. DOI: 10.3390/applbiosci3010002

Kenwright, B. (2018). Virtual reality: Ethical challenges and dangers [opinion] [</unknown>]. *IEEE Technology and Society Magazine*, *37*(4), 20–25. DOI: 10.1109/MTS.2018.2876104

Khalid, U., Naeem, M., Stasolla, F., Syed, M., Abbas, M., & Coronato, A. (2024). Impact of AI-Powered Solutions in Rehabilitation Process: Recent Improvements and Future Trends. *International Journal of General Medicine*, *17*, 943–969. DOI: 10.2147/IJGM.S453903 PMID: 38495919

Khalil, M., Teunissen, C. E., Lehmann, S., Otto, M., Piehl, F., Ziemssen, T., Bittner, S., Sormani, M. P., Gattringer, T., Abu-Rumeileh, S., Thebault, S., Abdelhak, A., Green, A., Benkert, P., Kappos, L., Comabella, M., Tumani, H., Freedman, M. S., Petzold, A., & Kuhle, J. (2024). Neurofilaments as biomarkers in neurological disorders—Towards clinical application. *Nature Reviews. Neurology*, *20*(5), 269–287. DOI: 10.1038/s41582-024-00955-x PMID: 38609644

Khan, F., Amatya, B., & Galea, M. (2014). Management of fatigue in persons with multiple sclerosis. *Frontiers in Neurology*, *5*, 177.

Khan, M. J., Kannan, P., Wong, T. W.-L., Fong, K. N. K., & Winser, S. J. (2022). A Systematic Review Exploring the Theories Underlying the Improvement of Balance and Reduction in Falls Following Dual-Task Training among Older Adults. *International Journal of Environmental Research and Public Health*, *19*(24), 16890. DOI: 10.3390/ijerph192416890 PMID: 36554771

Kiliçarslan, S., Adem, K., & Celik, M. (2021). An overview of the activation functions used in deep learning algorithms. *Journal of New Results in Science*, 75-88.

Kim, J., & André, E. (2008). Emotion recognition based on physiological changes in music listening. *IEEE Transactions on Multimedia, 10*(6), 1040–1053. PMID: 18988943

Kim, K.-T., Lee, J., Kim, H., Kim, C. H., & Lee, S. J. (2020). Classification of Selective Attention Within Steady-State Somatosensory Evoked Potentials From Dry Electrodes Using Mutual Information-Based Spatio-Spectral Feature Selection. *IEEE Access : Practical Innovations, Open Solutions, 8*, 85464–85472. DOI: 10.1109/ACCESS.2020.2990384

Kiranyaz, S., Ince, T., Hamila, R., & Gabbouj, M. (2014). Convolutional Neural Networks for patient- specific ECG classification. *Annual International Conference of the IEEE Engineering in Medicine and Biology Society, 2608-11*, 2608–2611. Advance online publication. DOI: 10.1109/EMBC.2015.7318926 PMID: 26736826

Kirasirova, L. A., Zakharov, A. V., Morozova, M. V., Kaplan, A. Y., & Pyatin, V. P. (2021). ERP Correlates of Emotional Face Processing in Virtual Reality. *Opera Medica et Physiologica, 8*(3), 3.

Kirschbaum, C., Pirke, K. M., & Hellhammer, D. H. (1993). The "Trier Social Stress Test" - A Tool for Investigating *Psychobiological Stress Responses in a Laboratory setting. Neuropsychobiology, 28*(1–2), 76–81. DOI: 10.1159/000119004 PMID: 8255414

Klingberg, T. (2010). Training and Plasticity of Working Memory. *Trends in Cognitive Sciences, 14*(7), 317–324. DOI: 10.1016/j.tics.2010.05.002 PMID: 20630350

Kołodziej, P., Piasecki, A. P., Piasecka, A. P., & Piasecki, M. (2024). Acquisition and Analysis of Facial Electromyographic Signals for Emotion Recognition. *Sensors (Basel), 24*(15), 4785. DOI: 10.3390/s24154785 PMID: 39123832

Krakauer, J. W., Carmichael, S. T., Corbett, D., & Wittenberg, G. F. (2012). Getting Neurorehabilitation Right: What Can Be Learned From Animal Models? *Neurorehabilitation and Neural Repair, 26*(8), 923–931. DOI: 10.1177/1545968312440745 PMID: 22466792

Krishnamoorthy, S., Zhang, Y., Kadry, S., & Yu, W. (2022). Framework to segment and evaluate multiple sclerosis lesion in MRI slices using VGG-UNet. *Computational Intelligence and Neuroscience, 2022*(1), 4928096. DOI: 10.1155/2022/4928096

Kumari, A. (2024). Security Aspects of Patient's Data in a Medical Diagnostic System. In *Machine Learning in Healthcare and Security* (pp. 195–210). CRC Press.

Kumar, J., Patel, T., Sugandh, F., Dev, J., Kumar, U., Adeeb, M., Kachhadia, M. P., Puri, P., Prachi, F. N. U., Zaman, M. U., Kumar, S., Varrassi, G., & Syed, A. R. S. (2023). Innovative approaches and therapies to enhance neuroplasticity and promote recovery in patients with neurological disorders: A narrative review. *Cureus*, *15*(7). Advance online publication. DOI: 10.7759/cureus.41914 PMID: 37588309

Lam, W. W., Tang, Y. M., & Fong, K. N. K. (2023). A systematic review of the applications of markerless motion capture (MMC) technology for clinical measurement in rehabilitation. *Journal of Neuroengineering and Rehabilitation*, *20*(1), 59. DOI: 10.1186/s12984-023-01186-9 PMID: 37131238

Lang, C. E., MacDonald, J. R., & Gnip, C. (2007). Counting Repetitions: An Observational Study of Outpatient Therapy for People with Hemiparesis Post-Stroke. *Journal of Neurologic Physical Therapy; JNPT*, *31*(1), 3–10. DOI: 10.1097/01.NPT.0000260568.31746.34 PMID: 17419883

Laver, K., George, S., Ratcliffe, J., & Crotty, M. (2011). Virtual reality stroke rehabilitation—Hype or hope?: VIEWPOINT. *Australian Occupational Therapy Journal*, *58*(3), 215–219. DOI: 10.1111/j.1440-1630.2010.00897.x PMID: 21599688

Laws, E., Palmer, J., Alderman, J., Sharma, O., Ngai, V., Salisbury, T., Hussain, G., Ahmed, S., Sachdeva, G., Vadera, S., Mateen, B., Matin, R., Kuku, S., Calvert, M., Gath, J., Treanor, D., McCradden, M., Mackintosh, M., Gichoya, J., & Liu, X. (2025). Diversity, inclusivity and traceability of mammography datasets used in development of Artificial Intelligence technologies: A systematic review. *Clinical Imaging*, *118*, 110369. DOI: 10.1016/j.clinimag.2024.110369

Leavy, B., Kwak, L., Hagströmer, M., & Franzén, E. (2017). Evaluation and implementation of highly challenging balance training in clinical practice for people with Parkinson's disease: Protocol for the HiBalance effectiveness-implementation trial. *BMC Neurology*, *17*(27), 27. Advance online publication. DOI: 10.1186/s12883-017-0809-2 PMID: 28173775

Lebedev, M. A., & Nicolelis, M. A. L. (2006). Brain–machine interfaces: Past, Present and Future. *Trends in Neurosciences*, *29*(9), 536–546. DOI: 10.1016/j.tins.2006.07.004 PMID: 16859758

LeCun, Y., Bengio, Y., & Hinton, G. (2015). Deep Learning. *Nature*, *521*(7553), 436–444. DOI: 10.1038/nature14539 PMID: 26017442

Lee, K. E., Choi, M., & Jeoung, B. (2022). Effectiveness of Rehabilitation Exercise in Improving Physical Function of Stroke Patients: A Systematic Review. *International Journal of Environmental Research and Public Health*, *19*(19), 12739. DOI: 10.3390/ijerph191912739 PMID: 36232038

Leemhuis E, Esposito RM, De Gennaro L, Pazzaglia M. (2021). GoVirtual to get real: Virtual reality as a resource for spinal cord treatment. Int J Environ Res Public Health; 18(4):1819. . https://doi.org/.DOI: 10.3390/ijerph18041819

Leonardi, S., Maggio, M. G., Russo, M., Bramanti, A., Arcadi, F. A., Naro, A., Calabrò, R. S., & De Luca, R. (2021). Cognitive recovery in people with relapsing/remitting multiple sclerosis: A randomized clinical trial on virtual reality-based neurorehabilitation. *Clinical Neurology and Neurosurgery*, *208*, 106828. DOI: 10.1016/j.clineuro.2021.106828 PMID: 34332269

Liao, Y., Tang, Z., Gao, K., & Trik, M. (2024). Optimization of resources in intelligent electronic health systems based on Internet of Things to predict heart diseases via artificial neural network. *Heliyon*, *10*(11), e32090. DOI: 10.1016/j.heliyon.2024.e32090 PMID: 38933933

Liao, Y.-Y., Chen, I.-H., Lin, Y.-J., Chen, Y., & Hsu, W.-C. (2019). Effects of virtual reality-based physical and cognitive training on executive function and dual-task gait performance in older adults with mild cognitive impairment: A randomized control trial. *Frontiers in Aging Neuroscience*, *11*, 162. DOI: 10.3389/fnagi.2019.00162 PMID: 31379553

Lilhore, U., Sharma, Y., Shukla, B., Vadlamudi, M. N., Simaiya, S., Alroobaea, R., Alsafyani, M., & Baqasah, A. M. (2025). Hybrid convolutional neural network and bi-LSTM model with EfficientNet-B0 for high-accuracy breast cancer detection and classification. *Scientific Reports*, *15*(1), 15. DOI: 10.1038/s41598-025-95311-4 PMID: 40204759

Liu, J., Zeng, M., Shan, K., & Tian, L. (2022). Loss Optimization Based Algorithm for Multi-classification of ECG Signal. In *Proceedings of the 3rd International Symposium on Artificial Intelligence for Medicine Sciences (ISAIMS '22)*. Association for Computing Machinery, New York, NY, USA, 537 541. DOI: 10.1145/3570773.3570856

Lopez-Larraz, E., Escolano, C., Robledo-Menéndez, A., Morlas, L., Alda, A., & Minguez, J. (2023). A Garment that Measures Brain Activity: Proof of Concept of an EEG Sensor Layer Fully Implemented with Smart Textiles. *Frontiers in Human Neuroscience*, *17*, 1135153. DOI: 10.3389/fnhum.2023.1135153 PMID: 37305362

Lotte, F., Bougrain, L., Cichocki, A., Clerc, M., Congedo, M., Rakotomamonjy, A., & Yger, F. (2018). A Review of Classification Algorithms for EEG-based Brain-Computer Interfaces: A 10-year Update. *Journal of Neural Engineering*, *15*(3), 031005. DOI: 10.1088/1741-2552/aab2f2 PMID: 29488902

Luck, S. J. (2014). *An Introduction to the event-related Potential Technique* (2nd ed.). MIT Press., https://mitpress.mit.edu/9780262525855/an-introduction-to-the-event-related-potential-technique/

Lustig, M., Donoho, D., & Pauly, J. M. (2007). Sparse MRI: The application of compressed sensing for rapid MR imaging. *Magnetic Resonance in Medicine*, *58*(6), 1182–1195. DOI: 10.1002/mrm.21391 PMID: 17969013

Luxton, D. D., McCann, R. A., Bush, N. E., Mishkind, M. C., & Reger, G. M. (2011). mHealth for Mental Health: Integrating Smartphone Technology in Behavioral Healthcare. *Professional Psychology, Research and Practice*, *42*(6), 505–512. DOI: 10.1037/a0024485

Lu, Y., Ge, Y., Chen, W., Xing, W., Wei, L., Zhang, C., & Yang, Y. (2022). The effectiveness of virtual reality for rehabilitation of Parkinson disease: An overview of systematic reviews with meta-analyses. *Systematic Reviews*, *11*(1), 115. DOI: 10.1186/s13643-022-01924-5 PMID: 35305686

Maciejasz, P., Eschweiler, J., Gerlach-Hahn, K., Jansen-Troy, A., & Leonhardt, S. (2014). A survey on robotic devices for upper limb rehabilitation. *Journal of Neuroengineering and Rehabilitation*, *11*(1), 3. DOI: 10.1186/1743-0003-11-3 PMID: 24401110

Madan, P., Singh, V., Singh, D. P., Diwakar, M., Pant, B., ... (2022). A Hybrid Deep Learning Approach for ECG-Based Arrhythmia Classification. Bioengineering 9, no. 2: 1-15. ISSN: 2306-5354.

Madduri, R., Li, Z., Nandi, T., Kim, K., Ryu, M., & Rodriguez, A. (2024, October). Advances in Privacy Preserving Federated Learning to Realize a Truly Learning Healthcare System. In *2024 IEEE 6th International Conference on Trust, Privacy and Security in Intelligent Systems, and Applications (TPS-ISA)* (pp. 273-279). IEEE. DOI: 10.1109/TPS-ISA62245.2024.00039

Maggio MG, Russo M, Foti Cuzzola M, Destro M, La Rosa G, Molonia F, Bramanti P, Lombardo G, De Luca R, Calabrò RS. Virtual reality in multiple sclerosis rehabilitation: A review on cognitive and motor outcomes. *Neurorehabilitation*. 2019;44(2):147-157. doi: . https://doi.org/.DOI: 10.3233/NRE-182477

Maggio, M. G., Luca, A., Cicero, C. E., Calabrò, R. S., Drago, F., Zappia, M., & Nicoletti, A. (2024). Effectiveness of telerehabilitation plus virtual reality (Tele-RV) in cognitive e social functioning: A randomized clinical study on Parkinson's disease. *Parkinsonism & Related Disorders*, *119*, 105970. DOI: 10.1016/j.parkreldis.2023.105970 PMID: 38142630

Mahadevan, K., Punitha, A., & Suresh, J. (2024). Automatic recognition of rice plant leaf diseases detection using deep neural network with improved threshold neural network. e-Prime-Advances in Electrical Engineering. *Electronics and Energy*, *8*, 100534.

Maheta, B., Kraft, A., Interrante, N., Fereydooni, S., Bailenson, J., Beams, B., Keny, C., Osborne, T., Giannitrapani, K., & Lorenz, K. (2025). Using virtual reality to improve outcomes related to quality of life among older adults with serious illnesses: Systematic review of randomized controlled trials. *Journal of Medical Internet Research*, *27*(1), e54452. https://www.jmir.org/2025/1/e54452. DOI: 10.2196/54452 PMID: 40009834

Mahmoud, H., Aljaldi, F., El-Fiky, A., Battecha, K., Thabet, A., Alayat, M., Abd Elkafy, E., Ebid, A., & Ibrahim, A. (2023). Artificial intelligence, machine learning, and conventional physical therapy for upper limb outcome in patients with stroke: A systematic review and meta-analysis. *European Review for Medical and Pharmacological Sciences*, *27*, 4812–4827. https://www.europeanreview.org/article/28267 PMID: 37318455

Mahmud, T., Barua, K., Habiba, S. U., Sharmen, N., Hossain, M. S., & Andersson, K. (2024). An explainable ai paradigm for alzheimer's diagnosis using deep transfer learning. *Diagnostics (Basel)*, *14*(3), 345. DOI: 10.3390/diagnostics14030345 PMID: 38337861

Malechka, T., Tetzel, T., Krebs, U., Feuser, D., & Graeser, A. (2015). sBCI-Headset—Wearable and Modular Device for Hybrid Brain-Computer Interface. *Micromachines*, *6*(3), 291–311. DOI: 10.3390/mi6030291

Mallat, S. G., & Zhang, Z. (1993). Matching pursuits with time-frequency dictionaries. *IEEE Transactions on Signal Processing*, *41*(12), 3397–3415. DOI: 10.1109/78.258082

Manogaran, P., Hanson, J. V., Olbert, E. D., Egger, C., Wicki, C., Gerth-Kahlert, C., Landau, K., & Schippling, S. (2016). Optical coherence tomography and magnetic resonance imaging in multiple sclerosis and neuromyelitis optica spectrum disorder. *International Journal of Molecular Sciences*, *17*(11), 1894. DOI: 10.3390/ijms17111894

Mao, Y., Chen, P., Li, L., & Huang, D. (2014). Virtual reality training improves balance function. *Neural Regeneration Research*, *9*(17), 1628–1634. DOI: 10.4103/1673-5374.141795

Markov, K., Elgendi, M. & Menon, C. EEG-based headset sleep wearable devices. *npj Biosensing 1, 12* (2024). https://doi.org/DOI: 10.1038/s44328-024-00013-y

Marouene, C., Malek, A., Mokhles, B., & Mouadh, F. (2025). Deep learning-driven predication in healthcare systems: Applying advanced CNNs for enhanced breast cancer detection. *Computers in Biology and Medicine*.

Martínez-Cid, S., Vallejo, D., Herrera, V., Schez-Sobrino, S., Castro-Schez, J. J., & Albusac, J. A. (2025). Explainable AI-driven decision support system for personalizing rehabilitation routines in stroke recovery. Progress in Artificial Intelligence, 1-23.

Marzbani, H., Marateb, H. R., & Mansourian, M. (2016). Methodological note: Neurofeedback: A Comprehensive Review on System Design, Methodology and Clinical Applications. *Basic and Clinical Neuroscience*, *7*(2), 143–148. DOI: 10.15412/J.BCN.03070208 PMID: 27303609

Maslova, O., Komarova, Y., Shusharina, N., Kolsanov, A., Zakharov, A., Garina, E., & Pyatin, V. (2023). Non-invasive EEG-based BCI spellers from the beginning to today: A mini-review. *Frontiers in Human Neuroscience*, *17*, 1216648. DOI: 10.3389/fnhum.2023.1216648 PMID: 37680264

Masooma, H., Andre, K., & Elizabeth, B. (2024). *Barriers to and Facilitators of Artificial Intelligence Adoption in Health Care: Scoping Review*. National Library of Medicine.

Meha, D., & Manan, S. (2021). An anatomization on breast cancer detection and diagnosis employing multi-layer perceptron neural network (MLP) and Convolutional Neural network (CNN). *Clinical eHealth*, 1-11.

Mehrholz, J., Pohl, M., Platz, T., Kugler, J., & Elsner, B. (2018). Electromechanical and robot-assisted arm training for improving activities of daily living, arm function, and arm muscle strength after stroke. *Cochrane Database of Systematic Reviews*, *9*(9), CD006876. Advance online publication. DOI: 10.1002/14651858.CD006876.pub5 PMID: 30175845

Meng, J. C., Shen, M. Q., Lu, Y. L., Feng, H. X., Chen, X. Y., Xu, D. Q., Wu, G.-H., Cheng, Q.-Z., Wang, L.-H., & Gui, Q. (2024). Correlation of glymphatic system abnormalities with Parkinson's disease progression: A clinical study based on non-invasive fMRI. *Journal of Neurology*, *271*(1), 457–471. DOI: 10.1007/s00415-023-12004-6 PMID: 37755462

Mennella, C., Maniscalco, U., De Pietro, G., & Esposito, M. (2023). The Role of Artificial Intelligence in Future Rehabilitation Services: A Systematic Literature Review. *IEEE Access : Practical Innovations, Open Solutions*, *11*, 11024–11043. DOI: 10.1109/ACCESS.2023.3236084

Miller, M. B., Watts, M. L., & Samuel, L. (2024). FDA's proposed rule for the regulation of laboratory-developed tests. *Journal of Clinical Microbiology, 62*(2), e01488–e23. DOI: 10.1128/jcm.01488-23 PMID: 38206042

Minghong, G., Yuejun, Z., Yongzhong, W., Guangpeng, A., Huihong, Z., Pengjun, W., & Guoqing, W. (2023). A lightweight convolutional neural network hardware implementation for wearable heart rate anomaly detection. *Computers in Biology and Medicine*. PMID: 36809696

Missiroli, F., Barsotti, M., Leonardis, D., Gabardi, M., Rosati, G., & Frisoli, A. (2019). Haptic Stimulation for Improving Training of a Motor Imagery BCI Developed for a Hand-Exoskeleton in Rehabilitation. *2019 IEEE 16th International Conference on Rehabilitation Robotics (ICORR)*, 1127–1132. DOI: 10.1109/ICORR.2019.8779370

Mittelstadt, B. D., Allo, P., Taddeo, M., Wachter, S., & Floridi, L. (2016). The ethics of algorithms: Mapping the debate. *Big Data & Society, 3*(2), 2053951716679679. Advance online publication. DOI: 10.1177/2053951716679679

Morone, G., Paolucci, S., Cherubini, A., De Angelis, D., Venturiero, V., Coiro, P., & Iosa, M. (2017). Robot-assisted gait training for stroke patients: Current state of the art and perspectives of robotics. *Neuropsychiatric Disease and Treatment, 13*, 1303–1311. DOI: 10.2147/NDT.S114102 PMID: 28553117

Mouatt, B., Smith, A. E., Mellow, M. L., Parfitt, G., Smith, R. T., & Stanton, T. R. (2020). The use of virtual reality to influence motivation, affect, enjoyment, and engagement during exercise: A scoping review. *Frontiers in Virtual Reality, 1*, 564664. Advance online publication. DOI: 10.3389/frvir.2020.564664

Mullen, T. R., Kothe, C. A. E., Chi, Y. M., Ojeda, A., Kerth, T., Makeig, S., Jung, T.-P., & Cauwenberghs, G. (2015). Real-time neuroimaging and cognitive monitoring using wearable dry EEG. *IEEE Transactions on Biomedical Engineering, 62*(11), 2553–2567. DOI: 10.1109/TBME.2015.2481482 PMID: 26415149

Murat, F., Yildirim, O., Talo, M., Demir, Y., Tan, R. S., ... (2021). Exploring Deep Features and ECG Attributes to Detect Cardiac Rhythm Classes. Knowledge-Based Systems 232: 1-12. ISSN: 0950-7051.

Muro-de-la-Herran, A., Garcia-Zapirain, B., & Mendez-Zorrilla, A. (2014). Gait Analysis Methods: An Overview of Wearable and Non-Wearable Systems, Highlighting Clinical Applications. *Sensors (Basel), 14*(2), 3362–3394. DOI: 10.3390/s140203362 PMID: 24556672

Murungi, N., Pham, M., Dai, X., Haverford, H., Qu, U., & Dai, C. (2023). Empowering Computer Science Students in Electroencephalography (EEG) Analysis: A Review of Machine Learning Algorithms for EEG Datasets. https://kdd.org/kdd2023/wp-content/uploads/2023/08/murungi2023trends.pdf

Musthafa, M. e., T R, M., v, V. K., & Guluwadi, S. (2024). Enhanced skin cancer diagnosis using optimized CNN architecture and checkpoints for automated dermatological lesion classification. *BMC Medical Imaging*, *24*(1), 24. DOI: 10.1186/s12880-024-01356-8 PMID: 39095688

Nabizadeh, F., Masrouri, S., Ramezannezhad, E., Ghaderi, A., Sharafi, A. M., Soraneh, S., & Moghadasi, A. N. (2022). Artificial intelligence in the diagnosis of multiple sclerosis: A systematic review. *Multiple Sclerosis and Related Disorders*, *59*, 103673. DOI: 10.1016/j.msard.2022.103673

Narayana, V. V., & Kodali, P. (2025). Enhanced epilepsy sensitivity and detection rate with improved specificity by integration of modified lstm networks. *IEEE Sensors Journal*.

Nasarudin, N. A., Al Jasmi, F., Sinnott, R. O., Zaki, N., Al Ashwal, H., Mohamed, E. A., & Mohamad, M. S. (2024). A review of deep learning models and online healthcare databases for electronic health records and their use for health prediction. *Artificial Intelligence Review*, *57*(9), 249. DOI: 10.1007/s10462-024-10876-2

Nasir, F., Rahman, S., & Nasir, N. (2025). Breast Cancer Detectiuon Using Convolutional Neural Network: A Deep Learning-Based Approach. *Cureus*, •••, 17.

Nath, D., Singh, N., Saini, M., Banduni, O., Kumar, N., Srivastava, M. V. P., Kumaran, S. S., & Mehndiratta, A. (2023). Clinical effectiveness of non-immersive virtual reality tasks for post-stroke neuro-rehabilitation of distal upper-extremities: A case report. *Journal of Clinical Medicine*, *12*(1), 92. DOI: 10.3390/jcm12010092 PMID: 36614892

Neurorights Foundation. (2024). Safeguarding brain data: assessing the privacy practices of consumer neurotechnology companies. https://perseus-strategies.com/wp-content/uploads/2024/04/FINAL_Consumer_Neurotechnology_Report_Neurorights_Foundation_April-1.pdf

Newman-Toker, D. E., Nassery, N., Schaffer, A. C., Yu-Moe, C. W., Clemens, G. D., Wang, Z., Zhu, Y., Saber Tehrani, A. S., Fanai, M., Hassoon, A., & Siegal, D. (2024). Burden of serious harms from diagnostic error in the USA. *BMJ Quality & Safety*, *33*(2), 109–120. DOI: 10.1136/bmjqs-2021-014130 PMID: 37460118

Peters, C., Currin, M., Tyson, S., Rogers, A., Healy, S., McPhail, S., Brauer, S. G., Heathcote, K., & Comans, T. (2012). A randomized controlled trial of an enhanced interdisciplinary community-based group program for people with Parkinson's disease: Study rationale and protocol. *Neurology International*, *4*(1), e3. DOI: 10.4081/ni.2012.e3 PMID: 22593807

Picard, R. W. (1997). *Affective computing*. MIT Press. DOI: 10.7551/mitpress/1140.001.0001

Pichierri, G., Wolf, P., Murer, K., & de Bruin, E. D. (2011). Cognitive and cognitive-motor interventions affecting physical functioning: A systematic review. *BMC Geriatrics*, *11*(1), 29. DOI: 10.1186/1471-2318-11-29 PMID: 21651800

Pisotta, I., Perruchoud, D., & Ionta, S. (2015). Hand-in-hand advances in biomedical engineering and sensorimotor restoration. *Journal of Neuroscience Methods*, *246*, 22–29. DOI: 10.1016/j.jneumeth.2015.03.003 PMID: 25769276

Polis, J. (2024). Protect Privacy of Biological Data Act. *Colorado Revised Statutes*. https://www.businessinsider.com/colorado-signs-bill-protect-privacy-rights-neurotechnology-neuralink-musk-2024-4

Popovic, M. R., Popovic, D. B., & Keller, T. (2002). Neuroprostheses for grasping. *Neurological Research*, *24*(5), 443–452. DOI: 10.1179/016164102101200311 PMID: 12117312

Pourbabaee, B., Roshtkhari, M. J., ... (2017). Deep Convolutional Neural Networks and Learning ECG Features for Screening Paroxysmal Atrial Fibrillation Patients." IEEE Transactions on Systems, Man, and Cybernetics: Systems 47, no. 12: 3128-3137. ISSN: 2168-2216.

Pradeep, A. K., Acharya, A., Chakravarty, R., & Dev, R. (2025). trendGPT–Discover Trends and Product Innovations Using neuroAi.

Preskill, J. (2018). Quantum Computing in the NISQ Era and Beyond. *Quantum : the Open Journal for Quantum Science*, *2*, 79. DOI: 10.22331/q-2018-08-06-79

Quick, K. M., Weiss, J. M., Clemente, F., Gaunt, R. A., & Collinger, J. L. (2020). Intracortical Microstimulation Feedback Improves Grasp Force Accuracy in a Human Using a Brain-Computer Interface. *2020 42nd Annual International Conference of the IEEE Engineering in Medicine & Biology Society (EMBC)*, 3355–3358. DOI: 10.1109/EMBC44109.2020.9175926

Rai, H. M., Tsoy, D., & Daineko, Y. (2024). MetaHospital: Implementing robust data security measures for an AI-driven medical diagnosis system. *Procedia Computer Science*, *241*, 476–481. DOI: 10.1016/j.procs.2024.08.067

Rajkumar, A., Ganesan, M., ... (2019). Arrhythmia Classification on ECG Using Deep Learning. 2019 5th International Conference on Advanced Computing & Communication Systems (ICACCS). ISSN: 2473-3571.

Ramaglia, V., Rojas, O., Naouar, I., & Gommerman, J. L. (2021). The ins and outs of central nervous system inflammation—Lessons learned from multiple sclerosis. *Annual Review of Immunology*, *39*(1), 199–226. DOI: 10.1146/annurev-immunol-093019-124155

Ramos-Murguialday, A., Broetz, D., Rea, M., Läer, L., Yilmaz, O., Brasil, F. L., Liberati, G., Curado, M. R., Garcia-Cossio, E., Vyziotis, A., Cho, W., Agostini, M., Soares, E., Soekadar, S., Caria, A., Cohen, L. G., & Birbaumer, N. (2013, July). Brain-machine interface in chronic stroke rehabilitation: A controlled study. *Annals of Neurology*, *74*(1), 100–108. DOI: 10.1002/ana.23879 PMID: 23494615

Rechtschaffen, A., & Kales, A. (1968). A manual of Standardized Terminology, Techniques and Scoring System for Sleep Stages of Human Subjects. *U.S. National Institute of Neurological Diseases and Blindness.* https://archive.org/details/RKManual

Reddy, A., Reddy, R. P., Roghani, A. K., Garcia, R. I., Khemka, S., Pattoor, V., Jacob, M., Reddy, P. H., & Sehar, U. (2024). Artificial intelligence in Parkinson's disease: Early detection and diagnostic advancements. *Ageing Research Reviews*, *99*, 102410. DOI: 10.1016/j.arr.2024.102410 PMID: 38972602

Rehák Bučková, B., Mareš, J., Škoch, A., Kopal, J., Tintěra, J., Dineen, R., Řasová, K., & Hlinka, J. (2023). Multimodal-neuroimaging machine-learning analysis of motor disability in multiple sclerosis. *Brain Imaging and Behavior*, *17*(1), 18–34. DOI: 10.1007/s11682-022-00737-3

Riemenschneider, M., Hvid, L. G., Ringgaard, S., Nygaard, M. K. E., Eskildsen, S. F., Petersen, T., Stenager, E., & Dalgas, U. (2021). Study protocol: Randomised controlled trial evaluating exercise therapy as a supplemental treatment strategy in early multiple sclerosis: The Early Multiple Sclerosis Exercise Study (EMSES). *BMJ Open*, *11*(1), e043699. DOI: 10.1136/bmjopen-2020-043699 PMID: 33436475

Ringeval, F., Sonderegger, A., Lingenfelser, M., Auberger, M., D'Errico, S., Baur, C., Bänninger, M., Schwaller, G., & Wicker, A. (2021). The HUME-VAM Dataset for Multimodal Spontaneous Emotion Recognition. *IEEE Transactions on Affective Computing*, *12*(3), 670–683.

Roach, B. J., & Mathalon, D. H. (2008). Event-related EEG Time-Frequency Analysis: An Overview of Measures and an Analysis of Early Gamma Band Phase Locking in Schizophrenia. *Schizophrenia Bulletin*, *34*(5), 907–926. DOI: 10.1093/schbul/sbn093 PMID: 18684772

Romania, T., Beatrice, P., Shlomit, A.-S., Matthew, B., Jocelyn, P., & Nina, S, V. (2025). The Current Scope of Artificial Intelligence in Breast US. *Applied Radiology*.

Rose, D. R., Amin, M., & Ontaneda, D. (2021). Prediction in treatment outcomes in multiple sclerosis: Challenges and recent advances. *Expert Review of Clinical Immunology*, *17*(11), 1187–1198. DOI: 10.1080/1744666X.2021.1986005

Rose, F. D., Brooks, B. M., & Rizzo, A. A. (2005). Virtual Reality in Brain Damage Rehabilitation [Review]. *Cyberpsychology & Behavior*, *8*(3), 241–262. DOI: 10.1089/cpb.2005.8.241 PMID: 15971974

Sadeghibakhi, M., Pourreza, H., & Mahyar, H. (2022). Multiple sclerosis lesions segmentation using attention-based CNNs in FLAIR images. *IEEE Journal of Translational Engineering in Health and Medicine*, *10*, 1–11. DOI: 10.1109/JTEHM.2022.3172025

Sahoo, S., Dash, M., Behera, S., & Sabut, S. (2020). Machine Learning Approach to Detect Cardiac Arrhythmias in ECG Signals: A Survey. IRBM 41, no. 4: 185-194. ISSN: 1959-0318.

Sajid, M., Malik, A. K., Tanveer, M., & Suganthan, P. N. (2024). Neuro-fuzzy random vector functional link neural network for classification and regression problems. *IEEE Transactions on Fuzzy Systems*, *32*(5), 2738–2749. DOI: 10.1109/TFUZZ.2024.3359652

Sanei, S., & Chambers, J. A. (2007). *EEG Signal Processing*. Wiley., DOI: 10.1002/9780470511923

Sannino, G., & De Pietro, G. (2018). A Deep Learning Approach for ECG-Based Heartbeat Classification for Arrhythmia Detection. Future Generation Computer Systems 86: 446-455. ISSN: 0167-739X.

Sarica, B., & Seker, D. Z. (2022). New MS lesion segmentation with deep residual attention gate U-Net utilizing 2D slices of 3D MR images. *Frontiers in Neuroscience*, *16*, 912000. DOI: 10.3389/fnins.2022.912000

Sarramone, L., Presso, M., Todorovich, E., Arlego, M., Zunino, A., Acosta, G., & Fernandez-Leon, J. A. (2025). Unlocking the potential of NeuroAI in Latin America. *AI & Society*, *40*(6), 1–11. DOI: 10.1007/s00146-025-02249-2

Sathian, K., Buxbaum, L. J., Cohen, L. G., Krakauer, J. W., Lang, C. E., Corbetta, M., & Fitzpatrick, S. M. (2011). Neurological Principles and Rehabilitation of Action Disorders: Common Clinical Deficits. *Neurorehabilitation and Neural Repair*, *25*(5, suppl), 21S–32S. DOI: 10.1177/1545968311410941 PMID: 21613535

Satyanarayanan, M. (2017). The Emergence of Edge Computing. *Computer*, *50*(1), 30–39. DOI: 10.1109/MC.2017.9

Saurabh, S., & Gupta, P. K. (2024). Deep learning-based modified bidirectional LSTM network for classification of ADHD disorder. *Arabian Journal for Science and Engineering*, *49*(3), 3009–3026. DOI: 10.1007/s13369-023-07786-w

Schiff, N. D. (2015). Cognitive Motor Dissociation following Severe Brain Injuries. *JAMA Neurology*, *72*(12), 1413–1415. DOI: 10.1001/jamaneurol.2015.2899 PMID: 26502348

Schuch, F. B., Vancampfort, D., Firth, J., Rosenbaum, S., Ward, P. B., Silva, E. S., Hallgren, M., Ponce De Leon, A., Dunn, A. L., Deslandes, A. C., Fleck, M. P., Carvalho, A. F., & Stubbs, B. (2018). Physical Activity and Incident Depression: A Meta-Analysis of Prospective Cohort Studies. *The American Journal of Psychiatry*, *175*(7), 631–648. DOI: 10.1176/appi.ajp.2018.17111194 PMID: 29690792

Segning, C. M., Ezzaidi, H., da Silva, R. A., & Ngomo, S. A. (2021). Neurophysiological pattern as a precursor of work-related musculoskeletal disorders using EEG combined with EMG. *International Journal of Environmental Research and Public Health*, *18*(4), 2001. DOI: 10.3390/ijerph18042001 PMID: 33669544

Sharifian, F., Schneider, D., Arnau, S., & Wascher, E. (2021). Decoding of cognitive processes involved in the continuous performance task. *International Journal of Psychophysiology*, *167*, 57–68. DOI: 10.1016/j.ijpsycho.2021.06.012 PMID: 34216693

Sharma, P., Dinkar, S. K., & Gupta, D. V. (2021) A Novel Hybrid Deep Learning Method with Cuckoo Search Algorithm for Classification of Arrhythmia Disease Using ECG Signals. Neural Computing and Applications 33, no. 14: 1-15. ISSN: 0941-0643.

Shevchenko, O., Yeremeieva, S., & Laschowski, B. (2024). *Comparative Analysis of Neural Decoding Algorithms for Brain-Machine Interfaces*. DOI: 10.1101/2024.12.05.627080

Shirolapov, I. V., Gribkova, O. V., Kovalev, A. M., Shafigullina, L. R., Ulivanova, V. A., Kozlov, A. V., Ereshchenko, A. A., Lyamin, A. V., & Zakharov, A. V. (2024). The Role of Interactions along the Brain–Gut–Microbiome Axis in the Regulation of Circadian Rhythms, Sleep Mechanisms, and Their Disorders. *Neuroscience and Behavioral Physiology*, *54*(8), 1177–1183. DOI: 10.1007/s11055-024-01712-9

Shirolapov, I. V., Zakharov, A. V., Bulgakova, S. V., Khivintseva, E. V., Sergeeva, M. S., Romanchuk, N. P., Pavlova, O. N., & Kazantsev, V. B. (2023). Glymphatic dysfunction in the pathogenesis of neurodegenerative diseases and pathological aging. *Genes to Cells*, *18*(4), 309–322. DOI: 10.23868/gc546022

Shi, W., Cao, J., Zhang, Q., Li, Y., & Xu, L. (2016). Edge computing: Vision and challenges. *IEEE Internet of Things Journal*, *3*(5), 637–646. DOI: 10.1109/JIOT.2016.2579198

Shruthi, M. (2022). Efficacy of virtual reality in physical therapy: A paradigm shift in patient engagement. *International Journal of Emerging Research in Engineering and Technology*, *3*(4), 1–6. DOI: 10.63282/3050-922X.IJERET-V3I4P101

Sikander, G., & Anwar, S. (2019). Driver Fatigue Detection Systems: A review. *IEEE Transactions on Intelligent Transportation Systems*, *20*(6), 2339–2352. DOI: 10.1109/TITS.2018.2868499

Sousa, A. S. P., Moreira, J., Silva, C., Mesquita, I., Macedo, R., Silva, A., & Santos, R. (2022). Usability of Functional Electrical Stimulation in Upper Limb Rehabilitation in Post-Stroke Patients: A Narrative Review. *Sensors (Basel)*, *22*(4), 1409. DOI: 10.3390/s22041409 PMID: 35214311

Spaulding, W., & Deogun, J. (2011). A Pathway to Personalization of Integrated Treatment: Informatics and Decision Science in Psychiatric Rehabilitation. *Schizophrenia Bulletin*, *37*(suppl 2), S129–S137. DOI: 10.1093/schbul/sbr080 PMID: 21860042

Spolaôr, N., Lee, H. D., Mendes, A. I., Nogueira, C. V., Parmezan, A. R. S., Takaki, W. S. R., Coy, C. S. R., Wu, F. C., & Fonseca-Pinto, R. (2024). Fine-tuning pre-trained neural networks for medical image classification in small clinical datasets. *Multimedia Tools and Applications*, *83*(9), 27305–27329. DOI: 10.1007/s11042-023-16529-w

Strelnik, A., Strelnik, S., Markina, E., Zakharov, A., Kolsanov, A., & Smirnova, D. (2022). The Effects of Transcranial Magnetic Stimulation on Cognitive Functioning in Bipolar Depression: A Systematic Review. *Psychiatria Danubina*, *34*(Suppl 8), 179–188. PMID: 36170725

Su, Z., Guo, Z., Wang, W., Liu, Y., Liu, Y., Chen, W., Zheng, M., Michael, N., Lu, S., Wang, W., & Xiao, H. (2022). The effect of telerehabilitation on balance in stroke patients: Is it more effective than the traditional rehabilitation model? A meta-analysis of randomized controlled trials published during the COVID-19 pandemic. *Frontiers in Neurology, 13*, 736645. Advance online publication. DOI: 10.3389/fneur.2022.736645 PMID: 37265467

Tabernig, C. B., Lopez, C. A., Carrere, L. C., Spaich, E. G., & Ballario, C. H. (2018). Neurorehabilitation therapy of patients with severe stroke based on functional electrical stimulation commanded by a brain computer interface. *Journal of Rehabilitation and Assistive Technologies Engineering, 5*, 2055668318789280. DOI: 10.1177/2055668318789280 PMID: 31191948

Taherdoost, H., & Ghofrani, A. (2024). *AI and the Evolution of Personalized Medicine in Pharmacogenomics*. Intelligent Pharmacy.

Tahghighi, P., Zhang, Y., Souza, R., & Komeili, A. (2024, October). Enhancing New Multiple Sclerosis Lesion Segmentation via Self-supervised Pre-training and Synthetic Lesion Integration. In *International Conference on Medical Image Computing and Computer-Assisted Intervention* (pp. 263-272). Cham: Springer Nature Switzerland. DOI: 10.1007/978-3-031-72111-3_25

Tanczak, N., Plunkett, T. K., Lin, S., Kuenzler, L., Lau, M., Kuah, W. K. C., Ng, C. Y., Gassert, R., Chua, K., & Lambercy, O. (2025). Feasibility of post-stroke hand rehabilitation supported by a soft robotic hand orthosis in-clinic and at-home. *Journal of Neuroengineering and Rehabilitation, 22*(1), 183. DOI: 10.1186/s12984-025-01717-6 PMID: 40842028

Tan, X., Wang, K., Sun, W., Li, X., Wang, W., & Tian, F. (2024). A Review of Recent Advances in Cognitive-Motor Dual-Tasking for Parkinson's Disease Rehabilitation. *Sensors (Basel), 24*(19), 6353. DOI: 10.3390/s24196353 PMID: 39409390

Tao, W., & Tan, X. (2023). A Survey on Affective Brain-Computer Interface: From Machine Learning to Deep Learning. *IEEE Transactions on Human-Machine Systems, 53*(2), 220–234.

TEAM. W. (2025). *Ethics and governance of artificial intelligence for health: Guidance on large multi-modal models.* Wold Health Organization.

Teplan, M. (2002). Fundamentals of EEG Measurement. *Measurement Science Review, 2*(2), 1–11. https://www.researchgate.net/publication/228599963_Fundamental_of_EEG_Measurement e Videman, M., Tokariev, A., Stjerna, S., Roivainen, R., Gaily, E., & Vanhatalo, S. (2016). Effects of Prenatal Antiepileptic Drug Exposure on Newborn Brain Activity. *Epilepsia, 57*(4), 608–619. https://doi.org/DOI: 10.1111/epi.13281

Torri, F., Vadi, G., Meli, A., Loprieno, S., Schirinzi, E., Lopriore, P., Ricci, G., Siciliano, G., & Mancuso, M. (2024). The use of digital tools in rare neurological diseases towards a new care model: A narrative review. *Neurological Sciences, 45*(10), 4657–4668. DOI: 10.1007/s10072-024-07631-4 PMID: 38856822

Tortora C, Di Crosta A, Mammarella N, La Malva P, Di Domenico A, Prete G, et al. (2024). Virtual reality and cognitive rehabilitation for older adults with mild cognitive impairment: A systematic review. Ageing Res Rev; 93:102146. .DOI: 10.1016/j.arr.2023.102146

Tsagkas, C., Magon, S., Gaetano, L., Pezold, S., Naegelin, Y., Amann, M., Stippich, C., Cattin, P., Wuerfel, J., Bieri, O., Sprenger, T., Kappos, L., & Parmar, K. (2018). Spinal cord volume loss: A marker of disease progression in multiple sclerosis. *Neurology, 91*(4), e349–e358. DOI: 10.1212/WNL.0000000000005853

Tsiara, A. A., Plakias, S., Kokkotis, C., Veneri, A., Mina, M. A., Tsiakiri, A., Kitmeridou, S., Christidi, F., Gourgoulis, E., Doskas, T., Kaltsatou, A., Tsamakis, K., Kazis, D., & Tsiptsios, D. (2025). Artificial Intelligence in the Diagnosis of Neurological Diseases Using Biomechanical and Gait Analysis Data: A Scopus-Based Bibliometric Analysis. *Neurology International, 17*(3), 45. DOI: 10.3390/neurolint17030045 PMID: 40137466

Ullah, A., Anwar, S. M., Bilal, M., & Mehmood, R. M. (2020). Classification of Arrhythmia by Using Deep Learning with 2-D ECG Spectral Image Representation. Remote Sensing 12, no. 10: 1685. ISSN: 2072-4292.

Valverde, S., Cabezas, M., Roura, E., González-Villà, S., Pareto, D., Vilanova, J. C., Ramió-Torrentà, L., Rovira, À., Oliver, A., & Lladó, X. (2017). Improving automated multiple sclerosis lesion segmentation with a cascaded 3D convolutional neural network approach. *NeuroImage, 155*, 159–168. DOI: 10.1016/j.neuroimage.2017.04.034

Vang, Y. S., Cao, Y., Chang, P. D., Chow, D. S., Brandt, A. U., Paul, F., . . . Xie, X. (2020, April). SynergyNet: a fusion framework for multiple sclerosis brain MRI segmentation with local refinement. In *2020 IEEE 17th international symposium on biomedical imaging (ISBI)* (pp. 131-135). IEEE. DOI: 10.1109/ISBI45749.2020.9098610

Vidaurre, C., Klauer, C., Schauer, T., Ramos-Murguialday, A., & Müller, K.-R. (2016). EEG-based BCI for the linear control of an upper-limb neuroprosthesis. *Medical Engineering & Physics*, *38*(11), 1195–1204. DOI: 10.1016/j.medengphy.2016.06.010 PMID: 27425203

Wang, H., Hou, Y., Zhan, S., Li, N., Liu, J., Song, P., Wang, Y., & Wang, H. (2023). EEG Biofeedback Decreases Theta and Beta Power While Increasing Alpha Power in Insomniacs: An Open-Label Study. *Brain Sciences*, *13*(11), 1542. DOI: 10.3390/brainsci13111542 PMID: 38002502

Wang, J., Wang, Z., & Liu, G. (2024). Recording brain activity while listening to music using wearable EEG devices combined with Bidirectional Long Short-Term Memory Networks. *Alexandria Engineering Journal*, *109*, 1–10. DOI: 10.1016/j.aej.2024.07.122

Wang, N., Zhang, X., Li, X., Zhang, H., Liu, W., Wang, C., Li, L., & Liu, P. (2022). Facial Electromyography for Assessment of Post-stroke Facial Paralysis: A Review. *Frontiers in Neurology*, *13*, 843232. 10.3389/fnins.2025.1646485/

Wang, Y., Nahon, R., Tartaglione, E., Mozharovskyi, P., & Nguyen, V.-T. (2023). Optimized preprocessing and Tiny ML for attention state classification. *arXiv*. https://arxiv.org/abs/2303.11371 DOI: 10.1109/SSP53291.2023.10207930

Waqar H, Tanveer F, Asadullah Arslan S, Ahmad A, Sarfraz S, Fatima K. (2022). Effects of sensorimotor stimulation program with and without routine physical therapy on balance and cognitive performance in patients with mild traumatic brain injury: A randomized controlled trial. *Pakistan Biomed J*; 5(7). .DOI: 10.54393/pbmj.v5i7.684

Warden, P., & Situnayake, D. (2019). TinyML: Machine learning with TensorFlow Lite on Arduino and ultra-low-power microcontrollers. *O'Reilly Media*. https://www.oreilly.com/library/view/tinyml/9781492052036/

Weiss, P. L., Kizony, R., Feintuch, U., & Katz, N. (2006). Virtual reality in neurorehabilitation. In Selzer, M., Clarke, S., Cohen, L., Duncan, P., & Gage, F. (Eds.), *Textbook of Neural Repair and Rehabilitation* (1st ed., pp. 182–197). Cambridge University Press., DOI: 10.1017/CBO9780511545078.015

Whitmore, A., Agarwal, A., & Xu, L. D. (2015). The Internet of Things - A Survey of Topics and Trends. *Information Systems Frontiers*, *17*(2), 261–274. DOI: 10.1007/s10796-014-9489-2

Wiltgen, T., McGinnis, J., Schlaeger, S., Kofler, F., Voon, C., Berthele, A., Bischl, D., Grundl, L., Will, N., Metz, M., Schinz, D., Sepp, D., Prucker, P., Schmitz-Koep, B., Zimmer, C., Menze, B., Rueckert, D., Hemmer, B., Kirschke, J., & Wiestler, B. (2024). LST-AI: A deep learning ensemble for accurate MS lesion segmentation. *NeuroImage. Clinical*, *42*, 103611. DOI: 10.1016/j.nicl.2024.103611

Wollesen, B., Janssen, T. I., Müller, H., & Voelcker-Rehage, C. (2022). Effects of cognitive-motor dual task training on cognitive and physical performance in healthy children and adolescents: A scoping review. *Acta Psychologica*, *224*, 103498. DOI: 10.1016/j.actpsy.2022.103498 PMID: 35091209

Wolpaw, J. R., Birbaumer, N., McFarland, D. J., Pfurtscheller, G., & Vaughan, T. M. (2002). Brain-Computer Interfaces for Communication and Control. *Clinical Neurophysiology*, *113*(6), 767–791. DOI: 10.1016/S1388-2457(02)00057-3 PMID: 12048038

Wolpaw, J. R., Millán, J. D. R., & Ramsey, N. F. (2020). Brain-computer interfaces: Definitions and principles. In *Handbook of Clinical Neurology* (Vol. 168, pp. 15–23). Elsevier., DOI: 10.1016/B978-0-444-63934-9.00002-0

Xia, Y., Zhang, H., Xu, L., Gao, Z., ... (2018). An Automatic Cardiac Arrhythmia Classification System with Wearable Electrocardiogram. IEEE Access 6: 16529-16538. ISSN: 2169-3536.

Xiao, Q., Lee, K., Mokhtar, S. A., Ismail, I., Pauzi, A. L. M., ... (2023) Deep Learning-Based ECG Arrhythmia Classification: A Systematic Review. Applied Sciences 13, no. 2: 1-20. ISSN: 2076-3417.

Xiao, Y., Yang, T., & Shang, H. (2023). The impact of motor-cognitive dual-task training on physical and cognitive functions in Parkinson's disease. *Brain Sciences*, *13*(3), 437. DOI: 10.3390/brainsci13030437 PMID: 36979247

Xiong, Z., Stiles, M. K., & Zhao, J. (2017). Robust ECG Signal Classification for Detection of Atrial Fibrillation Using a Novel Neural Network. 2017 Computing in Cardiology (CinC). ISSN: 2325-8861.

Xiong, X., Le-Wei, Z., Yu, D., Yu-Fei, C., Yu-Wen, C., Lei-Ping, W., & Ke-Da, Y. (2025). Breast cancer: Pathogenesis and treatments. *Signal Transduction and Targeted Therapy*, *10*(1), 49. DOI: 10.1038/s41392-024-02108-4 PMID: 39966355

Xu, X., & Liu, H. (2020). ECG Heartbeat Classification Using Convolutional Neural Networks. *IEEE Access : Practical Innovations, Open Solutions*, *8*, 8614–8619. DOI: 10.1109/ACCESS.2020.2964749

Yang, Z. Q., Wei, M. F., Chen, L., & Xi, J. N. (2022). Research progress in the application of motor-cognitive dual-task training in rehabilitation of walking function in stroke patients. *Journal of Neurorestoratology, 12*(1), 100028. DOI: 10.1016/j.jnrt.2022.100028

Yildirim, O., Baloglu, U. B., Tan, R. S., Ciaccio, E. J., ... (2019). A New Approach for Arrhythmia Classification Using Deep Coded Features and LSTM Networks." Computer Methods and Programs in Biomedicine 176: 121-133. ISSN: 0169-2607.

Yıldırım, Ö., Pławiak, P., Tan, R. S., & Acharya, U. R. (2018). Arrhythmia Detection Using Deep Convolutional Neural Network with Long Duration ECG Signals. Computers in Biology and Medicine 102: 411-420. ISSN: 0010-4825.

Yildirim, O., Talo, M., Ciaccio, E. J., & Ru, S. T. U Rajendra Acharya. (2020) Accurate deep neural network model to detect cardiac arrhythmia on more than 10,000 individual subject ECG records. Computer Methods and Programs in Biomedicine,Volume 197, 105740, ISSN 0169-2607, DOI: 10.1016/j.cmpb.2020.105740

Yizhou, C., Xiaoliang, S., Kuangyu, S., Axel, R., & Federico, C. (2025). AI in Breast Cancer Imaging: An Update and Future Trends. *Seminars in Nuclear Medicine*, •••, 358–370. PMID: 40011118

Yongshu, G., Jie, L., Weihan, L., Ming, H., Yang, L., & Huimin, Z. (2023). Augmented Grad-CAM++: Super-Resolution Saliency Maps for Visual Interpretation of Deep Neural Network. *Electronics (Basel)*, •••, 2023.

Yoo, Y. (2018). *Deep learning for feature discovery in brain MRIs for patient-level classification with applications to multiple sclerosis* (Doctoral dissertation, University of British Columbia).

Yoo, S. D., & Lee, H. H. (2023). The Effect of Robot-Assisted Training on Arm Function, Walking, Balance, and Activities of Daily Living After Stroke: A Systematic Review and Meta-Analysis. *Brain & Neurorehabilitation, 16*(3), e24. DOI: 10.12786/bn.2023.16.e24 PMID: 38047093

Yuste, R., Goering, S., Arcas, B. A. Y., Bi, G., Carmena, J. M., Carter, A., Fins, J. J., Friesen, P., Gallant, J., Huggins, J. E., Illes, J., Kellmeyer, P., Klein, E., Marblestone, A., Mitchell, C., Parens, E., Pham, M., Rubel, A., Sadato, N., & Wolpaw, J. (2017). Four ethical priorities for neurotechnologies and AI. *Nature, 551*(7679), 159–163. DOI: 10.1038/551159a PMID: 29120438

Zakharov, A. V., Vlasov, I. V., Poverennova, I. E., Khivintseva, E. V., & Antipov, O. I. (2014). [Posture disorders in patients with multiple sclerosis]. *Zhurnal Nevrologii I Psikhiatrii Imeni S.S. Korsakova, 114*(2 Pt 2), Article 2 Pt 2.

Zakharov, A. V., Bulanov, V. A., Khivintseva, E. V., Kolsanov, A. V., Bushkova, Y. V., & Ivanova, G. E. (2020). Stroke Affected Lower Limbs Rehabilitation Combining Virtual Reality With Tactile Feedback. *Frontiers in Robotics and AI, 7*, 81. https://www.frontiersin.org/articles/10.3389/frobt.2020.00081. DOI: 10.3389/frobt.2020.00081 PMID: 33501248

Zaltzhendler, M. (2015). *A deep-learning convolutional neural network framework for mulitple sclerosis lesion detection and segmentation in patient brain images.* McGill University.

Zander, T. O., & Kothe, C. (2011). Towards Passive Brain-Computer Interfaces: Applying Brain–Computer Interface Technology to Human–Machine Systems in General. *Journal of Neural Engineering*, *8*(2), 025005. DOI: 10.1088/1741-2560/8/2/025005 PMID: 21436512

Zeng, C., Gu, L., Liu, Z., & Zhao, S. (2020). Review of deep learning approaches for the segmentation of multiple sclerosis lesions on brain MRI. *Frontiers in Neuroinformatics*, *14*, 610967. DOI: 10.3389/fninf.2020.610967

Zhang J, Yang J, Xu Q, Xiao Y, Zuo L, Cai E. (2024). Effectiveness of virtual reality-based rehabilitation on the upper extremity motor function of stroke patients: A protocol for systematic review and meta-analysis. *PLoS ONE*; 19(11) e0313296. .: https://doi.org/.DOI: 10.1371/journal.pone.0313296

Zhang, J., Zuo, L., Dewey, B. E., Remedios, S. W., Hays, S. P., Pham, D. L., . . . Carass, A. (2024, April). Harmonization-enriched domain adaptation with light fine-tuning for multiple sclerosis lesion segmentation. In *Medical Imaging 2024: Clinical and Biomedical Imaging* (Vol. 12930, pp. 635-641). SPIE. DOI: 10.1117/12.3011291

Zhang, Y., Liu, S., He, Z., Zhang, Y., & Wang, C. (2022). A CNN Model for Cardiac Arrhythmias Classification Based on Individual ECG Signals. Cardiovascular Engineering and Technology 13, no. 2: 1-12. ISSN: 1869-408X.

Zhang, C., & Yu, S. (2024). The Technology to Enhance Patient Motivation in Virtual Reality Rehabilitation: A Review. *Games for Health Journal*, *13*(4), 215–233. DOI: 10.1089/g4h.2023.0069 PMID: 39159237

Zhang, H., Zhang, J., Li, C., Sweeney, E. M., Spincemaille, P., Nguyen, T. D., Gauthier, S. A., Wang, Y., & Marcille, M. (2021). ALL-Net: Anatomical information lesion-wise loss function integrated into neural network for multiple sclerosis lesion segmentation. *NeuroImage. Clinical*, *32*, 102854. DOI: 10.1016/j.nicl.2021.102854

Zhang, H., Zhang, J., Zhang, Q., Kim, J., Zhang, S., Gauthier, S. A., & Wang, Y. (2019). RSANet: recurrent slice-wise attention network for multiple sclerosis lesion segmentation. In *Medical Image Computing and Computer Assisted Intervention–MICCAI 2019: 22nd International Conference, Shenzhen, China, October 13–17, 2019* [Springer International Publishing.]. *Proceedings*, *22*(Part III), 411–419.

Zhang, Y. D., Pan, C., Sun, J., & Tang, C. (2018). Multiple sclerosis identification by convolutional neural network with dropout and parametric ReLU. *Journal of Computational Science*, *28*, 1–10. DOI: 10.1016/j.jocs.2018.07.003

Zhao, X., Wang, L., Zhang, Y., Han, X., Deveci, M., & Parmar, M. (2024). A review of convolutional neural networks in computer vision. *Artificial Intelligence Review*, *57*(4), 99. DOI: 10.1007/s10462-024-10721-6

Zhou, X., Liu, C., Wang, Z., Zhai, L., Jia, Z., Guan, C., & Liu, Y. (2023). Interpretable and robust AI in EEG systems: a survey. *arXiv*. https://arxiv.org/abs/2304.10755

Zhu, H., Cheng, C., Yin, H., Li, X., ... (2020). Automatic Multilabel Electrocardiogram Diagnosis of Heart Rhythm or Conduction Abnormalities with Deep Learning: A Cohort Study." The Lancet Digital Health 2, no. 1: e38-e48. ISSN: 2589-7500.

Ziegeldorf, J. H., Morchon, O. G., & Wehrle, K. (2014). Privacy in the internet of things: Threats and challenges. *Security and Communication Networks*, *7*(12), 2728–2742. DOI: 10.1002/sec.795

Ziyang, G., Yong, T., Shih-Chi, L., & Junghua, L. (2025). *A CT Image Classification Network Framework for Lung Tumors Based on Pre-trained MobileNetV2 Model and Transfer learning and Its Application and Market Analysis in the Medical field.*

Zuo, C., Jin, J., Yin, E., Saab, R., Miao, Y., Wang, X., Hu, D., & Cichocki, A. (2020). Novel hybrid brain–computer interface system based on motor imagery and P300. *Cognitive Neurodynamics*, *14*(2), 253–265. DOI: 10.1007/s11571-019-09560-x PMID: 32226566

About the Contributors

Adnène Arbi is a distinguished academic affiliated with the University of Carthage in Tunisia, where he has contributed significantly to the fields of mathematics and engineering. His tenure at the university spans over a decade, during which he has held various positions, including roles at the Ecole Polytechnique de Tunisie and the National Institute of Applied Sciences and Technology. He served as director of studies and vice-director in the National School of Advanced Sciences and Technologies from 2020 to 2024. His research interests primarily focus on neural networks, dynamical systems, and mathematical modeling, with a particular emphasis on the stability and controllability of complex systems. Arbi's recent publications reflect his commitment to advancing knowledge in applied mathematics, particularly through innovative approaches such as wavelet neural networks and the dynamics of nonlinear systems. His work has been published in reputable journals, contributing to the understanding of mathematical phenomena in both theoretical and practical contexts. In addition to his academic pursuits, Arbi has collaborated with various prestigious institutions globally, including the University of the Witwatersrand and Imperial College London, showcasing his dedication to fostering international research partnerships. His contributions to the academic community continue to inspire emerging scholars and practitioners in the field. Actually, Dr. Arbi served as editor of various journal: - Frontiers in Applied Mathematics and Statistics, - Journal of Algorithms & Computational Technology, Neural Computing and Applications, -Discover Artificial Intelligence, - Current Artificial Intelligence, - Journal of Innovative Applied Mathematics and Computational Sciences, - International Journal of Sustainable Business and Management, - Karshi Multidisciplinary International Scientific Journal. Besides, he is author of more than 40 scientific peer- reviewed papers in international journals and conference proceedings, and he served as reviewer for many international conferences, workshops.

Walid Ben Ameur earned his PhD from the University of Carthage. He currently serves as a teacher-researcher at the Department of Life Sciences, Faculty of Sciences of Gabès, Tunisia, and is a member of the Laboratory of Ecology of Terrestrial Fauna at the University of Gabès, Tunisia. Walid Ben Ameur has authored more than 20 peer-reviewed scientific papers published in international journals. His work has made useful contributions to the field of environmental chemistry, with a particular focus on persistent organic pollutants. He has developed analytical techniques for assessing emerging pollutants and evaluating their effects on both the environment and human health. His research spans a diverse range of samples, including those from environmental, biological, human, and food sources. Dr. Ben Ameur has mentored three Master's students and regularly serves as a reviewer for respected journals such as Science of the Total Environment, Chemosphere, Environmental Science and Pollution Research, Marine Pollution Bulletin, Environmental Pollution, Ecotoxicology and Environmental Safety, and Chemistry Africa.

***

Santi Kumari Behera is an esteemed Assistant Professor in the Department of Computer Science and Engineering at Veer Surendra Sai University of Technology (VSSUT), Burla, Odisha, India. With over 15 years of teaching and research experience, she specializes in image processing, wireless sensor networks, and machine learning applications in agriculture and healthcare. Dr. Behera earned her Master of Technology degree in Computer Science and Engineering from the National Institute of Technology (NIT), Rourkela. Her academic career includes positions at NIST Berhampur (2010–2012) and MNNIT Allahabad (2012–2015) before joining VSSUT. She has co-authored over 100 research publications, contributing significantly to areas such as disease detection in crops, fruit maturity classification, and medical diagnostics using deep learning. Notable works include studies on COVID-19 detection, rice leaf disease identification, and breast cancer detection using thermography images. Additionally, she holds a registered copyright for a literary work titled "IOT Based Management and Prediction of Currency Flow through UPI Transaction. Dr. Behera's contributions have been recognized with numerous citations, reflecting her impact in the fields of computer science and engineering. Email-b.santibehera@gmail.com

Khaoula Ben Ali As an Electrical Engineering PhD (INP-ENSEEIHT, 1999) with two decades of experience, Dr. Khaoula Ben Ali, Associate Professor at INSAT, and Researcher at Laboratory of Informatics for Industrial Systems (LISI), bridges foundational electromagnetics with cutting-edge industrial digitization. Her work, recently recognized by the Ministry of Research's 2024 Collaborative Research

Prize for the ARAFET project (an AI-powered platform for maternal health in rural areas), now centers on Certifiable Industrial IoT, developing robust solutions for the next generation of smart manufacturing.

S. Ida Evangeline, presently working as an Assistant Professor in the Department of Electrical and Electronics Engineering at the Government College of Engineering, Tirunelveli, Tamilnadu, India. She obtained her Bachelor's in Electrical and Electronics Engineering from Manonmaniam Sundaranar University in 2003, and Master's in Power Systems Engineering from Anna University, Chennai, Tamilnadu, India in 2005. She completed her PhD degree in 2023 at Anna University, Chennai, Tamilnadu, India. She has published six research papers in international journals. Her current research interests include optimal power flow, renewable energy, soft computing, machine learning, and deep learning.

Prabira Kumar Sethy is an accomplished academic and researcher in the field of Electronics and Communication Engineering. He currently serves as an Assistant Professor in the Department of Electronics at Sambalpur University Institute of Information Technology (SUIIT), Odisha, India, a position he has held since 2013. Dr. Sethy earned his Ph.D. in Electrical and Electronics Engineering from Sambalpur University, focusing his research on the study and analysis of paddy diseases using image processing techniques. He completed his M.Tech. in Electronics and Communication Engineering from the Indian Institute of Technology (ISM), Dhanbad, and his B.E. in Electronics and Telecommunication Engineering from Biju Patnaik University of Technology (BPUT), Odisha. Before joining academia, Dr. Sethy gained industry experience as an Engineer at Doordarshan, Prasar Bharati, Government of India, from 2009 to 2013. His research interests encompass image processing, machine learning, deep learning, signal processing, and medical imaging. He has published over 80 research papers in reputed journals and conferences, and holds two patents. Dr. Sethy has also guided several Ph.D. scholars, with

Affaan Shaikh is the Founder & CEO of Neuratia Labs. As an AI engineer, researcher and neuroscientist, he develops cutting-edge solutions at the intersection of artificial intelligence, neuroscience, and medical technology. His research spans neurodegenerative disease diagnosis, brain-computer interfaces (BCIs), and AI in aerospace. With over 10 peer-reviewed papers in journals like IEEE and Springer, Affaan is an active contributor to the tech community. He has mentored 20+ aspiring researchers and writers and is passionate about innovation, leadership, and public engagement.

Khalid Shaikh, is the Founder and CEO of Prognica Labs and Kountifi Innovations Inc. He is a researcher, author and business strategist. With over 20

years of experience spanning healthcare, finance, and technology, Khalid is an researcher, author, technocrat and business strategist. He has been honored as one of the "Most Creative People in Business 2023" and serves on the Harvard Business Review Advisory Council, and has received numerous awards for his innovations and contribution in healthcare and public health. He has delivered keynote sessions and participated in expert panels at events such as the Sharjah Investment Forum, St Petersburg Economic Forum, GITEX Global, and India Global Forum, Borsa del biomedicale Veneto in the Middle East and internationally. Throughout his journey, he have been actively contributed to various innovation ecosystems and have worked closely with academic institutions, research parks, and global forums. He have published and lectured extensively on business performance improvement, digitalization, and innovation.

Index

A

B

C

D

E

F

V

www.ingramcontent.com/pod-product-compliance
Lightning Source LLC
LaVergne TN
LVHW082051011026
849162LV00019B/455